PREP

PROGRAM REVIEW & EXAM PREPARATION

RADIOGRAPHY

2nd Edition

D. A. Saia, MA, RT(R)
Director, Radiography Program
The Stamford Hospital
Stamford, Connecticut

Appleton & Lange
Stamford, Connecticut

www.appletonlange.com

99 00 01 02 / 10 9 8 7 6 5 4 3 2 1

Prentice Hall of International (UK) Limited, *London*
Prentice Hall of Australia Pty. Limited, *Sydney*
Prentice Hall Canada, Inc., *Toronto*
Prentice Hall Hispanoamericana, S.A., *Mexico*
Prentice Hall of India Private Limited, *New Delhi*
Prentice Hall of Japan, Inc., *Tokyo*
Simon & Schuster Asia Pte. Ltd., *Singapore*
Editora Prentice Hall do Brasil Ltda., *Rio de Janeiro*
Prentice Hall, *Upper Saddle River, New Jersey*

Library of Congress Cataloging-in-Publication Data
Saia, D. A. (Dorothy A.)
    Radiography : PREP : program review & exam preparation / D. A.
Saia. — 2nd ed.
        p.   cm.
    Companion v. to: Appleton & Lange's review for the radiography
examination / D. A. Saia. 3rd ed. c1997.
    Includes bibliographical references and index.
    ISBN 0-8385-8262-1 (pbk. : alk. paper)
    1. Radiography, Medical Outlines, syllabl. etc. 1. Saia. D. A.
(Dorothy A.).   Appleton & Lange's review for the radiography
examination.   II. Title.
    (DNLM: 1. Radiography.   2. Technology, Radiologic.   WN 180 S132r
RC78.15.S255   1999
616.07'572'076—dc21
DNLM/DLC
for Library of Congress   99-17638
                                                              CIP

Editor-in-Chief: Cheryl L. Mehalik
Acquisitions Editor: Jessica M. Hirshon
Production Editor: Mary Ellen McCourt
Cover Designer: Libby Schmitz
Art Coordinator: Eve Siegel
Illustrations: Academy Artworks

PRINTED IN THE UNITED STATES OF AMERICA

ISBN 0-8385-8262-1

9 780838 582626   90000

Dedicated with love, to Tony

Reviewers

Mark E. Brown, RT(R) (M)
Evans Army Hospital
Fort Carson, Colorado

Carl F. Mayberry, RT(R)
Chief/Program Director
Academy of Health Sciences
Alamo Area Society of Radiologic Technologist
Order of Military Medical Merit
San Antonio, Texas

Connie L. Mitchell, BS, RT(R) (CT)
University of Nebraska Medical Center
Omaha, Nebraska

Susan Morison, M Ed, RT(R) (M)
University of Hartford
Enfield, Connecticut

Richard Terrass, M Ed, RT(R)
Education Coordinator,
Department of Radiology
Quality Management and Education
Massachusetts General Hospital
Boston, Massachusetts

Michael L. Walker, BA, RT(R)
Program Director
San Joaquin General Hospital
San Joaquin Delta College
Stockton, California

Contents

Preface

Radiography: Program Review and Exam Preparation (PREP), Second Edition, has been developed for use throughout all phases of radiography education. This text will be useful for regular course work, helping the student extract fundamental key concepts from reading assignments and class notes, and making study and test preparation easier and more productive.

PREP will also be useful for students preparing for their ARRT certification examination. It has been prepared to help students direct their study efforts toward exam-related material. This new edition includes registry-type multiple choice questions and a disk of review questions designed to help students practice computer-based test taking skills they will need for the ARRT radiography examination beginning the year 2000.

The ARRT's *Content Specifications for the Examination in Radiography* lists the exam's five content categories and provides a detailed list of the topics addressed in each category. *Radiography: PREP* is divided into five parts reflecting each of the five content categories. Part content reflects the material identified in the detailed list of category topics. Thus, study becomes more directed and focused on exam-related material. Used with its companion book, A&L's *Review for the Radiography Examination,* the *Radiography: PREP* provides a thorough preparation for the certification examination administered by the ARRT.

KEY FEATURES AND USE

- A *list of key terms* at the start of each section identifies important terms or phrases essential for the student to know. The student will find it helpful to write the definition of each term before beginning each section.
- Over 340 *illustrations* will appeal to the visual learner as well as the verbal learner. The essence of radiography is visual and *PREP's* graphics and radiographic images visually express the written words.
- The *summary boxes* serve to call the student's attention to the most important facts in a particular section. Students can use summary boxes as an overview of key information.
- *Endpapers* list a number of formulae, some drugs and their uses, and a brief list of processing chemicals and their functions. A "last minute cheat sheet" is provided for some things that students often forget because they don't use them on a regular basis.
- The *final review sections* allow students to assess chapter material in two ways. The first review section, *Chapter Exercises,* requires short essay answers; exact page references

follow each question, providing answers in chapter material. The second section, ***Chapter Review Questions,*** consists of registry-type multiple choice questions followed by detailed explanations.

Following completion of the chapter review questions, the student is ready for final self evaluation by answering more "registry-type" questions in the companion text, *Appleton & Lange's Review for the Radiography Examination.*

Acknowledgments

One of my most satisfying tasks is having the opportunity to thank those who have most generously contributed their insights, talents, and concerns to this project. Foremost among those are my teachers and colleagues who have contributed to my knowledge over the years and also my students on whom I have the privilege of sharpening my knowledge and skills. I am especially grateful to the professionals at Appleton & Lange who have been a source of guidance and encouragement. Marinita Timban, Editor, and Cheryl Mehalik, Editor-in-Chief, helped shape the *Radiography: PREP* concept. Eve Siegel, Art Coordinator, made the seemingly impossible task of reworking the art program and pulling everything together an almost painless experience. Deborah King, Editorial Assistant, could always be counted on for help whenever I needed it (which seemed quite often!). Sincerest appreciation is extended to Jessica Hirshon, Associate Editor; John Williams, Production Supervisor; Lynn Vail-Nagle, Buyer; and Libby Schmitz, Designer, for their part in seeing this second edition to fruition. Everyone at Appleton & Lange has been most supportive and helpful in the development of this project; it has been a pleasure to work with them.

Marinita Timban recruited an outstanding group of reviewers. Mark Brown, RT(R)(M), Carl F. Mayberry, RT(R), Connie Mitchell, BS, RT(R), Susan Morison, M Ed, RT(R)(M), Richard Terrass, M Ed, RT(R), and Michael Walker, BA, RT(R), are invaluable resources to the radiologic technology community. They reviewed the manuscript and offered suggestions to improve style and remove ambiguities and inaccuracies. Their participation on this project is deeply appreciated. A special thank you goes to Andrea Cornuelle for her encouragement and for preparing the *Foreword* to this book.

I wish to pay special acknowledgment to Thomas Piccoli, M.SC., D.A.B.R. for his contribution on Digital Imaging to this text. Tom is a Medical Physicist who has the unparalleled ability to make physics understandable and enjoyable.

I would like to thank the American College of Radiology for the use of many radiographs from their teaching file, and The Stamford Hospital Department of Radiology for permission to use many of their radiographs.

I wish to acknowledge and thank Bob Wong for permission to use several of his excellent teaching films throughout the text.

Several people were helpful in securing permission and providing photographs for illustration. Mr. Dick Burkhart at Burkhart Roentgen and Mr. Steve Schaaf, Marketing Administration Manager at Landauer, Inc. were very helpful and supportive. A special thank you goes to Mr. Artie Swayhoover, Advertising Manager at Nuclear Associates, for patiently answering questions and returning calls; his help is greatly appreciated. The multi-pattern shadow shield pictured in the radiation protection chapter was designed by the late William

Burger of C.B. Radiology Design, Inc, Jamestown, New York. I thank Janet H. Burger for her assistance in providing illustrations for use in this book.

A very special *thank you* is directed to faculty members of the department of education at Sacred Heart University in Fairfield, Connecticut. Dr. Lauren Kempton, Dr. Ed Murray, and Dr. Matt George were exceedingly supportive during the preparation of this second edition. Their understanding and advocacy is deeply appreciated.

The preparation of this text would have been a far more difficult task without the help and encouragement of my husband, Tony. His patience, support, and advice are lovingly appreciated.

Foreword

The traditional question-and-answer review book provides students with the opportunity to practice responding to questions written by someone other than their instructors and to identify their areas of weakness. Unfortunately, too many students believe they will be appropriately prepared to write the American Registry of Radiologic Technologist (ARRT) examination merely by answering questions in review books. Guessing correctly on review book questions does not mean the student understands the material and can give the student a false sense of security.

This review text is unique to the profession in that it presents the content to be tested on the ARRT examination in a narrative, summary format. The content is divided into the five topic categories identified by the ARRT. Ms. Saia's presentation of this content is clear, concise, and well organized. Diagrams and radiographic illustrations are used in each chapter to supplement the narrative. Summary boxes listing the important points are strategically placed throughout each chapter. Open-ended, self-test questions are included at the end of each chapter to help the reader assess learning and understanding of the content presented.

In addition to its obvious use, this review book has an additional application. While it was originally intended as preparation for the ARRT examination, it can also be used as a supplement to other books students use throughout their educational program. Many students have difficulty extracting the important points from traditional textbooks. Although new requirements have been added to the curriculum in the past 15 years, most programs are still two years in length. Students are often overwhelmed by the amount of content included in their texts and by the pace at which they must learn it. Regardless of the quality of instruction, some students need assistance in identifying the important points. This book serves to meet this need.

Ms. Saia is to be commended for tackling the task of summarizing the content included in a two-year, entry-level radiography program. This text is not intended to replace the traditional texts currently used. It is, however, comparable to a Registry review seminar in print. Like *Cliffs Notes* available in literature or review books available in the math and science disciplines, "Saia's Notes" provide a valuable resource for students studying radiologic technology.

Andrea Gauthier Cornuelle, MS RT(R)
Associate Professor and Director
Radiologic Technology Program
Northern Kentucky University
Highland Heights, Kentucky

part

I

Patient Care and Management

D. *Epistaxis*
E. *Postural Hypotension*
F. *Vertigo*
G. *Syncope*
H. *Convulsion*
I. *Unconsciousness*

J. *Acute Abdomen*
K. *Shock*
L. *Seizure*
M. *Respiratory Failure*
N. *Cardiopulmonary Arrest*
O. *Stroke*

Professional and Legal Obligations

KEY TERMS ◀

ASSAULT

BATTERY

BREACH

CATHARTIC

CONFIDENTIALITY

CONSENT

CONTRAST MEDIA

DEFAMATION

DIAGNOSIS

DUTY

INFECTION CONTROL

ISOLATION

LIBEL

LITIGATION

MALPRACTICE

PRIVACY

PRIVATE (CIVIL) LAW

PUBLIC LAW

RES IPSA LOQUITUR

RESPONDEAT SUPERIOR

SCOPE OF PRACTICE

SLANDER

STANDARD OF CARE

STATUTES

TORT

I. LEGAL CONSIDERATIONS IN RADIOLOGY

Practitioners of the profession of radiologic technology, like other health care professionals, have an ethical responsibility to adhere to principles of professional conduct and to provide the best services possible to the patients entrusted to their care. These principles are detailed in the American Registry of Radiologic Technologists (ARRT) Code of Ethics (Fig. 1–1) and the American Hospital Association (AHA) Patient's Bill of Rights (Fig. 1–2).

This Code shall serve as a guide by which Radiologic Technologists may evaluate their professional conduct as it relates to patients, colleagues, other members of the medical care team, health care consumers and employers. The Code is intended to assist radiologic technologists in maintaining a high level of ethical conduct.

1. The Radiologic Technologist conducts himself/herself in a professional manner, responds to patient needs and supports colleagues and associates in providing quality patient care.

2. The Radiologic Technologist acts to advance the principal objective of the profession to provide services to humanity with full respect for the dignity of mankind.

3. The Radiologic Technologist delivers patient care and service unrestricted by the concerns of personal attributes or the nature of the disease or illness, and without discrimination regardless of sex, race, creed, or socioeconomic status.

4. The Radiologic Technologist practices technology founded upon theoretical knowledge and concepts, utilizes equipment and accessories consistent with the purposes for which they have been designed, and employs procedures and techniques appropriately.

5. The Radiologic Technologist assesses situations, exercises care, discretion and judgment, assumes responsibility for professional decisions, and acts in the best interest of the patient.

6. The Radiologic Technologist acts as an agent through observation and communication to obtain pertinent information for the physician to aid in the diagnosis and treatment management of the patient, and recognizes that interpretation and diagnosis are outside the scope of practice for the profession.

7. The Radiologic Technologist utilizes equipment and accessories, employs techniques and procedures, performs services in accordance with an accepted standard of practice, and demonstrates expertise in limiting the radiation exposure to the patient, self, and other members of the health care team.

8. The Radiologic Technologist practices ethical conduct appropriate to the profession and protects the patient's right to quality radiologic technology care.

9. The Radiologic Technologist respects confidences entrusted in the course of professional practice, respects the patient's right to privacy, and reveals confidential information only as required by law or to protect the welfare of the individual or the community.

10. The Radiologic Technologist continually strives to improve knowledge and skills by participating in educational and professional activities, sharing knowledge with colleagues and investigating new and innovative aspects of professional practice. One means available to improve knowledge and skill is through professional continuing education.

Figure 1–1. The American Registry of Radiologic Technologists code of ethics. (Copyright 1993, The American Registry of Radiologic Technologists.)

A. PATIENT RIGHTS

All health care practitioners must recognize that their patients compose a community of people of all religions, races, and economic backgrounds and that each patient must be accorded their best efforts. Every patient should be treated with consideration of his or her worth and dignity. Patients must be provided **confidentiality** and **privacy.** They have the right to be informed, to make informed consent, and to refuse treatment. The Patient's Bill of Rights details 12 specific areas of patients' just due and the health professional is ethically (and often, legally) responsible to adhere to them.

Patient **consent** can be verbal, written, or implied. For example, if a patient arrived for emergency treatment alone and unconscious, implied consent would be assumed. A patient's previously granted or presumed consent can be withdrawn at any time. Written patient

Conditions for Valid Patient Consent

- The patient must be of legal age.
- The patient must be of sound mind.
- The patient must give consent freely.
- The patient must be adequately informed of the procedure about to take place.

Introduction

Effective health care requires collaboration between patients and physicians and other health care professionals. Open and honest communication, respect for personal and professional values, and sensitivity to differences are integral to optimal patient care. As the setting for the provision of health services, hospitals must provide a foundation for understanding and respecting the rights and responsibilities of patients, their families, physicians, and other caregivers. Hospitals must ensure a health care ethic that respects the role of patients in decision making about treatment choices and other aspects of their care. Hospitals must be sensitive to cultural, racial, linguistic, religious, age, gender, and other differences as well as the needs of persons with disabilities.

The American Hospital Association presents *A Patient's Bill of Rights* with the expectation that it will contribute to more effective patient care and be supported by the hospital on behalf of the institution, its medical staff, employees, and patients. The American Hospital Association encourages health care institutions to tailor this bill of rights to their patient community by translating and/or simplifying the language of this bill of rights as may be necessary to ensure that patients and their families understand their rights and responsibilities.

Bill of Rights

1. The patient has the right to considerate and respectful care.

2. The patient has the right to and is encouraged to obtain from physicians and other direct caregivers relevant, current, and understandable information concerning diagnosis, treatment, and prognosis.

   Except in emergencies when the patient lacks decision-making capacity and the need for treatment is urgent, the patient is entitled to the opportunity to discuss and request information related to the specific procedures and/or treatments, the risks involved, the possible length of recuperation, and the medically reasonable alternatives and their accompanying risks and benefits.

   Patients have the right to know the identity of physicians, nurses, and others involved in their care, as well as when those involved are students, residents, or other trainees. The patient also has the right to know the immediate and long-term financial implications of treatment choices, insofar as they are known.

3. The patient has the right to make decisions about the plan of care prior to and during the course of treatment and to refuse a recommended treatment or plan of care to the extent permitted by law and hospital policy and to be informed of the medical consequences of this action. In case of such refusal, the patient is entitled to other appropriate care and services that the hospital provides or transfer to another hospital. The hospital should notify patients of any policy that might affect patient choice within the institution.

4. The patient has the right to have an advance directive (such as a living will, health care proxy, or durable power of attorney for health care) concerning treatment or designating a surrogate decision maker with the expectation that the hospital will honor the intent of that directive to the extent permitted by law and hospital policy.

   Health care institutions must advise patients of their rights under state law and hospital policy to make informed medical choices, ask if the patient has an advance directive, and include that information in patient records. The patient has the right to timely information about hospital policy that may limit its ability to implement fully a legally valid advance directive.

5. The patient has the right to every consideration of privacy. Case discussion, consultation, examination, and treatment should be conducted so as to protect each patient's privacy.

6. The patient has the right to expect that all communications and records pertaining to his/her care will be treated as confidential by the hospital, except in cases such as suspected abuse and public health hazards when reporting is permitted or required by law. The patient has the right to expect that the hospital will emphasize the confidentiality of this information when it releases it to any other parties entitled to review information in these records.

7. The patient has the right to review the records pertaining to his/her medical care and to have the information explained or interpreted as necessary, except when restricted by law.

8. The patient has the right to expect that, within its capacity and policies, a hospital will make reasonable response to the request of a patient for appropriate and medically indicated care and services. The hospital must provide evaluation, service, and/or referral as indicated by the urgency of the case. When medically appropriate and legally permissible, or when a patient has so requested, a patient may be transferred to another facility. The institution to which the patient is to be transferred must first have accepted the patient for transfer. The patient must also have the benefit of complete information and explanation concerning the need for, risks, benefits, and alternatives to such a transfer.

Figure 1–2. Patient's Bill of Rights. *(Continued.)*

9. The patient has the right to ask and be informed of the existence of business relationships among the hospital, educational institutions, other health care providers, or payers that may influence the patient's treatment and care.

10. The patient has the right to consent to or decline to participate in proposed research studies or human experimentation affecting care and treatment or requiring direct patient involvement, and to have those studies fully explained prior to consent. A patient who declines to participate in research or experimentation is entitled to the most effective care that the hospital can otherwise provide.

11. The patient has the right to expect reasonable continuity of care when appropriate and to be informed by physicians and other caregivers of available and realistic patient care options when hospital care is no longer appropriate.

12. The patient has the right to be informed of hospital policies and practices that relate to patient care, treatment, and responsibilities. The patient has the right to be informed of available resources for resolving disputes, grievances, and conflicts, such as ethics committees, patient representatives, or other mechanisms available in the institution. The patient has the right to be informed of the hospital's charges for services and available payment methods.

The collaborative nature of health care requires that patients, or their families/surrogates, participate in their care. The effectiveness of care and patient satisfaction with the course of treatment depend, in part, on the patient fulfilling certain responsibilities. Patients are responsible for providing information about past illnesses, hospitalizations, medications, and other matters related to health status. To participate effectively in decision making, patients must be encouraged to take responsibility for requesting additional information or clarification about their health status or treatment when they do not fully understand information and instructions. Patients are also responsible for ensuring that the health care institution has a copy of their written advance directive if they have one. Patients are responsible for informing their physicians and other caregivers if they anticipate problems in following prescribed treatment.

Patients should also be aware of the hospital's obligation to be reasonably efficient and equitable in providing care to other patients and the community. The hospital's rules and regulations are designed to help the hospital meet this obligation. Patients and their families are responsible for making reasonable accommodations to the needs of the hospital, other patients, medical staff, and hospital employees. Patients are responsible for providing necessary information for insurance claims and for working with the hospital to make payment arrangements, when necessary.

A person's health depends on much more than health care services. Patients are responsible for recognizing the impact of their life-style on their personal health.

Conclusion

Hospitals have many functions to perform, including the enhancement of health status, health promotion, and the prevention and treatment of injury and disease; the immediate and ongoing care and rehabilitation of patients; the education of health professionals, patients, and the community; and research. All these activities must be conducted with an overriding concern for the values and dignity of patients.

Figure 1–2 *(continued)*. A patient's bill of rights. These rights can be exercised on the patient's behalf by a designated surrogate or proxy decision maker if the patient lacks decision-making capacity, is legally incompetent, or is a minor. (Reprinted with permission of the American Hospital Association, Copyright 1992.)

consent is required before any examination that involves greater than usual risk—for example, invasive vascular examinations requiring the use of injected iodinated contrast agents such as angiograms and arteriograms. For lower risk procedures, the consent given on admission to the hospital is generally sufficient.

It is imperative that the radiographer take adequate time to thoroughly explain the procedure or examination to the patient. An informed patient is a more cooperative patient, and a better examination is more likely to result. Patients should be clear about what will be expected of them and what they may expect from the radi- ▶ ographer. This must be considered the ***standard of care*** for each patient, not only to fulfill legal mandates, but to fulfill professional and humanistic obligations as well.

B. PROFESSIONAL LIABILITY

It is essential that radiographers, just like other health care professionals, be familiar with their **scope of practice** (Fig. 1–3). This ◀ document identifies educational and certification requirements and the range of the radiographer's responsibilities. Any radiographer who steps outside of these guidelines is making himself or herself vulnerable to legal retribution. Indeed, it is well for radiographers to recognize that they can be held legally liable for patient injury.

The four primary *sources of law* are the Constitution of the United States, statutory law, regulations and judgments of administrative bureaus, and court decisions.

The *Constitution* expresses the categorical laws of the country. Its impact with respect to health care and health care professionals lies, in part, in its insurance of the right to privacy. The right to privacy indicates that the patient's modesty and dignity will be respected. It also refers to the health care professional's obligation to respect the confidentiality of privileged information. Inappropriate communication of privileged information to anyone but the appropriate health care professionals is inexcusable.

Statutory law refers to laws enacted by congressional, state, or local legislative bodies. The enforcement of statutory laws is frequently delegated to administrative bureaus such as the Board of Health, the Food and Drug Administration, or the Internal Revenue Service. It is the responsibility of these agencies to enact *rules and regulations* that will serve to implement the statutory law.

Court decisions involve the interpretation of **statutes** and vari- ◀ ous regulations in decisions involving individuals. For example, the decision of an administrative bureau can be appealed and the court would decide if the agency acted appropriately and correctly. Court decisions are referred to as common law.

There are two basic kinds of law: **public law** and **private (civil)** ◀ **law.** *Public* laws are any that regulate the relationship between individuals and government. *Private,* or civil, law includes laws that regulate the relationships among people. **Litigation** involving a ◀ radiographer's professional practice is most likely to involve the latter.

A private (civil) injustice or injury is a **tort,** and the injured party ◀ may seek reparation for damage incurred. Torts are described as either *intentional* or *negligent*.

Examples of *intentional* torts include false imprisonment, **assault** ◀ and **battery,** defamation, and invasion of privacy. False imprison- ◀ ment is the illegal restriction of an individual's freedom. Holding a person against his or her will or using unauthorized restraints can constitute false imprisonment. Assault is to threaten harm; battery is to carry out the threat. A patient may feel sufficiently intimidated to claim assault by a radiographer who threatens to repeat a difficult examination if the patient does not try to cooperate better. A radiographer who performs an examination on a patient without his or her consent or after he or she has refused the examination may be guilty of battery. A charge of battery may also be made against a radiographer who treats a patient roughly or who performs an

---

For Liability for a Negligent Tort, Four Elements Must Be Present:

- Duty (what *should* have been done)
- *Breach* (deviation from duty)
- Injury sustained
- Cause (as a result of breach)

The practice of radiography is performed by a segment of healthcare professionals responsible for the administration of ionizing radiation to humans and animals for diagnostic, therapeutic or research purposes.

Credentials

1. State statutes may exist which define and/or delimit the scopes of practice for individuals who perform radiologic procedures.
2. The initials R.T.(R)(ARRT) indicates Registered Technologist Radiography with certification by the American Registry of Radiologic Technologists.
3. The initials R.T.(R)(CV)(ARRT) indicates Registered Technologist Radiography and Cardiovascular-Interventional Technology with certification by the American Registry of Radiologic Technologists.
4. The initials R.T.(R)(M)(ARRT) indicates Registered Technologist Radiography and Mammography with certification by the American Registry of Radiologic Technologists.
5. The initials R.T.(R)(MR)(ARRT) indicates Registered Technologist Radiography and Magnetic Resonance Imaging with certification by the American Registry of Radiologic Technologists.
6. The initials R.T.(R)(QM)(ARRT) indicates Registered Technologist Radiography and Quality Management with certification by the American Registry of Radiologic Technologists.

Scope of Practice

The practice of radiography includes, but is not limited to, the following:

1. Procedures or examinations performed upon the order of, or for diagnostic interpretation by a licensed practitioner.
2. Optimal patient care applying established and accepted protocols.
3. Supervision of peers and/or students where applicable.
4. Continued evaluation of responsibilities and methods with recommendations for expansion of the profession.

Three levels of practice are identified for radiography: comprehensive, extended, or limited.

Comprehensive Practice

Radiography is performed on any or all body organs, systems, or structures involving general radiographic procedures. Individuals demonstrate competency to meet state licensure, permit, or certification requirements defined by law for whole body radiography; or maintain the credential R.T.(R) ARRT, or equivalent.

Extended Practice

Radiography expertise is expanded beyond comprehensive practice. Individuals have obtained additional education and specific skills to enhance, expand, and demonstrate competency. Extended practice has been identified for the following disciplines:

• Cardiovascular-interventional technology
• Computed Tomography
• Mammography
• Magnetic Resonance Imaging
• Quality Management

Limited Practice

Radiography is limited to specific anatomical regions by particular state statutes. Individuals demonstrating competency are recognized by license, permit or certification requirements defined by law. Limited practice may include the following services:

• Chest/thorax
• Genitourinary
• Abdominal
• Skull
• Podiatric
• Pelvis
• Photofluorographic
• Chiropractic
• Extremities
• Orthopaedic
• Dental
• Musculoskeletal

Compendium of Learning

The art and science of radiography requires that the individual achieve specific knowledge and skills for a defined scope of practice.

Learning experiences, clinical practicum, and curriculum requirements shall be structured for the health care professional to successfully demonstrate the level of competency necessary for comprehensive, extended, or limited practice in the following areas:

• **Computer literacy and applications:** An understanding of generic terminology, keyboard operation, menu selection strategies, and logistics of program flow.
• **Human structure and function:** General anatomy, anatomical relationships, organ and system functions in order to perform accurate radiographic examination for the defined discipline and recognize the area of interest on desired images.

Figure 1–3. Radiography scope of practice. *(Continued)*

- **Medical ethics:** Legal considerations which impact upon the scope of practice, respecting an established code of ethics and risk management.
- **Medical terminology:** An understanding of disease descriptions, abbreviations, symbols, terms or phrases necessary to successfully communicate with other health care professionals.
- **Pathology:** Knowledge of disease and abnormalities which influence performance or outcome of a radiographic procedure.
- **Patient care:** Attention and concern for the physical and psychological needs of the patient. The individuals should recognize a life threatening condition and implement basic life sustaining actions.
- **Positioning:** Accurate placement of the body, respecting patient's comfort, ability and safety to achieve prescribed results and best demonstrate the anatomy of interest. Techniques to physically manipulate and apply radiographic equipment to produce various projections and/or desired image.
- **Principles of radiographic exposure:** Appropriate selection of all technical factors and equipment to produce a quality diagnostic image.
- **Quality control:** Preventive maintenance and knowledge of equipment capabilities, calibration of and care of equipment within operating standards, sensitometry characteristics, and monitoring of image processing systems for accuracy and consistency.
- **Radiation physics:** Atomic structure, beam quality, radiation interactions, and the function and operations of various generator components.
- **Radiation protection:** The use of beam restricting devices, patient shielding techniques, proper screen-film combinations, accurate assessment and implementation of appropriate exposure factors, and knowledge of applicable governmental regulations to minimize radiation exposure.
- **Radiobiology:** An understanding of beam formation and radiation interaction with matter as it relates to genetic and somatic effects.

Position Description

Discipline
Radiography

Position Title(s)
Radiographer (ASRT preferred term)
Radiologic Technologist
Diagnostic Medical Radiographer

Scope of Practice
Radiography—Practice Comprehensive

Position Summary

Provides health care services, applying x-ray energy to assist in diagnosis or treatment. Performs radiographic procedures and related techniques, producing images for the interpretation by; or at the request of a licensed practitioner. Exercises professional judgment in performance of services and maintains a demeanor complementary to medical ethics. Provides appropriate patient care and recognizes patient conditions essential for successful completion of the procedure.

Duties and Responsibilities

1. Performs diagnostic radiographic procedures.

   A. Corroborates patient's clinical history with procedure, assuring information is documented and available for use by a licensed practitioner.
   B. Prepares patient for procedures; providing instructions to obtain desired results, gain cooperation, and minimize anxiety.
   C. Selects and operates radiography equipment, imaging and/or associated accessories to successfully perform procedures.
   D. Positions patient to best demonstrate anatomic area of interest, respecting patient ability and comfort.
   E. Immobilizes patients as required for appropriate examination.
   F. Determines radiographic technique exposure factors.
   G. Applies principles of radiation protection to minimize exposure to patient, self and others.
   H. Evaluates radiographs or images for technical quality, assuring proper identification is recorded.
   I. Assumes responsibility for provision of physical and psychological needs of patients during procedures.
   J. Practices aseptic techniques as necessary.
   K. Understands methods and is capable of performing venipunctures.
   L. In agreement with state statute(s) and/or where institutional policy permits, prepares, identifies and /or administers contrast media and/or medications as prescribed by a licensed practitioner.
   M. Verifies informed consent for, and assists a licensed practitioner with interventional procedures.
   N. Assists licensed practitioner with fluoroscopic and specialized interventional radiography procedures.
   O. May perform non-interpretive fluoroscopic procedures as appropriate and consistent with applicable state statutes.
   P. Initiates basic life support action when necessary.

2. Provides patient education.

Figure 1–3 *(Continued).*

3. Assists in maintaining records, respecting confidentiality and established policy.

4. Assumes responsibility for assigned area and reports equipment malfunction.

5. Provides input for equipment purchase and supply decisions.

6. Provides practical instruction for students and/or other health care professionals.

7. Participates in the department's quality assessment and improvement plan. May be responsible for specific quality control duties in the assigned area.

8. May be responsible for control of inventory and purchase of supplies for the assigned area.

9. Maintains knowledge of and observes universal precautions.

10. Understands and applies patient relations skills.

11. Pursues appropriate continuing education.

Qualifications

1. Graduate of Joint Review Committee on Education in Radiologic Technology (JRCERT) accredited radiography program or equivalent.

2. Certification by the American Registry of Radiologic Technologists in radiography, or equivalent.

3. Possesses valid state credential, if applicable.

Figure 1–3 *(Continued).* Radiography scope of practice. (Reprinted with the permission of the American Society of Radiologic Technologists. All rights reserved, Copyright 1995.)

examination on the wrong patient. A radiographer who discloses confidential information to unauthorized individuals may be found ▶ guilty of invasion of privacy or ***defamation.*** A radiographer whose disclosure of confidential information is in some way detrimental to the patient (causing ridicule or loss of job, for example) may be ▶ accused of defamation. Spoken defamation is ***slander;*** written ▶ defamation is ***libel.***

▶   The assessment of ***duty*** (what *should* have been done) is determined by the professional *standard of care* (that level of expertise generally possessed by reputable members of the profession). The determination of whether or not the standard of care was met is usually made by determining what another reputable practitioner would have done in the same situation.

Examples of negligent torts may include patient injury as a result of a fall while unattended on an x-ray table, in a radiographic room, or on a stretcher without side rails or safety belt. Radiographing the wrong patient or opposite limb are other examples of negligence. ▶ The term ***malpractice*** is usually used with reference to negligence.

Three areas of frequent litigation in radiology involve patient falls and other positioning injuries, pregnancy, and errors or delays ▶ in ***diagnosis.***

Patient falls and other positioning injuries. Examples: A sedated patient left unattended in the radiographic room falls from the x-ray table; the radiographer moves the patient with a spinal injury to the x-ray table, resulting in irreversible damage to the spinal cord.

Pregnancy. Example: The radiographer fails to inquire about a possible pregnancy before performing a radiologic examination. Some time later, the patient calls expressing concern about the fetus.

Errors or delays in diagnosis. Example: The patient has an x-ray examination in the emergency room (ER) and is sent home. The radiologist reads the films and fails to notify the ER physician of findings; the physician gets a written report 2 days later. Meanwhile, the patient dies or suffers permanent damage from an untreated condition.

If patient injury results from misperformance of a duty in the routine scope of practice of the radiographer, most courts will apply **res ipsa loquitur,** that is, "the thing speaks for itself." If the patient ◄ is obviously injured as a result of the radiographer's actions, it becomes the radiographer's burden to *disprove* negligence. In many instances, the hospital and/or radiologist will also be held responsible according to **respondeat superior,** or, "the master speaks for ◄ the servant."

Summary

- ■ **The ARRT Code of Ethics details guidelines for the radiographer's professional conduct.**
- ■ **The AHA Patient's Bill of Rights details 12 specific areas of patient rights that the health care professional is obligated to respect.**
- ■ **The American Society of Radiologic Technologists (ASRT) Scope of Practice identifies the level of knowledge and skill required of a professional radiographer.**
- ■ **The two kinds of law are public law and private (civil) law. Litigation involving health care practitioners usually involves private (civil) law.**
- ■ **A civil injustice is a tort; a tort can be intentional or negligent.**
- ■ **Negligence litigation in radiology most frequently involves injuries from falls and other positioning injuries, pregnancy, and errors or delay in diagnosis.**

II. REQUISITION AND CONSULTATION CONSIDERATIONS

A. AUTHORIZATION

Request forms for radiologic examinations should be carefully reviewed by the radiographer prior to commencement of the examination. Many hospitals or radiology departments have specific rules about exactly what kind(s) of information must appear on the requisition.

The requisition is usually stamped with the patient's personal information (name, address, age, admitting physician's name, and the patient's hospital identification number). The requisition should also include the patient's mode of travel to the radiology department (eg, wheelchair versus stretcher), the type of examination to be performed, pertinent diagnostic information, and any **infection control** ◄ or **isolation** information. Many institutions now have computerized, ◄ paperless systems that accomplish the same information transmittal. The healthcare professional generally has access to the system via personal password to ensure confidentiality of patient information. X-ray examinations can be requested only by a physician.

The radiographer should carefully review the patient information before bringing the patient into the radiographic room. This will enable the radiographer to have the x-ray room prepared, having all necessary cassettes and other radiographic accessories readily available.

B. ACCURATE TERMINOLOGY AND APPROPRIATE REQUEST

The radiographer must be certain to understand and, if necessary, clarify the information provided, for example, any abbreviations used, any vague terms such as "leg" or "arm" (versus femur or humerus). The radiographer must also be alert for, and obtain clarification of, conflicting information, for example, a request for a left ankle examination when the patient complains of, or has obvious injury to, the right ankle. Computerized systems or department policy may require that there be appropriate and accurate diagnosis information accompanying every request for diagnostic procedure.

C. ADEQUATE PATIENT HISTORY

It is important that the radiologist obtain a short, pertinent patient history of why the examination has been requested. Since patients are rarely examined or interviewed by the radiologist, observations and information obtained by the radiographer can be a significant help in making an accurate diagnosis.

D. VERIFICATION OF PATIENT IDENTITY

Care must be taken when making the initial patient identification. If the radiographer calls out a name at the door of a rather full waiting room, or asks a patient if he or she is Mr. or Ms. so-and-so, an anxious patient may readily respond in the affirmative without actually having heard his or her name called. It is always advisable to ask a patient to tell you his or her name or, if an inpatient, check his or her wristband.

E. MODIFIED AND ADDITIONAL PROJECTIONS

If a patient is unable to assume or maintain the routine position used for a particular examination, the radiographer should be able to modify the projection to provide the required information. It is not within the radiographer's scope of practice to supply additional, unrequested positions, but the radiographer should advise the physician of other projections or modifications that might enable him or her to better visualize the affected area.

F. SCHEDULING AND PREPARATION CONSIDERATIONS

When the patient must be scheduled for multiple x-ray examinations, ▶ each requiring the use of a ***contrast medium,*** the examinations must be scheduled in the correct sequence. For example, if a particular patient must be scheduled for a gallbladder series (GB), upper gastrointestinal (UGI) series, barium enema (BE), and intravenous pyelogram (IVP), what sequence will permit optimal visualization of the required structures? Remember, it will be important that residual barium not overlie structures of interest.

Generally speaking, those examinations with a contrast medium that is excreted quickly and completely should be scheduled first.

Sequence and Combining of Contrast Exams
Sequence
IVP
GB
BE
GI
Exams that can be performed together
GB and IVP
IVP and BE
GB and GI

Therefore, the IVP should be scheduled first, then the GB. If the UGI series were scheduled next, residual barium would be in the large bowel the next day, thus preventing adequate investigation. So the BE should be scheduled third; any residual barium should not interfere with an UGI examination, although a preliminary scout film should first be taken in each case.

If it is desired to expedite the studies, perhaps to reduce the length of hospital stay, some examinations can be performed on the same day. For example: GB and IVP. If the patient's GB is studied first and a fatty meal is used to evaluate its emptying function, there should be little contrast medium left to obscure the right collecting system. Another example of paired examinations is the IVP and BE. IVP contrast medium is excreted rapidly by the kidneys and should not interfere with visualization of the barium and air filled large bowel.

Patient preparation is somewhat different for each of these examinations. An iodinated contrast agent, usually in the form of several pills, is taken by the patient the evening before the scheduled GB examination and only water is allowed the morning of the examination. The patient scheduled for an UGI series must be npo (receive nothing by mouth) after midnight. A barium enema (lower GI) requires that the large bowel be very clean prior to the administration of barium; this requires the administration of **cathartics** (lax- ◀ atives) and cleansing enemas. Preparation for an IVP requires that the patient be npo after midnight; many institutions also require that the large bowel be cleansed of gas and fecal material. Aftercare for barium examinations is very important. Patients are typically instructed to take milk of magnesia, increase their intake of fiber, drink plenty of water, to expect change in stool color until all barium is evacuated, and to call their physician if they do not have a bowel movement within 24 hours. Since water is removed from the barium sulfate suspension in the large bowel, it is essential to make patients understand the importance of these instructions to avoid barium impaction in the large bowel.

The use of barium sulfate suspensions is contraindicated when ruling out visceral perforation. Barium could enter the peritoneal cavity and cause the very serious condition, *peritonitis*. When performing examinations on patients suspected or known to have stomach or intestinal perforation, *water-soluble iodinated contrast media* should be used instead of barium sulfate. If this water-soluble medium leaks through a perforation into the peritoneal cavity, it will simply be absorbed and excreted by the kidneys.

Diabetic patients who are scheduled for an UGI series are generally instructed to withhold their morning insulin until the meal following the examination. Should the patient take insulin before the examination and remain npo, a reaction might occur, especially if the examination was delayed for any reason. Upper GI examinations on diabetic patients should be among the first examinations scheduled each day and priority should be given these patients.

> ## Patient Preparation
>
> ### *GB*
> Iodinated contrast evening before exam; water only in AM
> ### *UGI*
> NPO after midnight
> ### *BE*
> Cathartics, cleansing enemas
> ### *IVP*
> NPO after midnight, cleansing enemas, empty bladder before scout film

Summary

- **Radiologic examinations can be requested only by a physician.**
- **The radiographer should examine the requisition carefully prior to bringing the patient to the radiographic room.**

■ Most radiology departments require that examination requests include pertinent diagnostic information and any infection control or isolation information.

■ The patient should be identified by asking his or her name and/or checking the wristband.

■ It is the radiographer's responsibility to clarify any vague or conflicting information found on the requisition.

■ Multiple radiologic examinations must be scheduled in a sequence that will allow prompt and adequate visualization of structures of interest.

■ Patients must be appropriately prepared for the contrast examination(s) for which they are scheduled.

Chapter Exercises

⭐ *Congratulations!* You have completed this chapter. If you are able to answer the following group of very comprehensive questions, you should feel confident that you have really mastered this section. You will then be ready to go on to the "Registry-type" questions that follow. For greatest success, do not go to these multiple choice questions without first completing the short answer questions below.

1. Discuss the ARRT Code of Ethics with respect to legal considerations pertinent to radiology *(p. 4)*.

2. Discuss the AHA Patient's Bill of Rights with respect to legal considerations pertinent to radiology *(pp. 5–6)*.

3. Discuss the ASRT Scope of Practice for the Radiographer with respect to legal considerations pertinent to radiology *(pp. 8–10)*.

4. List the conditions necessary for valid consent *(pp. 4–7)*.

5. Explain the importance of explaining the procedure to the patient *(p. 7)*.

6. Define the listed terms and/or correctly identify their definitions *(p. 3)*.

7. Discuss public versus private (civil) law *(p. 7)*.

8. Differentiate between assault and battery; slander and libel *(pp. 7–10)*.

9. Give examples of intentional and unintentional torts *(pp. 7–10)*.

10. List the four elements of a negligent tort *(p. 10)*.

11. Identify the three areas of litigation that most frequently involve radiology *(pp. 10–11)*.

12. Explain the importance of reviewing the examination request and other patient information prior to bringing the patient to the radiographic room *(p. 12)*.

13. List the patient information usually found on examination request forms *(pp. 12–13)*.

14. Identify the kinds of clarification that may be required prior to starting the examination *(p. 12)*.

15. Explain the importance of obtaining a patient history *(p. 12)*.

16. Discuss the best way(s) to ensure correct identification of a patient *(p. 12).*

17. Explain how best to correctly schedule multiple contrast examinations on the same patient; identify which examinations can be performed together *(pp. 12–13).*

18. Explain the appropriate patient preparation for GB, UGI, BE, and IVP *(pp. 13–14).*

19. Explain why diabetic patients that are required to be npo should be scheduled as the first AM appointment *(p. 13).*

A&U Chapter Review Questions

1. An informed consent is required before performing which of the following examinations?
   (A) upper GI
   (B) lower GI
   (C) sialogram
   (D) renal arteriogram

2. In what order should the following examinations be performed?
   1. UGI
   2. IVP
   3. barium enema
   (A) 3, 1, 2
   (B) 1, 3, 2
   (C) 2, 1, 3
   (D) 2, 3, 1

3. The usual patient preparation for an upper GI examination is:
   (A) npo 8 hours before the exam
   (B) light breakfast only, the morning of the exam
   (C) clear fluids only, the morning of the exam
   (D) 2 ounces of castor oil and enemas until clear

4. When a GI series has been requested on a patient with a suspected perforated ulcer, the type contrast medium that should be used is:
   (A) thin barium sulfate suspension
   (B) thick barium sulfate suspension
   (C) water-soluble iodinated medium
   (D) oil base iodinated medium

5. A radiographer who discloses confidential information to unauthorized individuals may be found guilty of:
   (A) assault
   (B) battery
   (C) intimidation
   (D) defamation

6. Patients' rights include which of the following?
    1. the right to refuse treatment
    2. the right to confidentiality
    3. the right to possess one's radiographs
    (A) 1 only
    (B) 1 and 2 only
    (C) 1 and 3 only
    (D) 1, 2, and 3

7. Which of the following examinations require(s) restriction of the patient's diet?
    1. GI series
    2. abdominal survey
    3. pyelogram
    (A) 1 only
    (B) 1 and 2 only
    (C) 1 and 3 only
    (D) 2 and 3 only

8. Which of the following instructions should the patient be given following a barium enema examination?
    1. increase fluid and fiber intake for a few days
    2. changes in stool color will occur until all barium is evacuated
    3. contact your physician if you do not have a bowel movement within 24 hours
    (A) 1 only
    (B) 2 only
    (C) 1 and 3 only
    (D) 1, 2, and 3

9. What is the best way to be sure you have the correct patient for an x-ray examination?
    (A) ask the receptionist to identify the patient
    (B) call the patient's name
    (C) check the patient's hospital identification
    (D) ask the radiologist to identify the patient

10. The threat to do harm is referred to as:
    (A) assault
    (B) battery
    (C) slander
    (D) libel

Answers and Explanations

1. (D) Written patient consent is required before any examination that involves greater than usual risk. This includes invasive vascular examinations requiring the use of iodinated contrast agents, such as renal arteriograms. For lower risk procedures, such as sialography and upper and lower GI series, the consent given on admission to the hospital is generally sufficient.

2. (D) When scheduling patient examinations, it is important to avoid the possibility of residual contrast medium overlying areas of interest of later examinations. The IVP should be scheduled first because the contrast medium used is excreted very rapidly. The barium enema should be scheduled next. The UGI is scheduled last. Any barium remaining from the previous BE is unlikely to interfere with the stomach or duodenum—though a preliminary scout film should be taken in each case.

3. (A) Patient preparation differs for various contrast examinations. To obtain a diagnostic examination of the stomach, it must first be empty. The usual *UGI* preparation is npo (nothing by mouth) after midnight (approximately 8 hours before the exam). Any material in the stomach can simulate the appearance of disease. An iodinated contrast agent, usually in the form of several pills, is taken by the patient the evening before a scheduled *GB* examination and only water is allowed the morning of the examination. The patient scheduled for a *barium enema* (lower GI) requires a large bowel that is very clean prior to the administration of barium; this requires the administration of cathartics (laxatives) and cleansing enemas. Preparation for an *IVP* requires that the patient be npo after midnight; many institutions also require that the large bowel be cleansed of gas and fecal material. *Aftercare* for barium examinations is also very important. Patients are typically instructed to take milk of magnesia and to drink plenty of water. Since water is removed from the barium sulfate suspension in the large bowel, it is essential to make patients understand the importance of these instructions to avoid barium impaction in the large bowel.

4. (C) The use of barium sulfate suspensions is contraindicated when ruling out visceral perforation. Barium could enter the peritoneal cavity and cause the very serious condition, *peritonitis.* When performing examinations on patients suspected or known to have stomach or intestinal perforation, *water-soluble iodinated contrast media* (such as Gastrografin or Oral Hypaque) should be used instead of barium sulfate. If this water-soluble medium leaks through a perforation into the peritoneal cavity, it will simply be absorbed and excreted by the kidneys. Water-soluble contrast agents may also be used in place of barium sulfate when the possibility of barium impaction exists.

5. (D) A radiographer who discloses confidential information to unauthorized individuals may be found guilty of *invasion of privacy* or *defamation.* A radiographer whose disclosure of confidential information is in some way detrimental to the patient may be accused of defamation. Spoken defamation is *slander;* written defamation is *libel. Assault* is to threaten harm; *battery* is to carry out the threat.

6. (B) The American Hospital Association identifies twelve important areas in their "Patient's Bill of Rights." These include the right to refuse treatment (to the extent allowed by law), the right to confidentiality of records and communication, and the right to continuing care. Other patient rights identified are the right to informed consent, privacy, respectful care, *access* to personal records, refusal to participate in research projects, and an explanation of one's hospital bill.

7. (C) A patient having a GI series is required to be npo for at least 8 hours prior to the exam; food or drink in the stomach can simulate diasase. A patient scheduled for a pyelogram must have the preceding meal withheld to avoid the possibility of aspirating vomitus in case of an allergic reaction. An abdominal survey does not require the use of contrast media, and no patient preparation is necessary.

8. (D) A mild laxative is often recommended to aid in the elimination of barium sulfate. The patient may also be instructed to increase dietary fiber and fluid and monitor bowel movement (should have at least one within 24 hours, or physician should be notified). Patients should also be aware of the white-colored appearance of the stool. It will be present until all barium is expelled.

9. (C) The best way to be sure you have the correct patient is to check the name on their wristband (hospital identification). Calling out the patient's name in the waiting room can have less accurate results. If a patient has been anxiously awaiting the x-ray exam, he or she may *expect* to hear his or her name next and unintentionally respond to another name. It is always wise to double check the patient's hospital ID.

10. (A) *Assault* is to threaten harm; *battery* is to carry out the threat. A patient may feel sufficiently intimidated to claim assault by a radiographer who threatens to repeat a difficult examination if the patient doesn't try to cooperate better. A radiographer who performs an examination on a patient without his or her consent or after he or she has refused the examination, may be guilty of battery. A charge of battery may also be made against a radiographer who treats a patient roughly or who performs an examination on the wrong patient. A radiographer who discloses confidential information to unauthorized individuals may be found guilty of *invasion of privacy* or *defamation*. A radiographer whose disclosure of confidential information is in some way detrimental to the patient may be accused of defamation. Spoken defamation is *slander;* written defamation is *libel.*

Patient Education and Assessment

2

I. COMMUNICATION SKILLS AND PATIENT INSTRUCTION

The importance of effective patient and professional ***communica-*** ◀
tion skills cannot be overstressed; the interaction between patient
and radiographer generally leaves a lasting impression of the
patient's health care experience. Of course, communication refers
not only to the spoken word but also to unspoken communication.
Facial expression, for example, can convey caring and reassurance or
impatience and disapproval. Similarly, a radiographer's touch can
convey his or her commitment to considerate care, or it can convey
a rough, uncaring, impersonal attitude.

A. VERBAL AND NONVERBAL COMMUNICATION

Consider the nonverbal messages communicated to a patient brought into a disorderly radiographic room, or by a radiographer presenting a sloppy, poorly groomed appearance. What about the grim-faced professional who brings the patient along to the radiographic room, gives rapid-fire instructions on what to do while searching about for missing markers and cassettes, then tosses the patient about on the x-ray table, and finally dismisses the patient with a curt "you can go now"?

Another patient is greeted by a smiling professional who introduces himself or herself and brings the patient to a neat and orderly radiographic room, where everything is in readiness for the procedure. The radiographer explains the procedure and answers the patient's questions. At the end of the examination, the patient is escorted back to the waiting area and clear instructions are given for appropriate post-procedural care.

Which patient has a more comfortable, anxiety-free examination? Which leaves the hospital or clinic environment with a more favorable impression of his or her healthcare experience? Which experience would *you* prefer as a patient?

The volume of the radiographer's voice and his or her rate of speech are extremely important factors to consider in effective communication. Loud, rapid speech is particularly uncomfortable for the sick patient. A conscious effort should be made to use a well-modulated tone. The radiographer should face the patient and make direct eye contact during communication.

Gaining the patient's confidence and trust through effective communication is an essential part of the radiographic examination. Some patients will require a greater use of the radiographer's communication skills. Patients who are seriously ill or injured; traumatized patients; patients who have impaired vision, hearing, or speech; pediatric patients; nonEnglish-speaking patients; the elderly and infirm; the physically or mentally impaired; alcohol and drug abusers—the radiographer must adapt his or her communication skills to meet the needs of many types of individuals.

Elderly patients, for example, dislike being pushed or hurried about. They appreciate the radiographer who is compassionate enough to take the extra few minutes necessary for comfort. Some elderly patients are easily confused; it is best to address them by their full name and to keep instructions simple and direct. The elderly deserve the same courteous, dignified care as all other patients.

B. EXPLANATION OF PROCEDURE

The radiographer requires the cooperation of the patient throughout the course of the examination. Effective communication skills will help to ensure this cooperation. It is particularly important that the patient understand the procedure about to take place. A thorough explanation will alleviate the patient's anxieties and permit fuller cooperation.

C. EXPLANATION OF AFTERCARE

Radiographers must be certain to provide patients with appropriate aftercare instructions (eg, plenty of fluids following barium examinations). Patients sometimes need to repeat explanations or instructions (to the radiographer) to be certain they understand; some have an additional question or two they must ask to clarify their thoughts. The radiographer's patience and understanding at these times is greatly appreciated by the anxious patient or relative.

Summary

- **Communication may be verbal or nonverbal. Verbal communication involves the tone and rate of speech as well as what is being said. It involves personalization and respect. Nonverbal communication involves facial expression, professional appearance, orderliness of the radiographic room, and the preparation and efficiency of the radiographer.**
- **A thorough explanation of procedures reduces the patient's anxiety, increases cooperation, and results in a better examination.**

II. EVALUATING PATIENT CONDITION

The radiographer must **assess** a patient's condition prior to bringing the patient to the radiographic room, and as the examination progresses. A good place to begin is with a review of the patient's chart. Other useful information includes the admitting diagnosis and recent nurses' notes including information regarding the patient's degree of ambulation, any preparation for the x-ray procedure and how it was tolerated, notes regarding laboratory tests, and saving the patient's urine.

A. PHYSICAL SIGNS

When the patient is first approached, and as the examination progresses, the radiographer should be alert to the patient's appearance and condition, and any subsequent changes in them. Notice the color, temperature, and moistness of the patient's skin. Paleness frequently indicates weakness; the **diaphoretic** patient has pale, cool skin. Fever is frequently accompanied by hot, dry skin. "Sweaty" palms may indicate **anxiety.** A patient who becomes **cyanotic** (bluish lips, mucous membranes, or nail beds) needs oxygen and requires immediate medical attention.

B. VITAL SIGNS

If a medical emergency arises, the radiographer may be required to assist by obtaining the patient's vital signs. Although checking vital signs is not a routine function, the radiographer should be proficient and confident if and when the need arises. Practicing vital signs during "slow" periods will benefit the patient who needs those skills during an emergency; also, those on whom you practice will learn their vital signs—valuable information for all.

Obtaining vital signs involves the measurement of body temperature, pulse rate, respiratory rate, and arterial blood pressure. Increased body temperature, or **fever,** usually signifies infection. Symptoms of fever include general **malaise,** increased pulse and respiratory rates, flushed skin that is hot and dry to the touch, and occasional chills. Very high, prolonged fevers can cause irreparable brain damage.

Normal Body Temperatures

Adult	
Oral	98.6
Rectal	99.1–99.6
Axillary	97.6–98.1
Infant–3 years	99–99.7
Children 5–13 years	97.8–98.6

Common Pulse Points

Artery	Location
Radial	wrist; at base of thumb
Carotid	neck; just lateral to midline
Temporal	in front of upper ear
Femoral	inguinal region; groin
Popliteal	posterior knee

Normal Pulse Rates (beats/min)

Men	70–72
Women	78–82
Children	90–100
Infants	120

Normal body temperature varies from person to person depending on several factors, including age. A normal adult body temperature taken orally is 98.6°F (37°C). Rectal temperature is generally 0.5 to 1.0° higher, whereas axillary temperature is usually 0.5 to 1.0° lower. Variation of 0.5 to 1.0° is generally considered within normal limits. Body temperature is usually lowest in the early morning and highest at night. Infants up to 3 years of age have normal body temperatures of between 99° and 99.7°. Children ages 5 to 13 years have a normal range of 97.8 to 98.6°.

Body areas having superficial arteries are best suited for determination of a patient's pulse rate. The five most readily palpated pulse points are the radial, carotid, temporal, femoral, and popliteal pulse. Of these, the radial pulse is the most frequently used. The apical pulse, at the apex of the heart, may be readily evaluated with the use of a stethoscope.

Pulse rate depends on the person's age, sex, body exertion and position, and general state of health. The very young and very old have higher pulse rates. The pulse rate increases in the standing position and after exertion. The pulse rate also increases with certain conditions, such as fever, organic heart disease, **shock,** and alcohol and drug use. Certain variations in the regularity and strength of the pulse are characteristic of various maladies. Pulse rates vary between men and women and among adults, children, and infants.

The act of respiration serves to deliver oxygen to all the body's cells and rid the body of carbon dioxide. The radiographer must be able to recognize abnormalities or changes in patient respiration. The general term used to describe difficult breathing is **dyspnea.** More specific terms used to describe abnormal respirations include uneven, **spasmodic, strident** (shrill, grating sound), **stertorous** (labored, eg, snoring), **tachypnea** (abnormally rapid breathing), **orthopnea** (difficulty breathing while recumbent), **oligopnea** (abnormally shallow, slow).

A patient's respirations should be counted after counting the pulse rate, while still holding the patient's wrist. Respiratory action may become more deliberate and less natural in the patient who is aware that his or her respirations are being counted. The normal respiratory rate is 12 to 18 breaths per minute. The respiratory rate of young children is somewhat higher, up to 30 breaths per minute. While the radiographer is counting respirations, he or she should be assessing the respiratory pattern (even, uneven) and depth (normal, shallow, deep) as well.

Blood encounters a degree of resistance as it travels through the peripheral vascular system; thus, a certain amount of pressure exists within the walls of the vessels. Blood pressure among individuals varies with age, sex, fatigue, mental or physical stress, disease, and trauma. The blood pressure within vessels is greatest during ventricular **systole** (contraction) and lowest during **diastole** (relaxation). Blood pressure measurements are recorded with the systolic pressure on top and the diastolic pressure on the bottom, as in 100/80 (read: "one hundred over eighty"). Normal adult systolic pressure ranges between 100 and 140 mm Hg; the normal diastolic range is between 60 and 90 mm Hg. Blood pressure consistently above 140/90 is considered **hypertension.** Hypertension is easily treated. Left undiagnosed, it can lead to renal, cardiac, or brain damage. Hypotension is characterized by a systolic pressure of less than 90 mm Hg. Hypotension is seen in individuals with a decreased blood volume as a result of hemorrhage, infection, fever, and anemia. ***Orthostatic*** hypoten- ◀ sion occurs in some individuals when they rise quickly from a recumbent position.

Blood pressure is measured using a ***sphygmomanometer*** and ◀ stethoscope. The patient may be recumbent or seated with the arm supported. The cuff of the sphygmomanometer is wrapped snugly around the arm, with its lower edge just above the ***antecubital*** ◀ ***fossa.*** With the stethoscope earpieces in place, the brachial artery pulse is palpated in the antecubital fossa and the bell (diaphragm) of the stethoscope is placed over the brachial artery. The valve on the bulb pump is closed and the cuff inflated enough to collapse the brachial artery (about 180 mm Hg). The valve is then opened very slowly. The first sound heard is the systolic pressure; as the valve pressure is slowly released, the sound becomes louder, then suddenly gets softer—this is the diastolic pressure. After the blood pressure measurements are recorded, the stethoscope earpieces and bell should be cleaned.

Summary

- Patient condition may be assessed through chart information, observation, questioning, and vital signs.
- A patient's vital signs are temperature, pulse and respiration rate, and blood pressure.
- A normal adult oral body temperature is 98.6°F, axillary temperatures are 0.5 to 1° lower, and rectal temperatures are 0.5 to 1° higher.
- The arterial pulse points include radial, carotid, temporal, femoral, and popliteal.
- The normal adult pulse rate is 70 to 80 beats per minute; infant and children pulse rates are higher.
- The normal adult respiratory rate is 12 to 18 breaths per minute, with children's respirations being higher (up to 30 per minute).
- Dyspnea refers to difficulty breathing; other terms are used to describe specific respiratory abnormalities.
- Blood pressure is measured using a sphygmomanometer and stethoscope.
- The average normal adult blood pressure is 120/80; blood pressure varies with a person's age, sex, fatigue and stress level, disease, and with trauma.
- Systolic pressure (contraction) is the top number, diastolic pressure (relaxation) is the bottom number.

III. PATIENT TRANSPORTATION AND TRANSFER

Radiographers work with many patients whose capacities for ***ambu-*** ◀ ***lation*** vary greatly. Outpatients are usually ambulatory, that is, able to walk and not confined to bed. Ambulatory inpatients generally travel by wheelchair, while patients confined to bed must travel by stretcher. It is essential for the radiographer to use proper technique and body mechanics when transferring patients, for the safety of the patient and the radiographer.

Other Rules of Good Body Mechanics

1. When carrying a heavy object, hold it close to the body.
2. The back should be kept straight; avoid twisting.
3. When lifting an object, bend the knees and use leg and abdominal muscles to lift (rather than back muscles).
4. Whenever possible, push or roll heavy objects (rather than lifting or pulling).

To transfer the patient with maximum safety for the patient and himself or herself, the radiographer must correctly use certain concepts of body mechanics. First, a broad base of support lends greater stability; therefore, the radiographer should stand with his or her feet about 12 inches apart and with one foot slightly forward. Secondly, stability is achieved when the body's center of gravity (center of the pelvis) is positioned over its base of support. For example, leaning away from the central axis of the body makes the body more vulnerable to losing balance; if the feet are close together, balance is even more difficult to keep.

Even the ambulatory outpatient may be somewhat unsteady, so a ready, supporting hand at the elbow can be very helpful. The radiographer should keep a watchful eye on the patient and assist him or her as needed. Not all patients need, or want, well-intentioned assistance. Many prefer to manage on their own. The radiographer should recognize this but be ever alert and watchful should the patient need assistance. Other patients find it reassuring and feel an added sense of security with an attentive radiographer. The professional radiographer develops a sense of awareness of each patient's needs and concerns.

Before helping a patient into or out of a wheelchair, it must first be locked. Then, the footrests must be moved aside to avoid tripping over them or tilting the wheelchair forward. Once the patient is seated, the footrests should be lowered into place for the patient's comfort.

When transferring a patient between the x-ray table and a stretcher, it is essential that it, too, is first securely locked. Often a smooth piece of plastic, placed partially under the patient and used in conjunction with the drawsheet, is used to facilitate patient transfer. Patient transfer should involve pulling, not pushing; pushing increases friction and makes the transfer more difficult. Use the biceps muscles for pulling; do not bend at the waist and pull, as this motion increases back strain.

▶ It is essential that someone be responsible for keeping any IV tubing, *catheters,* oxygen lines, or other equipment free from entanglement during wheelchair and/or stretcher transfers.

The patient may be adjusted into the Fowler's position (head higher than feet) for comfort or ease of breathing. The radiographer must be certain that safety belts and/or side rails are appropriately used for any patient on a stretcher.

IV. PATIENT SAFETY AND COMFORT

It is the health care practitioner's responsibility to ensure patient safety and comfort while the patient is in his or her care. The radiographer should make mental notes of what the patient has when he or she enters the department, such as glasses or a purse. Patient belongings should be properly secured according to institution or department policy. The radiographer must be certain that the radiographic room is hazard free, that all equipment and accessories are used properly and safely, and that the patient is as comfortable as possible.

When moving to or from the wheelchair or stretcher, patients should always be assisted or, at least, given careful attention. It is exceedingly unwise to finish a radiographic examination and say "OK, you can get off the x-ray table now," or something to that effect. The x-ray tube must be moved away from the x-ray table, a footstool must be in place to assist the patient from the table, and the radiographer must be there to guide or assist the patient safely to the correct dressing room. Should an injured patient require assistance with dressing and undressing, it is important to remember that clothing should be *removed* from the *un*injured side first and *placed* on the *injured* side first.

Special consideration must be given to each patient according to his or her condition. The elderly, very thin patients, and those who will be required to lie on the x-ray table for a lengthy period of time benefit greatly from a foam pad between them and the x-ray table. Lumbar strain is relieved by a strategically placed pillow or positioning sponge under the knees. An extra pillow for the head or cushioning under the heels or ischial tuberosities can make a big difference in patient care. Special care and attention should be given to the skin of the elderly, as it bruises and bleeds easily.

Patients that are sedated, senile, in shock, or under the influence of alcohol or drugs must never be left unattended. Patients who arrive in the radiology department with restraints in place must never be left alone on the x-ray table, since they are usually active, disoriented, and occasionally, combative. Indeed, many radiology departments have rules stating that *no* patient may *ever* be left unattended in the radiographic room.

Just as health care practitioners provide for patient safety and comfort, they must ensure their own safety by practicing good body mechanics, infection control, and universal precautions.

Should an accident ever occur and a patient or health care practitioner be injured, no matter how small or insignificant the injury seems, it must be reported to the supervisor and an incident report completed. The risk management team, or similar group, requires all such information for legal documentation and as a means of identifying and resolving potential hazards.

Summary

- Modes of patient transportation include ambulation, wheelchair, and stretcher.
- Patient and radiographer safety require the use of proper and safe body mechanics.
- Wheelchairs and stretchers must be locked and wheelchair footrests positioned out of the way prior to patient transfer.
- One person should be responsible for the safe transport of IV lines, catheters, and other tubes.
- Patient transfer between the radiographic table and stretcher should involve pulling, not pushing; a smooth plastic board often helps.
- The knees should be bent when lifting heavy objects; leg and abdominal muscles are used instead of back muscles.
- Heavy objects should be carried close to the body.
- The back should be kept straight and twisting motions should be avoided.
- Heavy objects should be pushed or rolled (instead of pulled or lifted) whenever possible.

- Patient belongings should be properly secured according to policy while the patient is in the radiographer's care.
- The radiographer must be alert for patient safety and comfort at all times; patients should not be left unattended in the radiographic room.
- Should an accident occur involving the patient and/or radiographer, an incident report should be completed regardless how minor the incident.

Chapter Exercises

 Congratulations! *You have completed your review of this chapter. If you are able to answer the following group of very comprehensive questions, you should feel confident that you have really mastered this section. You are then ready to go on to "Registry-type" questions that follow. For greatest success, do not go to these multiple choice questions without first completing the short answer questions below.*

1. Define the key terms listed at the beginning of this chapter and/or correctly identify their definitions *(p. 21)*.

2. Discuss five ways in which the radiographer can send nonverbal messages to the patient *(pp. 21–22)*.

3. Discuss some qualities of verbal communication likely to evoke a positive response from the patient; a negative response *(p. 22)*.

4. Explain the value of making as many preparations as possible prior to bringing the patient into the radiographic room *(p. 22)*.

5. Discuss five types of patients who might require special communication efforts on the part of the radiographer *(pp. 22–23)*.

6. List five benefits of effective communication skills *(pp. 22–23)*.

7. Discuss the importance of being alert to initial patient condition and any subsequent changes in condition *(p. 23)*.

8. Identify the following with respect to body temperature:

   A. normal adult, infant, and child temperature *(p. 24)*.

   B. the significance of fever, that is, what it usually indicates *(p. 23)*.

   C. symptoms usually associated with fever *(p. 23)*.

   D. difference among oral, rectal, and axillary temperatures *(p. 24)*.

9. Identify the following with respect to pulse rate:

   A. the normal, average adult pulse rate for men and women *(p. 24)*.

   B. normal and abnormal conditions under which pulse rate will vary or change *(p. 24)*.

C. the usual site of pulse determination; other possible sites *(p. 24)*.

10. Identify the following with respect to respiration:

    A. its function *(p. 24)*.

    B. the ideal time to determine patient respiration rate; why *(p. 24)*.

    C. the normal, average adult respiratory rate *(p. 24)*.

11. Identify the following with respect to blood pressure:

    A. equipment necessary *(p. 25)*.

    B. position of patient *(p. 25)*.

    C. position of cuff and bell *(p. 25)*.

    D. first and second sounds heard *(p. 25)*.

12. Discuss three modes of patient transport *(p. 25)*.

13. Identify, with respect to body mechanics and patient transfer:

    A. position of radiographer's feet (as base of support) *(p. 26)*.

    B. the body's center of gravity (versus stability) and when moving heavy objects: push versus pull; use of knees, legs, and back; proximity of object to body *(p. 26)*.

    C. position of footrests and locks during wheelchair transfers *(p. 26)*.

    D. position of locks, use of drawsheet and plastic mover, push versus pull in stretcher transfer. *(p. 26)*.

    E. care of IV lines, catheters, O_2, safety belts, side rails *(p. 26)*.

14. Identify the manner in which patients should be directed onto, and removed from, the x-ray table *(p. 26)*.

15. Explain how clothing should be removed from a patient with unilateral injury *(p. 27)*.

16. Identify techniques used to reduce patient discomfort of elderly and/or thin patients recumbent on the radiographic table *(p. 27)*.

17. Discuss the types of patients likely to be at greater risk left unattended on the radiographic table *(p. 27)*.

A&U Chapter Review Questions

1. Which of the following can communicate specific messages to the patient?
   1. tone of voice
   2. eye contact
   3. appearance of radiographer
   (A) 1 only
   (B) 1 and 2 only
   (C) 3 only
   (D) 1, 2, and 3

2. An ambulatory patient is one who:
   (A) has difficulty breathing
   (B) arrives by ambulance
   (C) is able to walk
   (D) is unable to walk

3. What number of breaths per minute represents the average rate of respiration for a normal adult?
   (A) 8 to 15
   (B) 10 to 20
   (C) 30 to 60
   (D) 60 to 90

4. The normal adult oral temperature is:
   (A) higher than rectal temperature
   (B) lower than rectal temperature
   (C) the same as rectal temperature
   (D) the same as axillary temperature

5. The period of relaxation of the heart is termed:
   (A) systole
   (B) diastole
   (C) hypertension
   (D) dyspnea

6. A patient who is diaphoretic has:
   (A) pale, cool, clammy skin
   (B) hot, dry skin
   (C) dilated pupils
   (D) warm, moist skin

7. The pulse can be detected only by the use of a stethoscope in which of the following locations?
   (A) wrist
   (B) neck
   (C) groin
   (D) apex of the heart

8. Rules for good body mechanics when transferring patients include:
    1. the radiographer's feet should be about 12″ apart
    2. the radiographer's trunk should lean toward the patient
    3. the radiographer's pelvis should be positioned over his or her feet
    (A) 1 only
    (B) 1 and 2 only
    (C) 1 and 3 only
    (D) 2 and 3 only

9. To reduce the back strain associated with transferring patients from stretcher to x-ray table, you should:
    (A) pull the patient
    (B) push the patient
    (C) hold the patient away from your body and lift
    (D) bend at the waist and pull

10. Instruments needed to assess vital signs include:
    1. tongue blade
    2. watch with second hand
    3. thermometer
    (A) 1 only
    (B) 1 and 2 only
    (C) 2 and 3 only
    (D) 1, 2, and 3

Answers and Explanations

1. (D) The interaction between patient and radiographer generally leaves a lasting impression of the patient's health care experience. Communication may be verbal or nonverbal. Verbal communication involves tone and rate of speech as well as what is being said. It involves personalization and respect. Nonverbal communication involves facial expression, professional appearance, orderliness of radiographic room, and preparation and efficiency of the radiographer.

2. (C) Radiographers work with many patients whose capacities for ambulation vary greatly. Outpatients are usually *ambulatory,* that is, able to walk and not confined to bed. Ambulatory inpatients generally travel by wheelchair, while patients confined to bed must travel by stretcher. It is essential for the radiographer to use proper technique and body mechanics when transferring patients, for the safety of the patient and the radiographer.

3. (B) A patient's respirations should be counted after counting the pulse rate, while still holding the patient's wrist. Respiratory action may become more deliberate, or less natural, in the patient who is aware that his or her respirations are being counted. The normal respiratory rate is 12 to 18 breaths per minute. The respiratory rate of young children is somewhat higher, up to 30 breaths per minute. While the radiographer is counting respirations, he or she should be assessing the respiratory pattern (even, uneven) and depth (normal, shallow, deep) as well.

4. (B) Obtaining vital signs involves the measurement of body temperature, pulse rate, respiratory rate, and arterial blood pressure. Increased body temperature, or fever, usually signifies infection. Symptoms of fever include general malaise, increased pulse and respiratory rates, flushed skin that is hot and dry to the touch, and occasional chills. Very high, prolonged fevers can cause irreparable brain damage.

Normal body temperature varies from person to person depending on several factors, including age. Normal adult body temperature taken orally is 98.6°F (37°C). Rectal temperature is generally 0.5 to 1.0° higher, whereas axillary temperature is usually 0.5 to 1.0° lower. Variation of 0.5 to 1.0° is generally considered within normal limits. Body temperature is usually lowest in the early morning and highest at night. Infants up to three years of age have normal body temperatures of between 99° and 99.7°F. Children ages 5 to 13 years have a normal range of 97.8 to 98.6°F.

5. (B) Blood pressure within vessels is greatest during ventricular *systole* (contraction) and lowest during *diastole* (relaxation). Blood pressure measurements are recorded with the systolic pressure on top and the diastolic pressure on the bottom, as in 100/80 (read: "one hundred over eighty"). Normal adult systolic pressure ranges between 100 and 140 mm Hg; the normal diastolic range is between 60 and 90 mm Hg. Blood pressure consistently above 140/90 is considered *hypertension. Dyspnea* is the medical term used to describe difficulty in breathing.

6. (A) The radiographer should be alert to the patient's appearance and condition, and any subsequent changes in them. Notice the color, temperature, and moistness of the patient's skin: paleness frequently indicates weakness; the *diaphoretic* patient has pale, cool skin; fever is frequently accompanied by hot, dry skin; "sweaty" palms may indicate *anxiety,* a patient who becomes *cyanotic* (bluish lips, mucous membranes, nail beds) needs oxygen and requires immediate medical attention.

7. (D) Body areas having superficial arteries are best suited for determination of a patient's pulse rate. The five most readily palpated pulse points are the radial, carotid, temporal, femoral, and popliteal pulse. Of these, the radial pulse is the most frequently used. *The apical pulse, at the apex of the heart, may be readily evaluated with the use of a stethoscope.*

8. (B) It is essential for the radiographer to use proper technique and body mechanics when transferring patients, for the safety of the patient and the radiographer. In order to transfer the patient with maximum safety to the patient and himself or herself, the radiographer must correctly utilize certain concepts of body mechanics. First, a broad base of support lends greater stability; therefore, the radiographer should stand with *his or her feet about 12 inches apart* and with one foot slightly forward. Second, stability is achieved when the body's center of gravity (center of the *pelvis*) *is positioned over its base of support.* For example, leaning away from the central axis of the body makes the body more vulnerable to losing balance; if the feet are close together, balance is even more difficult to keep.

9. (A) Patient transfer should involve *pulling,* not pushing; pushing increases friction and makes the transfer more difficult. Use the biceps muscles for pulling; do not bend at the waist and pull, as this motion increases back strain.

When transferring a patient from stretcher to x-ray table, several rules apply that will help reduce back strain. Pull, do not push the patient; pushing increases friction and makes the transfer more difficult. Use the biceps muscles for pulling; do not bend at the waist and pull, as this motion increases back strain.

10. (C) Obtaining vital signs involves the measurement of *body temperature,* pulse rate, *respiratory rate,* and *arterial blood pressure.* A thermometer is used to take the patient's temperature. A watch with a second hand is required to time the patient's pulse rate and respirations. To measure blood pressure, a sphygmomanometer and stethoscope are required. A tongue blade is used to depress the tongue for inspection of the throat and is not part of vital sign assessment.

Infection Control and Prevention

I. MODES OF TRANSMISSION

The control and prevention of infection must be a hospital-wide effort; each department is required to have its own infection-control protocol, designed according to the risks unique to the services provided. Because radiography often involves exposure to sickness and disease, the radiographer must be aware of, and conscientiously practice, infection control and effective preventative measures.

Infectious microorganisms can be transmitted from one patient to other patients or to health care workers. They are transmitted by means of either direct or indirect contact. *Direct contact* involves touch. The polite act of handshaking is a simple way of transmitting infection from one individual to another. Diseases transmitted by direct contact include skin infections such as boils, and sexually transmitted diseases such as syphilis and AIDS. Direct contact with droplets of nasal or oral secretions from a sneeze or cough is referred to as droplet contact.

Indirect contact involves transmission of microorganisms via *airborne* contamination, ▶ *fomites,* and *vectors. Pathogenic microor-* ▶ *ganisms* expelled from the respiratory tract through the mouth or nose can be carried as evaporated droplets through the air or on dust and settle on clothing, utensils, or food. Patients with respiratory infections or disease transported to the radiology department, therefore, should wear a mask to prevent such transmission during a cough or sneeze; it is not necessary for the health care professional or transporter to wear a mask (as long as the patient does). Many such microorganisms can remain infectious while awaiting transmission to another host. A contaminated inanimate object such as a food utensil, doorknob, or IV pole is referred to as a *fomite.* A *vector* is an insect or animal carrier of infectious organisms, such as a rabid animal, a mosquito that carries malaria, or a tick that carries Lyme disease.

It is somewhat surprising, yet understandable, that many infections are acquired in the hospital; surprising because hospitals are places where people go to regain their health, yet understandable because individuals weakened by illness or disease are more susceptible to infection than healthy individuals. Infections acquired in hospitals, especially by patients whose resistance to infection has ▶ been diminished by their illness, are termed *nosocomial.* The most common nosocomial infection is the urinary tract infection (UTI), related to the use of urinary catheters, which allow passage of pathogens into the patient's body. Other types of nosocomial infections include wound and respiratory infections.

Health care practitioners must exercise strict infection-control precautions so that their equipment and/or technique will not be the ▶ source of nosocomial infection. *Contaminated* waste products, soiled linen, and improperly sterilized equipment are all means by which microorganisms can travel. Not every patient will come in contact with these items; however, the health care professional is in constant contact with patients and is therefore a constant threat to spread infection. Microorganisms are most commonly spread by way of the hands; spread of infection can be effectively reduced by proper disposal of contaminated objects and proper hand washing ▶ before and after each patient. *Disinfectants,* or *germicides,* are used in many hand-washing liquids to kill microorganisms.

II. STANDARD PRECAUTIONS

Exposure to infectious microorganisms is a daily concern for health care professionals, especially with the rapid spread of human ▶ immunodeficiency virus *(HIV)* and acquired immunodeficiency syn- ▶ drome *(AIDS),* and the hazard of hepatitis B virus *(HBV)* infection. ▶ HIV-infected individuals may be symptomless and go undiagnosed for as long as 10 years, yet they are carriers of the infection and have ▶ the potential to spread the disease. *Epidemiologic* studies indicate that HIV infection can be transmitted only by intimate contact with blood or body fluids of an infected individual. This can occur through the sharing of contaminated needles, through sexual contact, from mother to baby at childbirth, and from transfusion of contaminated blood. HIV cannot be transmitted by inanimate objects such as water fountains, telephones, and toilet seats. Hepatitis B is another bloodborne infection and affects the liver. It is thought that over one million people in the United States have chronic hepatitis B and, as such, can transmit the disease to others.

Since no symptoms may be evident in patients infected with particular diseases, such as HIV, AIDS, and HBV, all patients must be treated as potential sources of infection from blood and other body fluids. The practices associated with this concept are called ***standard*** ◀ ***precautions.*** This rationale treats *all* body fluids and substances as infectious and serves to prevent the spread of microorganisms to other patients by the radiographer as well as to protect the radiographer from contamination. Body fluids and substances that may be considered infectious include blood, breast milk, vaginal secretions, amniotic fluid, semen, peritoneal fluid, synovial fluid, cerebrospinal fluid, feces, urine, secretions from the nasal and oral cavities, and secretions from the lacrimal and sweat glands.

It is essential, then, that the radiographer make the practice of blood and body fluid precautions *standard*, that is, they must be practiced on all patients without exception. Special precautions must also be taken with the disposal of biomedical waste, such as laboratory and pathology waste, all sharp objects, and liquid waste from suction, bladder catheters, chest tubes, and IV tubes, as well as drainage containers. Biomedical waste is generally packaged in easily identifiable impermeable bags and removed from the premises by an approved biomedical waste hauler.

Summary

- **Infectious microorganisms are transmitted by either direct or indirect contact. Direct contact involves touch. Indirect contact includes airborne contamination, fomites, and vectors.**
- **Infections acquired in hospitals are called nosocomial infections; the most common nosocomial infection is the UTI.**
- **Disinfectants (germicides) are used in hand-washing liquids to kill microorganisms.**
- **Since no symptoms may be evident in patients afflicted with certain diseases such as HIV, AIDS, and hepatitis B, all patients must be treated as potential sources of infection from blood and other body fluids; this is the standard precautions concept.**
- **The practice of standard precautions helps prevent transmission of infection to the health care professional and to other patients.**
- **The health care professional is legally and ethically responsible for adhering to standard precautions principles.**
- **Standard precautions must be practiced on all patients at all times without exception.**
- **Biomedical waste (body substances and their containers) must be disposed of in carefully controlled circumstances.**

Guidelines for Standard Precautions

The radiographer is now legally, as well as ethically, responsible for strict adherence to standard precaution principles identified in the following guidelines.

- Shielding for the face and eyes must be in place whenever the possibility of blood or body fluid splashes may occur near the face.
- Plastic aprons must be worn whenever the possibility of blood or body fluid splashes may occur on the clothing.
- Gloves must be worn whenever touching blood or body fluids is possible, and whenever handling equipment or touching surfaces contaminated with blood or body fluids is possible.
- Gloves must be changed and the hands washed after every patient contact.
- Blood and body fluid spills should be carefully cleaned and disinfected using a solution of one part bleach to ten parts water.
- Used needles must not be separated from the syringe and must be placed in designated puncture-proof containers.
- Prescribed procedures must be followed and sufficient care and attention given risky tasks to avoid needle sticks and other skin penetrations from cutting instruments.
- Emergency cardiopulmonary resuscitation (CPR) equipment must include resuscitation bags and mouthpieces.

III. MEDICAL VERSUS SURGICAL ASEPSIS

▶ *Antisepsis* is a practice that retards the growth of pathogenic bacteria but does not necessarily kill them. Alcohol is an example of an
▶ antiseptic. *Medical asepsis* refers to the destruction of pathogenic microorganisms through the process of *disinfection*. Examples of dis-
▶ infectants are hydrogen peroxide, chlorine, and boric acid. *Surgical asepsis (sterilization)* refers to the removal of all microorganisms *and* their spores (reproductive cells) and is practiced in the surgical suite. Health care practitioners must practice medical asepsis at all times.

The most important precaution in the practice of aseptic technique is proper hand washing. The radiographer's hands should be thoroughly washed with soap and warm, running water after each patient examination. If the faucet cannot be operated with the knee, it should be opened and closed using paper towels (to avoid contamination of or by the faucet). The radiographer's uniform should not touch the sink. The hands and forearms should always be kept lower than the elbows; care should be taken to wash all surfaces and between fingers. Hand lotions should be used to prevent hands from chapping; broken skin permits the entry of microorganisms. Disinfectants, or germicides, are substances used to kill pathogenic bacteria; they are frequently used in hand-washing substances.

Uniforms are recommended because clothing that is worn in patient areas should not be worn elsewhere. Since clothing becomes contaminated in the patient area, a clean uniform should be worn daily. Microorganisms can find safe harbor in jewelry, especially rings with stones and other crevices, and in cracked nail polish. It is always recommended that the only jewelry a health care practitioner wears is a wristwatch and unadorned wedding band. Remember, many microorganisms can remain infectious while awaiting transmission to another host.

Sterile technique is employed during invasive procedures, such as arthrography, and for the administration of contrast media via the
▶ intravenous and *intrathecal* routes (eg, angiography and myelography). When radiography is required in the surgical suite, every precaution must be made to maintain the surgical asepsis required in surgical procedures. This requires proper dress, cleanliness of equipment, and restricted access to certain areas. One example of a restricted area is the "sterile corridor," the area between the draped patient and the instrument table. This area is occupied only by the surgeon and the instrument nurse.

IV. ISOLATION

Adherence to standard blood and body fluids and substances precautions in the care of all patients will minimize the risk of transmission of HIV and other blood and body-substance–borne pathogens from the patient to the radiographer and from the radiographer to patient. The use of standard precautions also minimizes the need
▶ for other isolation categories, except in the cases of *strict isola-*
▶ *tion* and *respiratory isolation* (when controlled air circulation is required).

Medical asepsis and blood and body fluids precautions are used when performing radiographic examinations on all patients, but additional precautions may be required when a patient is suspected or known to have a particular communicable disease. For example, *acid-fast-bacillus* **(AFB)** *isolation* is employed with patients sus- ◄ pected or known to be infected with the tubercle bacillus (TB). AFB isolation requires the patient to wear a mask to avoid the spread of acid-fast bacilli (in bronchial secretions) during coughing. If the patient is unable or unwilling to wear a mask, the radiographer must. The radiographer should wear gloves, but a gown is required only if flagrant contamination is likely. Patients infected with AFB require a private, specially ventilated room.

A private room is indicated for all patients on *respiratory isola-tion*. Measles, mumps, and meningitis are among those diseases spread by *droplet contact* and also require respiratory isolation. Because these diseases are communicable via droplet contact, a pri-vate room is required for the patient, and health care practitioners must use gown and gloves. Any diseases spread by direct or close contact, such as streptococcal and staphylococcal viruses, conjunc-tivitis, and influenza, require **contact isolation.** Contact isolation ◄ procedures require the use of gloves, masks, and gown for anyone coming in close contact with the infected individual.

Patients in respiratory or contact isolation occasionally have to be transported to the radiology department for examination. When this is the case, the wheelchair or stretcher should first be covered with a clean sheet, followed by a second sheet or thin blanket. After transferring the patient to the wheelchair or stretcher, the inner sheet is wrapped around the patient, and the outer sheet over it (thus, the inner sheet is the contaminated one). The radiographic room should be available and ready for the patient to be taken in directly. The x-ray table should be covered with a clean sheet before the patient is transferred to it. One radiographer (wearing gloves) must be respon-sible for patient positioning and the other for equipment controls and operation (to avoid contamination of equipment and possible transmission of disease to others via indirect contact or fomites).

Once the examination is completed, the patient is transferred to the wheelchair or stretcher and wrapped in the same way. Any con-taminated linens should be placed in a plastic bag and contaminated disposables such as tissues are placed in a separate bag; both are returned with the patient to the isolation unit.

The radiographic table and other equipment should be cleaned with a disinfectant and hands should be washed carefully when the task is completed.

The use of a procedure known as *strict isolation* is required for patients having diseases communicated via the airborne or contact routes. An example of this kind of disease is chickenpox, a highly contagious disease whose spread is difficult to control. Health care practitioners caring for these patients are required to wear gloves, mask, and gown. The patient requires a private room or a room shared with another chickenpox patient.

Mobile radiography performed on patients in strict isolation gen-erally requires special precautions and the teamwork of two people. The radiographer dons gown, gloves (being certain that gloves cover gown cuffs), and mask, usually available just outside the patient's room. The necessary cassette(s) must be placed in a plastic bag to protect them from contamination. The "clean" radiographer must remember to bring an extra pair of gloves into the patient room. The mobile x-ray unit is brought into the room, and all possible adjustments must be made before the radiographer touches anything else. Once the equipment is in position, the cassette and patient are adjusted properly. *At this point, the mobile x-ray unit must not be touched* until the "clean" radiographer properly disposes of the gloves he or she has on, and replaces them with the clean extra pair. The exposure is then made; the covered cassette is removed from the patient and brought to the door. The radiographer slides the plastic cover away from the cassette and the second member of the team (generally a second, or "dirty," radiographer) grasps the unveiled portion. Just inside the patient room door, the contaminated gloves should be removed properly and the hands washed thoroughly. The mask and gown ties are then untied with clean hands; the gown is removed by placing a clean hand under the cuff and pulling the arm down from underneath. The other sleeve is also removed by touching only the inside of the gown. The gown is slipped off and folded forward with the contaminated surfaces touching. The discarded garments must be placed in the container provided. The radiographer should then carefully rewash his or her hands, dry them with paper towels, and take care not to touch the faucets. After leaving the room, *the mobile unit must be thoroughly cleaned* with a disinfectant and the hands carefully washed once again. It should be noted that patients in strict isolation may feel ostracized and relegated to a kind of solitary confinement. The radiographer must remember that isolation patients have the same needs as other patients (indeed, perhaps greater needs) and be certain to treat them with dignity and care.

Protective, or reverse, isolation is used to keep the susceptible patient from becoming infected. Burn patients who have lost their means of protection, their skin, have increased susceptibility to bacterial invasion. Patients whose immune systems are depressed are unable to combat infection and are more susceptible to infection. These patients are treated with strict isolation technique, taking care to protect the *patient* from contamination (Table 3–1).

Table 3–1. Category-specific Isolation

CATEGORY	NECESSARY PROTECTION
Drainage–secretion Examples: burn infection, conjunctivitis, wound infection	Gloves, gown (if necessary) Handwashing (2 minutes)
Enteric (fecal material) Examples: coxsackievirus, viral meningitis, gastroenteritis	Gloves and gown if possible contact with infectious material Thorough handwashing
Acid-fast bacillus (AFB) Example: tuberculosis	Mask Handwashing Gown if gross contamination possible
Respiratory Examples: measles, mumps, bacterial meningitis	Mask Handwashing
Contact Examples: herpes simplex, influenza in young children	Mask, gloves, gown Handwashing
Strict Examples: chickenpox, pneumonic plague	Mask, gloves, gown Handwashing

Summary

- Antiseptics retard the growth of bacteria.
- Medical asepsis refers to the destruction of bacteria through the use of disinfectants.
- Surgical asepsis refers to the destruction of all microorganisms and their spores through sterilization.
- The practice of medical asepsis is required at all times, while surgical asepsis is required for invasive procedures.
- The single most important component of medical asepsis is proper and timely hand washing.
- A clean uniform must be worn daily; uniforms become contaminated and should not be worn elsewhere; pathogenic microorganisms thrive in jewelry crevices and cracked nail polish.
- Medical asepsis and standard (blood and body fluid) precautions are employed for all patients; additional precautions are required for patients with certain communicable diseases.
- AFB isolation requires that the patient wear a mask and be admitted to a private, specially ventilated room.
- Respiratory isolation and a private room are also required for measles, mumps, and meningitis; the radiographer requires gown and gloves (and mask if the patient is not wearing one).
- Communicable diseases spread by direct or close contact (conjunctivitis, streptococcal or staphylococcal infections) require that the radiographer use mask, gown, and gloves.
- Strict isolation (as for chickenpox) requires a private room and the wearing of mask, gloves, and gown.
- Mobile radiography on a patient in strict isolation requires that one radiographer positions the patient and cassette, while the other handles the equipment.
- Protective, or reverse, isolation is used to keep the susceptible patient from being infected.

Chapter Exercises

 Congratulations! *You have completed your review of this chapter. If you are able to answer the following group of very comprehensive questions, you should feel confident that you have really mastered this section. You are then ready to go on to "Registry-type" questions that follow. For greatest success, do not go to these multiple choice questions without first completing the short answer questions below.*

1. Define the key terms listed at the beginning of this chapter and/or correctly identify their definitions *(p. 35)*.

2. Identify and differentiate between the two basic means of transmitting infectious microorganisms *(pp. 35–36)*.

3. List three means of indirect transmission of pathogenic microorganisms *(p. 36)*.

4. Identify the most common type of hospital-acquired infection *(p. 36)*.

5. List five possible sources of nosocomial infection in the radiology department *(p. 36)*.

6. Describe the type protection required for patients with respiratory infections *(p. 36)*.

7. Identify the means by which microorganisms are spread *(p. 36)*.

8. What substances are added to hand-washing liquids to kill microorganisms *(p. 36)*?

9. Discuss the rationale of body fluid and substance (standard) precautions *(p. 37)*.

10. Discuss each of the following with respect to standard precautions *(p. 37)*:

    A. when a face shield should be used

    B. when a plastic apron should be used

    C. when hands should be washed

    D. when gloves should be used

    E. how body fluid and substance spills should be cleaned

    F. care of used needles

G. special devices available for CPR

H. on whom standard precautions should be practiced

11. Differentiate between medical and surgical asepsis *(pp. 37–38).*

12. Identify and explain the most important practice in good aseptic technique *(p. 38).*

13. Discuss the function of uniforms worn by health care practitioners; the hazards of jewelry and nail polish *(p. 38).*

14. Explain the precautionary measures taken in AFB isolation, ie, apparel (and for whom), patient room *(pp. 38–39).*

15. List three communicable diseases spread by droplet contact that require respiratory isolation *(p. 39).*

16. Identify circumstances when strict isolation must be employed and special apparel is required by the radiographer *(p. 39).*

17. Describe the method of performing mobile chest radiography on patients in strict isolation, to include: *(pp. 38–39)*

    A. number of persons needed

    B. radiographer's apparel

    C. how to protect cassettes from contamination

    D. why an extra pair of gloves is needed in the patient room

    E. role played by the second individual

    F. how protective clothing should be removed

    G. care of x-ray machine at completion of exam

18. Describe the proper method of transporting an isolation patient to the radiology department *(p. 39).*

19. Describe the purpose of reverse isolation *(pp. 40–41).*

20. Discuss any special needs the isolation patient may have *(pp. 40–41).*

A&U Chapter Review Questions

1. Diseases that can be transmitted by direct contact include:
    1. skin infections
    2. syphilis
    3. rabies
    (A) 1 only
    (B) 1 and 2 only
    (C) 2 and 3 only
    (D) 1, 2, and 3

2. Which of the following can be transmitted via infected blood?
    1. tuberculosis
    2. AIDS
    3. HBV
    (A) 1 only
    (B) 1 and 2 only
    (C) 2 and 3 only
    (D) 1, 2, and 3

3. Which of the following are means of indirect transmission of microorganisms?
    1. vector
    2. fomite
    3. airborne
    (A) 1 only
    (B) 1 and 2 only
    (C) 3 only
    (D) 1, 2, and 3

4. What is the most effective means of controlling the spread of infectious microorganisms?
    (A) wearing gloves
    (B) wearing masks
    (C) handwashing
    (D) sterilization

5. What technique is practiced when all patients are treated as potential sources of infection from blood and other body fluids?
    (A) standard precautions
    (B) sterilization
    (C) disinfection
    (D) contamination precautions

6. What is the name of the practice that serves to retard the growth of pathogenic bacteria?
    (A) antisepsis
    (B) bacteriogenesis
    (C) sterilization
    (D) disinfection

7. Which of the following diseases require respiratory isolation?
    1. meningitis
    2. mumps
    3. measles
    (A) 1 only
    (B) 1 and 2 only
    (C) 3 only
    (D) 1, 2, and 3

8. The radiographer must perform the following procedure(s) prior to entering a strict isolation room with a mobile x-ray unit:
    1. wear gown and gloves
    2. wear gown, mask, gloves, and cap
    3. clean the mobile x-ray unit
    (A) 1 only
    (B) 2 only
    (C) 1 and 3 only
    (D) 2 and 3 only

9. Lyme disease is a condition caused by bacteria carried by deer ticks. The tick bite may cause fever, fatigue, and other associated symptoms. This is an example of transmission of an infection by:
    (A) droplet contact
    (B) the airborne route
    (C) a vector
    (D) a vehicle

10. With which of the following conditions is protective or reverse isolation associated?
    1. tuberculosis
    2. burns
    3. leukemia
    (A) 1 only
    (B) 1 and 2 only
    (C) 2 and 3 only
    (D) 1, 2, and 3

Answers and Explanations

1. (B) Infectious microorganisms can be transmitted from one patient to other patients or to health care workers. They are transmitted by means of either direct or indirect contact. *Direct contact* involves touch. Diseases transmitted by direct contact include skin infections such as boils and sexually transmitted diseases such as syphilis.

Indirect contact involves transmission of microorganisms via airborne contamination, fomites, and vectors. Pathogenic microorganisms expelled from the respiratory tract through the mouth or nose can be carried as evaporated droplets through the air or on dust and settle on clothing, utensils, or food. Patients with respiratory infections and disease transported to the radiology department, therefore, should wear a mask to prevent such transmission during a cough or sneeze; it is not necessary for the health care professional or transporter to wear a mask (as long as the patient does). Many such microorganisms can remain infectious while awaiting transmission to another host. A contaminated inanimate object such as a food utensil, doorknob, or IV pole is referred to as a fomite. A vector is an insect or animal carrier of infectious organisms, such as a rabid animal (rabies), a mosquito that carries malaria, or a tick that carries Lyme disease.

2. (C) Epidemiologic studies indicate that HIV/*AIDS* can be transmitted only by intimate contact with blood or body fluids of an infected individual. This can occur through the sharing of contaminated needles, through sexual contact, from mother to baby at childbirth, and from transfusion of contaminated blood. HIV/AIDS cannot be transmitted by inanimate objects. Hepatitis B virus *(HBV)* is another bloodborne infection and affects the liver. It is thought that over one million people in the US have chronic hepatitis B and, as such, can transmit the disease to others. Acid-fast-bacillus (AFB) isolation is employed with patients suspected or known to be infected with the tubercle bacillus *(TB)*. AFB isolation requires that the patient wear a mask to avoid the spread of acid-fast bacilli (in bronchial secretions) during *coughing.*

3. (D) *Indirect* contact involves transmission of microorganisms via *airborne* contamination, *fomites,* and *vectors.* Pathogenic microorganisms expelled from the respiratory tract through the mouth or nose can be carried as evaporated droplets through the air or on dust and settle on clothing, utensils, or food. A contaminated inanimate object such as a pillowcase, x-ray table, or IV pole is referred to as a *fomite.* A *vector* is an insect or animal carrier of infectious organisms, such as a rabid animal (rabies), a mosquito that carries malaria, or a tick that carries Lyme disease.

4. (C) Health care practitioners must exercise strict infection-control precautions so that they or their equipment will not be the source of nosocomial infection. Contaminated waste products, soiled linen, and improperly sterilized equipment are all means by which microorganisms can travel. Not every patient will come in contact with these items; however, the health care professional is in constant contact with patients and is therefore a constant threat to spread infection. *Microorganisms are most commonly spread by way of the hands; therefore handwashing before and after each patient is the most effective means of controlling the spread of microorganisms.* Disinfectants or germicides are used in many hand-washing liquids to kill microorganisms.

5. (A) Standard precautions treats *all* body fluids and substances as infectious. Its use prevents the spread of microorganisms to other patients and protects the radiographer from contamination. Body fluids and substances that may be considered infectious include blood, breast milk, vaginal secretions, amniotic fluid, semen, peritoneal fluid, synovial fluid, cerebrospinal fluid, feces, urine, secretions from the nasal and oral cavities, and secretions from the lacrimal and sweat glands.

Sterilization (surgical asepsis) refers to the removal of all microorganisms and their spores (reproductive cells) and is practiced in the surgical suite. The destruction of pathogenic microorganisms is the process of *disinfection* (medical asepsis). Examples of disinfectants are hydrogen peroxide, chlorine, and boric acid.

6. (A) *Antisepsis* retards the growth of pathogenic bacteria but does not necessarily kill them. Alcohol is an example of an antiseptic. Medical asepsis refers to the destruction of pathogenic microorganisms through the process of *disinfection.* Examples of disinfectants are hydrogen peroxide, chlorine, and boric acid. Surgical asepsis *(sterilization)* refers to the removal of all microorganisms *and* their spores (reproductive cells) and is practiced in the surgical suite. Bacteriogenesis refers to the formation of bacteria.

7. (D) Measles, mumps, and meningitis are among those spread by droplet contact and require respiratory isolation. Because these diseases are communicable via droplet contact a private room is required for the patient and health care practitioners must use gown and gloves.

8. (B) When performing bedside radiography in an isolation room, the radiographer should wear a gown, gloves, mask, and cap. The cassettes are prepared for the examination by placing a pillowcase over them to protect them from contamination. Whenever possible, one person should manipulate the portable unit and remain "clean," while the other handles the patient. The portable unit should be cleaned with a disinfectant before exiting the patient's room.

9. (C) Lyme disease is a condition that results from transmission of an infection by a vector (deer tick). Vectors are insects and animals carrying disease. Droplet contact involves contact with secretions (from the nose, mouth) that travel via a sneeze or cough. Airborne route involves evaporated droplets in the air that transfer disease.

10. (C) Protective or reverse isolation is used to keep the susceptible patient from becoming infected. Patients who have suffered burns have lost a very important means of protection, their skin, and therefore have increased susceptibility to infection. Active tuberculosis requires AFB (acid-fast bacilli) isolation.

Contrast Media

KEY TERMS ◀

Allergic	Ionic	Parenteral
Anaphylactic Reaction	Ingestion	Side Effects
Anaphylaxis	Inspissation	Subcutaneous
Antihistamine	Intradermal	Topical
Cardiopulmonary Arrest	Intramuscular	Toxic
Contraindication	Intrathecal	Urticaria
Dysphagia	Intravenous	Viscosity
Dyspnea	Miscibility	Viscous
Edema	Nausea	
Hypotension	Nonionic	

I. CHARACTERISTICS AND NOMENCLATURE

Although radiographic contrast media are usually administered orally or intravenously, there are a number of routes and methods of *drug administration* (see table of commonly used medications and their application, page 52). Drugs and medications may be administered either *orally* or *parenterally*. **Parenteral** refers to any ◀ route other than via the digestive tract (orally) and includes: ***topi-*** ◀ ***cal, subcutaneous, intradermal, intramuscular, intravenous,*** and ***intrathecal.*** ◀

Methods of Administration

Oral
PO (by mouth), through digestive system
Parenteral
topical
subcutaneous
intradermal
intramuscular
intravenous
intrathecal

Qualities of Iodinated Contrast Agents that Contribute to Discomfort, Side Effects, and Reactions

Viscosity More viscid (thick, sticky) agents are more difficult to inject and produce more heat and vessel irritation; the higher the concentration, the greater the viscosity.

Toxicity Potential toxicity is greater with higher-concentration agents and ionic agents; viscosity also increases as room temperature decreases.

Miscibility Contrast agents should be readily *miscible* (able to mix) with blood.

Osmolality Low osmolality agents have fewer number of particles in a given amount of solution and are less likely to provoke an allergic reaction.

The purpose of contrast media is to artificially increase subject contrast in body tissues and areas where there is little natural subject contrast. The abdominal viscera, for example, have very little subject contrast, that is, it is very difficult to identify specific organs or distinguish one organ from another. However, if a contrast agent is introduced into a particular organ such as the kidney or stomach, or into a vessel such as the aorta or one of its branches, we may more readily visualize these anatomic structures as well as evaluate physiologic activity.

Contrast media can be described as either positive (radiopaque) or negative (radiolucent). *Positive,* or *radiopaque,* contrast agents have a higher atomic number than the surrounding soft tissue, resulting in a greater attenuation or absorption of x-ray photons. They therefore produce a higher radiographic contrast. Examples of positive contrast media are iodinated agents (both water and oil-based) and barium sulfate suspensions. The inert characteristics of barium sulfate render it the least *toxic* contrast medium. On the other hand, iodinated contrast media have characteristics that increase their likelihood of producing *side effects* and reactions.

Negative, or *radiolucent, contrast agents* used are air and various gases. Since the atomic number of air is also quite different from that of soft tissue, an artificially high subject contrast can be produced. The advantage of carbon dioxide over air is that it is absorbed more rapidly by the body.

Negative contrast is often used with positive contrast in examinations termed "double contrast" studies. The function of the positive agent is usually to coat the various parts under study, while the air fills the space and permits visualization through the gaseous medium. Examinations that frequently use double-contrast technique are a barium enema (BE), upper gastrointestinal (GI) series, and arthrography.

II. USES AND CONTRAINDICATIONS

Radiopaque contrast media are most frequently employed for radiographic procedures. *Barium sulfate* is one type of radiopaque contrast agent that is used to visualize the GI tract. Mixed with water, it forms a suspension that is generally administered orally for demonstration of the upper GI tract (esophagus; fundus, body, and pylorus of stomach; and progression through the small intestine), and rectally for demonstration of the lower GI tract (large intestine).

Barium sulfate is *contraindicated* if a perforation is suspected somewhere along the course of the GI tract (eg, a perforated diverticulum or gastric ulcer). Barium could escape into the peritoneal cavity in this case and result in peritonitis. A water-soluble (absorbable) iodinated contrast medium is generally used instead. These preparations are available as a ready-mixed liquid or as a powder requiring appropriate dilution with water. A patient with a nasogastric (NG) tube can have the contrast medium administered through it for the purpose of locating and studying the site of obstruction. This procedure is called *enteroclysis.*

Patients often experience constipation following a GI or BE examination unless proper aftercare instructions are given to the patient upon completion of the examination. Barium preparations in the large bowel become thickened as a result of absorption of its fluid

content, a process called ***inspissation,*** causing symptoms from mild ◄
constipation to bowel obstruction. Constipation can be a serious
problem, particularly in the elderly, and fecal impaction or obstruction
can result. It is, therefore, essential that the radiographer provide clear
instructions for follow-up care, especially to outpatients. Patients are
usually advised to expect light-colored stools for the next few days, to
drink plenty of fluids, increase their intake of fiber, and to take a mild
laxative such as milk of magnesia following a barium study.

Iodinated contrast agents are another type of radiopaque contrast media. They may be *oil-based* or *water-based.* Oil-based contrast media are infrequently used. They are not water soluble, and
are therefore not readily absorbed by the body and so remain in
body tissues for lengthy periods of time. Examinations that employ
the use of oil-based contrast agents, though infrequently performed,
are lymphangiograms, sialograms, and bronchograms. Water-based
contrast materials may be ***ionic*** or ***nonionic*** (low osmolality). These ◄
agents are principally used to delineate the urinary and vascular systems, the gallbladder (GB), and the GI tract when barium sulfate is
contraindicated.

Ionic contrast media have a higher osmolality, that is, a greater
number of particles in a given amount of solution. Nonionic, or low
osmolality, contrast agents are used with children, the elderly, patients
with renal disease, patients having a history of ***allergic*** reaction to ◄
contrast media, or patients having multiple allergies. Side effects and
allergic reactions are less likely and less severe with these media.
Nonionic contrast agents are associated with less injection discomfort, and a lower incidence of ***nausea,*** vomiting, and cardiovascular ◄
complications. Their only disadvantage is their cost, which is many
times that of ionic contrast agents.

Iodinated contrast agents can become more ***viscous*** at normal ◄
room temperatures, making injection more difficult. Warming the
contrast to body temperature reduces ***viscosity,*** permitting an easier ◄
and more comfortable injection. The vial of contrast material can be
placed in a special warming oven.

III. REACTIONS AND EMERGENCY SITUATIONS

Anaphylaxis can result from the body's sensitivity and allergic reac- ◄
tion to certain foods, insect bites, drugs, and anesthetics. The reaction can be the result of ***ingestion,*** *injection,* or *absorption* of the ◄
sensitizing agent.

Since iodinated contrast media are potentially toxic, the radiographer must be knowledgeable and alert to the possible adverse
effects of their use (although the risk of a life-threatening reaction is
relatively rare). Reactions to contrast media generally occur within
2 to 10 minutes following injection and can affect all body systems.
The body's response to the introduction of contrast material is the
production of histamines, which brings about various symptoms.
Symptoms of a mild reaction include a flushed appearance, nausea,
a metallic taste in the mouth, nasal congestion, a few hives
(urticaria), and occasionally, vomiting. Treatment of these minor ◄
symptoms generally consists of administration of either an ***antihis-*** ◄
tamine such as diphenhydramine (Benadryl), which blocks the
action of the histamine and reduces the body's inflammatory
response, or epinephrine to raise the blood pressure and relax the

bronchioles (see the table of commonly used medications and their application below).

Potentially life-threatening responses include respiratory failure, shock, and death within minutes. A very serious and life-threatening

▶ response is an ***anaphylactic reaction.*** Early symptoms of an anaphylactic reaction include itching of the palms and soles, wheezing,

▶ constriction of the throat (possibly due to laryngeal ***edema***) ***dyspnea, dysphagia, hypotension,*** and ***cardiopulmonary arrest.*** The

▶ radiographer must maintain the patient's airway, summon the radiologist, and call a "code." The radiographer should then be prepared to stay with the patient and assist in any way possible until the arrival of the code team.

COMMON MEDICATIONS AND THEIR APPLICATION

TYPE	EFFECT	EXAMPLE
Adrenergic	Vasopressor, stimulates sympathetic nervous system: increases BP, relaxes smooth muscle of respiratory system	epinephrine (Adrenalin)
Analgesic	Relieves pain	aspirin, acetaminophen (Tylenol), codeine, meperidine (Demerol)
Antiarrhythmic	Relieves cardiac arrythmia	quinidine sulfate, lidocaine (Xylocaine)
Antibacterial	Stops growth of bacteria	penicillin, tetracycline, erythromycin
Anticholinergic	Depresses parasympathetic system	atropine, scopolamine, belladonna
Anticoagulant	Inhibits blood clotting; keeps IV lines and catheters free of clots	heparin, warfarin
Antihistamine	Relieves allergic symptoms	diphenhydramine hydrochloride (Benadryl)
Antipyretic	Reduces fever	aspirin, acetaminophen
Barbiturate	Depresses CNS, decreases BP and respiration, induces sleep	phenobarbital, secobarbital sodium (Seconal)
Cardiac stimulant	Increases cardiac output	digitalis
Cathartic	Laxative, relieves constipation, prepares colon for diagnostic tests	bisacodyl (Dulcolax), castor oil
Diuretic	Stimulates urine	furosemide (Lasix)
Emetic	Stimulates vomiting	ipecac
Hypoglycemic	Lowers blood sugar	insulin, chlorpropamide (Diabinese)
Narcotic	Sedative/analgesic; potentially addictive	morphine, codeine, meperidine (Demerol)
Vasodilator	Relaxes and dilates blood vessels, decreases BP	nitroglycerine, verapamil

Summary

- Drugs and medications may be administered orally or parenterally.
- Parenteral administration includes topical, oral, subcutaneous, intradermal, intramuscular (IM), intravenous (IV), and intrathecal.
- Artificial contrast media function to increase insufficient subject contrast.
- Artificial contrast media can be positive (radiopaque) or negative (radiolucent).
- Positive contrast media include barium sulfate and iodinated (oil or water-based) agents.
- Qualities of iodinated contrast media that contribute to its risk include viscosity, toxicity, and miscibility.
- Negative and positive contrast agents are often used together in "double contrast" studies.
- Water soluble (absorbable) contrast agents are used in place of barium sulfate when visceral perforation is suspected.
- Patients require clear and complete post-procedural instructions, particularly following barium examinations.
- Nonionic iodinated contrast agents produce far fewer side effects than do their ionic counterparts; ionic contrast agents are far more expensive.
- Reactions to ionic agents usually occur within 2 to 10 minutes following injection.
- Symptoms of a mild reaction include mild urticaria, flushing, nausea, nasal congestion, metallic taste; an antihistamine is usually given to the patient.
- Side effects that are potentially life-threatening include wheezing, throat constriction, dyspnea, dysphagia, hypotension; the emergency code team should be summoned.

Chapter Exercises

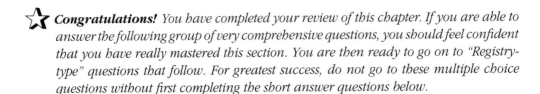 ***Congratulations!*** *You have completed your review of this chapter. If you are able to answer the following group of very comprehensive questions, you should feel confident that you have really mastered this section. You are then ready to go on to "Registry-type" questions that follow. For greatest success, do not go to these multiple choice questions without first completing the short answer questions below.*

1. Define the key terms listed at the beginning of this chapter and/or correctly identify their definitions *(p. 49)*.

2. Describe the difference between oral and parenteral drug administration; list five types of parenteral administration *(pp. 49–50)*.

3. Explain the purpose of contrast medium *(pp. 49–50)*.

4. Identify the two types of contrast media, describe their characteristics, and give examples of each *(p. 50)*.

5. Describe the risks associated with iodinated contrast media and identify the type of iodinated media associated with less risk *(p. 51)*.

6. Describe three qualities of iodinated contrast media that contribute to the production of side effects *(p. 50)*.

7. Explain how double contrast examinations can serve to better demonstrate certain anatomic parts *(p. 50)*.

8. Describe contraindications to the use of barium sulfate; identify the alternative contrast medium *(p. 50)*.

9. Explain the importance of aftercare explanations, especially following barium examinations *(pp. 50–51)*.

10. Distinguish between oil and water-based iodinated contrast media, their uses and characteristics *(p. 51)*.

11. Identify the basic difference between ionic and nonionic contrast media and identify when use of nonionic agents is indicated *(p. 51)*.

12. Identify the major disadvantage of nonionic contrast media *(p. 51)*.

13. Describe symptoms a patient having a mild reaction to iodinated contrast media might experience and their usual treatment *(p. 51)*.

14. Describe the symptoms of a possible impending anaphylactic reaction and the radiographer's responsibilities *(pp. 51–52).*

A&U Chapter Review Questions

1. Rapid onset of severe respiratory or cardiovascular symptoms after ingestion or injection of a drug, vaccine, contrast agent; or food; or after an insect bite, best describes:
   (A) rhinitis
   (B) myocardial infarct
   (C) anaphylaxis
   (D) asthma

2. Which of the following is a vasopressor and may be used for an anaphylactic reaction or cardiac arrest?
   (A) digitoxin
   (B) hydrocortisone
   (C) epinephrine
   (D) nitroglycerine

3. Which of the following drugs is considered a bronchodilator?
   (A) verapamil
   (B) nitroglycerine
   (C) lidocaine
   (D) epinephrine

4. Parenteral administration of drugs may be performed:
   1. intrathecally
   2. intravenously
   3. orally
   (A) 1 only
   (B) 1 and 2 only
   (C) 3 only
   (D) 1, 2, and 3

5. That quality of a substance that renders it poisonous is referred to as its:
   (A) toxicity
   (B) miscibility
   (C) viscosity
   (D) osmolality

6. Symptoms of a mild reaction to contrast media include:
   1. few hives
   2. nausea
   3. flushed appearance
   (A) 1 only
   (B) 1 and 2 only
   (C) 1 and 3 only
   (D) 1, 2, and 3

7. Early symptoms of anaphylactic reaction include:
   1. diaphoresis
   2. dyspnea
   3. hypotension
   (A) 1 only
   (B) 1 and 2 only
   (C) 2 and 3 only
   (D) 1, 2, and 3

8. Which of the following is appropriate to administer for treatment of minor symptoms following intravenous injection of contrast media?
   (A) histamine
   (B) antihistamine
   (C) emetic
   (D) cathartic

9. Types of positive contrast agents include:
   1. barium sulfate suspension
   2. water base iodinated media
   3. carbon dioxide
   (A) 1 only
   (B) 2 only
   (C) 1 and 2 only
   (D) 1 and 3 only

10. The advantages of using nonionic, water-soluble contrast media include:
    1. less patient discomfort
    2. low toxicity
    3. cost containment benefits
    (A) 1 only
    (B) 1 and 2 only
    (C) 2 and 3 only
    (C) 1, 2, and 3

Answers and Explanations

1. (C) *Anaphylaxis* is an acute reaction characterized by sudden onset of urticaria, respiratory arrest, vascular collapse, or systemic shock, and sometimes leads to death. It is caused by ingestion or injection of a sensitizing agent such as a drug, vaccine, contrast agent, food, or after an insect bite. *Asthma* and *rhinitis* are examples of allergic reactions.

Myocardial infarct (heart attack) describes failure of the myocardium to receive adequate blood supply, usually as a result of an occluded vessel.

2. (C) *Epinephrine* (trade name Adrenalin) is the vasopressor used to treat an anaphylactic reaction or cardiac arrest. *Nitroglycerine* is a vasodilator. *Hydrocortisone* is a steroid that may be used to treat bronchial asthma, allergic reactions, and inflammatory reactions. *Digitoxin* is used to treat cardiac fibrillation.

3. (D) *Epinephrine* is a bronchodilator. Bronchodilators may be administered in a spray mister, such as for asthma, or injection form to relieve severe bronchospasm. *Lidocaine* (xylocaine) is an antiarrhythmic used to prevent or treat cardiac arrhythmias (dysrhythmia). *Nitroglycerine* and *verapamil* are vasodilators. Vasodilators permit increased blood flow by relaxing the walls of the blood vessels.

4. (B) Although radiographic contrast media are usually administered orally or intravenously, there are a number of routes or methods of drug administration. Drugs and medications may be administered either *orally* or *parenterally*. *Parenteral* refers to any route other than via the digestive tract (orally) and includes: *topical, subcutaneous, intradermal, intramuscular, intravenous,* and *intrathecal*.

5. (A) A *toxic* substance is a poisonous substance. Our contrast agents must have low toxicity. *Viscosity* refers to the degree of thickness or stickiness of a substance. More viscid contrast agents are more difficult to inject, and produce more heat and vessel irritation; the higher the agent's concentration, the greater its viscosity. *Miscibility* refers to the contrast agent's ability to mix with the blood. Contrast agents should be readily miscible. *Osmolality* refers to the number of particles in a given amount of solution. Low osmolality agents are less likely to provoke an allergic reaction.

6. (D) The body's response to the introduction of contrast material is the production of histamines, which brings about various symptoms. Symptoms of a mild reaction include a flushed appearance, nausea, a metallic taste in the mouth, nasal congestion, a few hives *(urticaria)*, and occasionally vomiting. Treatment of these minor symptoms generally consists of administration of either an *antihistamine* such as diphenhydramine (Benadryl), which blocks the action of the histamine and reduces the body's inflammatory response, or epinephrine to raise the blood pressure and relax the bronchioles.

7. (C) Potentially life-threatening responses to contrast agents include respiratory failure, shock, and death within minutes. A very serious and life-threatening response is an *anaphylactic reaction* whose early symptoms include itching of the palms and soles, wheezing, constriction of the throat (possibly due to laryngeal edema), dyspnea, dysphagia, hypotension, and cardiopulmonary arrest. The radiographer's responsibilities include maintaining the patient's airway, summoning the radiologist, and calling a "code." The radiographer should then be prepared to stay with the patient and assist in any way possible until the arrival of the code team. Diaphoresis refers to profuse sweating and is unrelated to an anaphylactic reaction.

8. (B) Symptoms of a mild reaction include a flushed appearance, nausea, a metallic taste in the mouth, nasal congestion, a few hives *(urticaria)*, and occasionally vomiting. Treatment of these minor symptoms generally consists of administration of either an *anti-*

histamine such as diphenhydramine (Benadryl), which blocks the action of *histamine* and reduces the body's inflammatory response, or epinephrine to raise the blood pressure and relax the bronchioles. An emetic is used to induce vomiting; a cathartic is a laxative.

9. (C) Contrast media may be described as either positive (radiopaque) or negative (radiolucent). *Positive, or radiopaque, contrast agents* have a higher atomic number than the surrounding soft tissue, resulting in a greater attenuation/absorption of x-ray photons, and thereby producing a higher radiographic contrast. Examples of positive contrast media are iodinated agents (both water and oil-based) and barium sulfate suspensions. *Negative, or radiolucent, contrast agents* used are air and various gases. Since the atomic number of air is also quite different from that of soft tissue, an artificially high subject contrast can be produced. The advantage of carbon dioxide over air is that it is absorbed more rapidly by the body.

10. (B) The relatively new low-osmolality and nonionic, water-soluble contrast media available to radiology departments have outstanding advantages, especially for patients with a history of allergic reaction. They were originally used for intrathecal injections (myelography), but were quickly accepted for intravascular injections. Side effects and allergic reactions are less likely and less severe with these media. Their one very significant disadvantage is their huge cost compared to ionic media. Many institutions are choosing to use nonionic media in select procedures and with patients at greater risk of allergic reaction.

Managing Acute Situations

KEY TERMS ◄

APHASIA	EXTRAVASATION	INFUSION
ASPIRATE	FOWLER'S POSITION	LUMEN
ASTHMA	GAUGE	NASAL CANNULA
CONVULSION	HEIMLICH MANEUVER	OCCLUSION
CVA	HEMATOMA	SEIZURE
CYANOSIS	HEMIPARESIS	STROKE
DIAPHORESIS	HEMORRHAGE	SYNCOPE
DYSPHASIA	HYPERTENSION	THROMBUS
EMPHYSEMA	HYPOTENSION	TIA
EPISTAXIS	HYPOXIA	VERTIGO

I. PATIENT SUPPORT EQUIPMENT

One of a human being's most basic physiologic needs is an adequate supply of oxygen. Diminished oxygen supply *(hypoxia)* can result ◄ from an airway obstructed by aspirated material, laryngeal edema as a result of anaphylaxis, or a pathologic process such as *emphy-* ◄ *sema.* The radiographer must be knowledgeable enough to recognize symptoms and respond appropriately. The proper response might be to perform the *Heimlich maneuver,* summon the code ◄ team, or to check the flow of oxygen already in place.

Oxygen is taken into the body and supplied to the blood to be delivered to all body tissues. Any tissue(s) lacking in, or devoid of, an adequate blood supply will die or suffer permanent damage. Oxygen may be required in cases of severe anemia, pneumonia, pulmonary edema, and shock.

Symptoms of inadequate oxygen supply include dyspnea, ▶ ***cyanosis, diaphoresis,*** and distention of the veins of the neck. The patient who experiences some or all of these symptoms will be very anxious and must not be left unattended. The radiographer must *call* ▶ for help, assist the patient to a sitting or semi-***Fowler's position*** (the recumbent position makes breathing more difficult), and have oxygen and emergency drugs available.

In areas that patients will occupy for extended periods (eg, patient rooms, operating room, emergency room, and radiology department), oxygen is available through wall outlets at a pressure of 60 to 80 psi (pounds per square inch) equipped with an easily adjustable flowmeter to regulate the administration of oxygen. It is important to administer *humidified* oxygen to avoid drying and irritation of the mucosa. In other areas, oxygen will be available in tanks having one valve to regulate its flow and another to indicate the amount of oxygen remaining in the tank.

There are various devices available to deliver oxygen to the patient. Their use is determined by the amount of oxygen required by the patient. They are frequently classified as *low* or *high flow*. ▶ The ***nasal cannula*** is the most frequently used device and is used to supplement the oxygen in room air. The nasal cannula is a low-flow oxygen device. It is convenient and fairly comfortable for the patient, although it can be somewhat easily moved out of position, during sleep for example.

There are various types of oxygen *masks* available for delivery of oxygen. The *simple face mask* (low-flow) is best suited for short-term oxygen therapy. With extended use, the plastic becomes warm and sticky. Communication is difficult, the mask is easily displaced, and it must be removed at mealtime. The *partial rebreathing mask* (low-flow) and *nonrebreathing mask* (low-flow) deliver more precise concentrations of oxygen to the patient.

Mechanical ventilators (high-flow) are most frequently encountered in a hospital critical care unit. Patients on ventilators have an artificial airway in place, while the ventilator controls the respiratory rate and volume.

Although oxygen is not a flammable substance, it does support combustion, so care must be taken to avoid spark or flame where oxygen is in use.

The use of a *suction* device is occasionally required to maintain ▶ a patient's airway by ***aspirating*** (removing) secretions, blood, or other fluids when the patient is unconscious or otherwise unable to do so. Suction is available from a wall outlet, similar to oxygen, or as a mobile apparatus. It is unlikely that the radiographer would be required to suction a patient, but he or she might be needed to assist with the procedure. Suction tubing must have a disposable catheter attached to its end for collection of airway secretions. The radiographer should be familiar with the location of suction equipment and replacement disposable catheters.

Intravenous equipment includes needles, syringes, fluids such as normal saline or D5W (a solution of dextrose in water), IV catheters, heparin locks, IV poles, and infusion sets.

The diameter of a needle is identified as its ***gauge.*** As the diam- ◀
eter of its bore increases, the gauge decreases. Hence, an 18-gauge
needle has a larger diameter bore than a 23-gauge needle. Hypodermic needles are generally used for phlebotomy (ie, blood samples),
while butterflies and IV catheters are used more frequently for injections such as contrast media. If an ***infusion*** injection is required, an ◀
IV catheter is generally preferred. The hub of the hypodermic needle is attached to a syringe, while the hub of the butterfly tubing or
IV catheter may be attached to a syringe or an IV bottle or bag via
an IV infusion set.

Medication or contrast material is often mixed with normal
saline or D5W. Some intravenous medications are given at intervals
through an established heparin lock. A *heparin lock* consists of a
venous catheter established for a certain length of time to make a
vein available for medications that have to be administered at frequent intervals. This helps prevent the formation of scarred, sclerotic
veins as a result of frequent injections at the same site.

The IV bottle or bag should be hung 18 to 24 inches *above the
level of the vein.* If placed lower than the vein, the solution will stop
flowing and blood will return into the tubing. If hung too high, the
solution can run too fast. Occasionally, the position of the needle or
catheter in the vein will affect the flow rate. If the bevel is adjacent
to the vessel wall, flow may decrease or stop altogether. Usually, just
changing the position of the patient's arm will remedy the situation.

Extravasation occurs when medication or contrast medium is ◀
introduced into the tissues surrounding a vein rather than into the
vein itself. It can occur when the patient's veins are particularly deep
or small. The needle should be removed, pressure applied to prevent
formation of a ***hematoma,*** and warm moist heat applied to relieve ◀
pain.

The *antecubital* vein is the most commonly used injection site
for contrast medium administration. It is not used for infusions that
take longer than 1 hour due to its location at the bend of the elbow.
The basilic vein, located on the dorsal surface of the hand, is used
when the antecubital vein is inaccessible. The cephalic vein may also
be used. Strict aseptic technique must be used for all intravenous
injections.

Following thoracic surgery, *chest tubes* may be put in place for
the purpose of removing air and/or fluid from the pleural space. The
chest drainage system usually has three compartments; one is the suction control chamber, another is the collection chamber, and the
third is the water seal chamber, which prevents atmospheric air from
entering the chest cavity. The drainage system must always be kept
below the level of the patient's chest. Radiographers generally
encounter chest drainage systems when performing mobile radiographic examinations on postsurgical patients. The radiographer
must be exceedingly careful not to disturb the chest tubes during
patient or equipment manipulation.

Nasogastric (NG) and *nasointestinal* (NI) *tubes* are frequently
employed following digestive tract surgery to remove gastric fluids
and air. NG and NI tubes may be single or double ***lumen*** and can ◀
sometimes be temporarily disconnected for radiographic exams. The
single-lumen NG or NI tube can be clamped, but the double-lumen
tube must never be clamped. If clamped, the walls of the double-
lumen tube could adhere permanently. Instead, the tip of a syringe
is inserted into the lumen and the syringe and tube then pinned

(open side up) to the patient's gown. Care must be taken not to disturb the placement of the NG or NI tube.

Urinary catheterization may be employed postsurgically to assist in the healing of tissues or to assist the incontinent patient in the elimination of urine. It is essential that equipment used for the catheterization procedure is sterile, and that subsequent care is given to the catheterized patient to prevent infection, as UTIs account for the greatest number of nosocomial infections. Urinary catheters are made of plastic, rubber, and silicone. The type selected is dependent on how long it is expected to remain in the bladder. Plastic and rubber are generally employed for short-term use, while a silicone catheter may be in place for up to 3 months. The urine collection bag must be kept below the level of the bladder; backflow of urine into the bladder can lead to infection. When transporting or transferring the catheterized patient, the radiographer must be careful that the catheter does not become entangled or dislodged.

II. MEDICAL AND LIFE-THREATENING EMERGENCIES

The importance of the radiographer's careful evaluation of his or her patient is never more obvious than when an emergency arises. An emergency is defined as a sudden change in a patient's condition requiring immediate medical intervention. Most patients arrive in the radiology department in a stable condition; a few arrive for diagnostic evaluation of a medical crisis. The radiographer must note the patient's condition on arrival and be alert to any subsequent sudden change in that condition. The radiographer must recognize the value of continual review of the knowledge and skills required for emergency situations. Many of these emergencies can occur with little or no warning. Many can be life-threatening if not dealt with immediately and correctly.

A. VOMITING

Patients who are seated or standing should be provided with a basin, tissues, and water for rinsing their mouth. It is essential that the recumbent patient have his or her head turned to the side to prevent choking from aspiration of vomitus. A patient who reports feeling nauseous is often apprehensive, as well, and may get some relief by breathing slowly and deeply through his or her mouth.

B. FRACTURES

An unsplinted fracture should be moved with great care and areas proximal and distal to the fracture site should be adequately supported. Any motion is very painful and can result in further injury to the tissues surrounding the fracture. Muscle spasm will cause additional pain and can interfere with proper reduction of the fracture. A splint should never be removed from an extremity except by or under the direct supervision of the physician. Some splinting devices are not radiolucent and removal may be required before the radiographic examination.

Rib fractures may be associated with lung trauma, and sternum fractures with heart lacerations. Rib fractures can be very painful—

the patient experiences pain just from breathing. Pelvic fractures are often associated with injuries to pelvic and abdominal viscera, and extreme care must be taken to avoid ***hemorrhage.***   ◀

C. SPINAL INJURIES

Patients arriving for radiographic evaluation with possible spinal injuries must not be moved. The position of any sandbags or other supportive mechanisms must not be changed. A horizontal (cross-table) lateral projection should be evaluated by a physician first to determine the extent of injury and necessity for further radiographs. If the patient must be placed in a lateral position, the logrolling method is usually advised. *A physician must be present whenever the patient's position is changed.*

D. EPISTAXIS

A nosebleed ***(epistaxis)*** may be a result of any one of many ◀ causes, including ***hypertension,*** dry nasal mucous membranes, ◀ sinusitis, or trauma. The patient should be seated or in a Fowler's position. The radiographer should place cold cloths over the patient's nose and back of the neck. Compressing the sides of the nose against the nasal septum for 6 to 8 minutes is also helpful. Continued hemorrhage should be brought to the attention of the physician, since cautery or nasal packs may be required.

E. POSTURAL HYPOTENSION

Orthostatic, or postural, ***hypotension*** is a decrease in blood pres- ◀ sure that occurs on rising to the erect position. It can be severe enough to cause fainting in individuals who have been confined to bed for several days. The radiographer should assist patients slowly and be watchful for signs of weakness.

F. VERTIGO

Objective ***vertigo*** is the sensation of having *objects* (or "the room") ◀ spinning about the person; *subjective* vertigo is the sensation of the *person* spinning about. It is usually associated with an inner-ear disturbance. Patients experiencing true vertigo (as opposed to dizziness or lightheadedness) are often very nauseous and must be protected from falls by the use of siderails and/or safety belts.

G. SYNCOPE

A patient who reports feeling dizzy or faint should be immediately assisted to a chair. Bending forward and placing the head between the knees will often help relieve the lightheadedness as blood flow to the brain increases. In more severe cases, a patient who cannot be assisted to a chair should be *lowered to a recumbent position.* Elevation of the lower legs or use of the Trendelenburg position is helpful. If the patient loses consciousness, the radiographer should make certain that the airway is open and that clothing, especially at the collar, is loose. Once the patient is recumbent, recovery is usually swift; however, a physician should be notified and the cause of ***syn-*** ◀ ***cope*** identified.

H. CONVULSION

Involuntary muscular contractions and relaxations, often associated
▶ with epilepsy, characterize a ***convulsion.*** Febrile convulsions are
associated with fever, especially in children. No attempt must be made
to restrain the patient's movements. The radiographer's responsibility
here is to keep the patient from injuring himself or herself. Tight
clothing can be loosened and objects that could harm the patient
should be moved out of the way. A padded tongue blade or other
suitable object should be placed between the patient's teeth to prevent biting the tongue.

I. UNCONSCIOUSNESS

The unconscious patient is unaware of and unresponsive to his or
her surroundings. Unconsciousness can be caused by a wide variety
of conditions including insulin overdose, uremia, concussion, heat
▶ ***stroke,*** and intoxication.

There are various levels of consciousness and the condition of
an acutely ill patient can rapidly deteriorate from being fully aware
and responsive, to diminished or inappropriate responsiveness, to
complete unresponsiveness. The unconscious patient must never be
left unattended and the radiographer must be alert to changes in the
patient's level of consciousness and notify the physician immediately
of any deterioration.

J. ACUTE ABDOMEN

Patients arriving for radiographic evaluation having a diagnosis of
"acute abdomen" are usually suffering severe abdominal pain, are
nauseous and vomiting, and are frequently close to being in shock.
These are indeed very sick patients. The radiographer must perform
the examination swiftly and efficiently and remain alert for any sudden changes in patient condition.

K. SHOCK

Shock is a general term and is characterized by diminished peripheral blood flow and insufficient oxygen supply to body tissues.
Shock can be caused by a number of conditions including allergic
reaction, trauma, hemorrhage, myocardial infarction, and infection.
The patient is pale and may become cyanotic; the pulse is rapid and
weak, breathing is shallow and rapid, and blood pressure drops
sharply. The radiographer should keep the patient warm and flat, or
in the Trendelenburg position, and be prepared to assist with emergency procedures.

L. SEIZURE

▶ The type of ***seizure*** known as *petit mal* is so subtle as to go unno-
ticed by the patient and observer. It is characterized by brief loss of
consciousness (10 to 30 seconds) and accompanied by eye or muscle flutterings. A *grand mal* seizure is characterized by loss of consciousness and falling, followed by generalized muscle spasms. The
radiographer should remove any objects in the area that could harm
the patient and loosen any tight clothing. The patient's head should
be turned to the side to allow any secretions to flow from the mouth.

A padded tongue blade should be placed between the patient's teeth to help avoid biting the tongue.

M. RESPIRATORY FAILURE

The inability of the lungs to perform ventilating functions is respiratory distress and may be described as *acute* or *chronic.* Acute respiratory distress can be due to impaired gas exchange processes (requiring positive-pressure ventilation) or airway obstruction (requiring the Heimlich maneuver). Chronic respiratory failure is a result of a disease process that impairs breathing, such as emphysema, bronchitis, **asthma,** or cystic fibrosis. ◄

The radiographer should be able to distinguish between respiratory arrest (absence of chest movement and breathing sounds) and cardiopulmonary arrest (absence of pulse and respiration with loss of consciousness) and be able to initiate life-saving actions.

N. CARDIOPULMONARY ARREST

The sudden cessation of productive ventilation and circulation is called cardiopulmonary arrest. The radiographer should be trained in the ABCs (airway, breathing, and circulation) of CPR and be able to initiate the appropriate care until the arrival of the emergency team.

Many radiology departments require their employees to be certified in basic life saving (BLS) skills, but even if not required by their employer, it is wise for radiographers to be familiar with skills such as the Heimlich maneuver (abdominal thrust) and CPR should the need arise outside of the hospital environment.

O. STROKE

A **stroke,** or cerebrovascular accident **(CVA),** is an interference with ◄ blood supplied to the brain as a result of occlusion or rupture of a cerebral vessel. If the condition results from a partial vessel occlusion, the interference is usually mild and temporary and is referred to as a *transient ischemic attack* **(TIA).** The patient may experience ◄ temporary blindness in one eye, **dysphasia** or **aphasia, hemi-** ◄ **paresis** or hemiplegia, or anesthesia.

If the cerebral vessel is totally occluded or ruptures into the brain or subarachnoid space, a much more serious event has occurred. The patient frequently experiences sudden loss of consciousness and one-sided paralysis (hemiparesis), although the onset can be slower if the **occlusion** is caused by **thrombus** formation. ◄ Other symptoms include speech disturbances and cool, sweaty skin. The patient should have his or her head and shoulders elevated or be in the lateral recumbent position; an open airway must be maintained. Since a stroke can occur without warning at any time, the radiographer should be familiar with the signs of an impending stroke and be able to provide appropriate immediate care. Radiographers will frequently encounter stroke patients while performing mobile radiography in intensive care units.

Summary

- ■ **Symptoms of inadequate oxygen supply include dyspnea, cyanosis, diaphoresis, and neck vein distention.**
- ■ **Seated or semi-Fowler's positions are most helpful for the dyspneic patient.**

- Oxygen is usually available through wall outlets having adjustable flowmeters, or in tanks having a flow-regulation valve and an indicator showing the quantity of oxygen left in the tank.
- Oxygen can be administered via nasal cannula, masks, and mechanical ventilators.
- Oxygen supports combustion so it must be used away from flame.
- Suction devices are used for aspiration of secretions, frequently from unconscious patients; suction is available from wall outlets or portable suction mechanisms.
- Needle size is indicated by gauge; the larger the gauge, the smaller the needle bore.
- Butterfly sets or IV catheters are generally used for IV injection of contrast medium.
- A heparin lock makes a vein accessible for medications administered at frequent intervals.
- IV solutions should be elevated 18 to 24 inches above the injection site.
- The antecubital vein is generally used for injection of contrast material; occasionally the basilic or cephalic vein will be used.
- Chest tubes function to remove fluids or air from the thoracic cavity following surgery; care must be taken not to disturb these tubes during radiographic procedures.
- NG and NI tubes assist in the removal of gastric secretions or air following GI surgery and/or for the administration of water-soluble (absorbable) contrast material for the purpose of locating and studying the site of obstruction.
- Urinary collection bags must be kept below the level of the bladder; catheterization procedures must be sterile in order to prevent UTIs.
- It is essential that the radiographer be alert for any sudden changes in patient condition; how well the radiographer recognizes and is prepared to meet the challenges of emergency situations can largely determine the outcome of the emergency.

Chapter Exercises

 Congratulations! *You have completed your review of this chapter. If you are able to answer the following group of very comprehensive questions, you should feel confident that you have really mastered this section. You are then ready to go on to "Registry-type" questions that follow. For greatest success, do not go to these multiple choice questions without first completing the short answer questions below.*

1. Define the key terms listed at the beginning of this chapter and/or identify their definitions *(p. 59)*.

2. Identify illnesses and conditions that might require supplemental oxygen *(p. 59)*.

3. List the subjective symptoms of inadequate oxygen; identify the body position frequently helpful for the dyspneic patient *(p. 60)*.

4. Describe four methods of oxygen therapy and identify when each might be indicated *(p. 60)*.

5. Identify any hazards involved in the use of oxygen *(p. 60)*.

6. Describe the circumstance(s) in which suction might be required; identify types of suction devices available *(p. 60)*.

7. Identify how needle bore changes with increasing gauge *(pp. 60–61)*.

8. Describe the function and uses of a heparin lock *(p. 61)*.

9. Identify the height at which IV bottles and bags should be hung *(p. 61)*.

10. Explain how contrast medium extravasation should be treated *(p. 61)*.

11. Identify the vein(s) frequently used for introduction of contrast medium *(p. 61)*.

12. Explain the function of chest tubes and precautions that should be taken by the radiographer *(p. 61)*.

13. Describe the function of NG and NI tubes and any precautions that should be taken by the radiographer *(pp. 61–62)*.

14. Describe the function of urinary catheters and any precautions that should be taken by the radiographer *(p. 62)*.

15. Identify the level at which urinary collection bags should be kept *(p. 62)*.

16. Discuss the importance of observing initial patient condition and any subsequent changes *(p. 62)*.

17. Describe care provided to the nauseous or vomiting patient; identify the body position required for the recumbent patient *(p. 62)*.

18. Describe precautions the radiographer should take when examining a patient with a fracture *(pp. 62–63)*.

19. Discuss precautions that should be taken with patients having suspected spinal injuries *(p. 63)*.

20. Describe first aid for epistaxis *(p. 63)*.

21. Distinguish between postural hypotension, vertigo, and syncope; discuss precautions taken and care given by the radiographer *(p. 63)*.

22. Describe any precautions that should be taken with the unconscious patient *(p. 64)*.

23. Describe symptoms of acute abdomen and shock; indicate any precautions that should be taken by the radiographer *(p. 64)*.

24. Distinguish between grand mal and petit mal seizures; discuss the care appropriate for a patient experiencing a grand mal seizure *(p. 64)*.

25. Distinguish between respiratory arrest and cardiopulmonary arrest; discuss the responses appropriate to the radiographer *(p. 65)*.

26. Describe "stroke," to include some symptoms and responses appropriate for the radiographer *(p. 65)*.

A&U Chapter Review Questions

1. Which of the following is/are symptoms of inadequate oxygen supply?
    1. diaphoresis
    2. cyanosis
    3. dyspnea
    (A) 1 only
    (B) 1 and 2 only
    (C) 2 and 3 only
    (D) 1, 2, and 3

2. A patient's IV bottle or bag should be hung:
   (A) 18–24″ above the vein
   (B) 18–24″ below the vein
   (C) 18–24″ above the heart
   (D) 18–24″ below the heart

3. Which of the following gauge needles has the largest bore?
   (A) 12
   (B) 18
   (C) 20
   (D) 23

4. Proper treatment for contrast media extravasation into tissues around a vein includes:
       1. application of cold wet towel to affected area
       2. application of moist heat to affected area
       3. application of pressure to injection site
   (A) 1 only
   (B) 2 only
   (C) 1 and 2 only
   (D) 2 and 3 only

5. What is the most frequently used site for intravenous injection of contrast agents?
   (A) basilic vein
   (B) cephalic vein
   (C) antecubital vein
   (D) femoral vein

6. What precaution should be taken with a vomiting patient?
   (A) place the patient in the Trendelenburg position
   (B) place the patient in Fowler's position
   (C) turn the patient's head to the side
   (D) turn the patient prone

7. A decrease in blood pressure which occurs on suddenly arising from the recumbent position is called:
   (A) orthostatic hypotension
   (B) epistaxis
   (C) vertigo
   (D) syncope

8. What is the correct response by the radiographer when a patient suffers a convulsion?
       1. gently restrain the patient
       2. keep the patient from injuring himself
       3. loosen tight clothing
   (A) 1 only
   (B) 1 and 2 only
   (C) 2 and 3 only
   (D) 1, 2, and 3

9. The Heimlich maneuver may be used for:
   (A) chronic pulmonary obstruction
   (B) acute pulmonary obstruction
   (C) cardiopulmonary arrest
   (D) shock

10. All of the following statements are true, EXCEPT:
    (A) A heparin lock makes a vein accessible for medications administered at frequent intervals.
    (B) Aseptic technique is employed for catheterization of the urinary bladder.
    (C) Oxygen may be administered via nasal cannula, masks, and mechanical ventilators.
    (D) Oxygen supports combustion so it must be used away from flame.

Answers and Explanations

1. (D) Symptoms of inadequate oxygen supply include dyspnea, *cyanosis, diaphoresis,* and distention of the veins of the neck. The patient who experiences some or all of these symptoms will be very anxious and must not be left unattended. The radiographer must *call* for help, assist the patient to a sitting or semi-Fowler's position (the recumbent position makes breathing more difficult), and have oxygen and emergency drugs available.

2. (A) The IV bottle or bag should be hung 18 to 24 inches *above the level of the vein.* If placed lower than the vein, solution will stop flowing and blood will return into the tubing. If hung too high, solution can run too fast. Occasionally, the position of the needle or catheter in the vein will affect the flow rate. If the bevel is adjacent to the vessel wall, flow may decrease or stop altogether. Usually just changing the position of the patient's arm will remedy the situation.

3. (A) The diameter of a needle is identified as its *gauge.* As the diameter of its *bore* increases the gauge decreases. Hence, an 18-gauge needle has a larger diameter bore than a 23-gauge needle. Hypodermic needles are generally used for phlebotomy (ie, blood samples), while butterflies and IV catheters are used more frequently for injections such as contrast media. If an infusion injection is required, an IV catheter is generally preferred. The hub of the hypodermic needle is attached to a syringe, while the hub of the butterfly tubing or IV catheter may be attached to a syringe or an IV bottle or bag via an IV infusion set.

4. (D) *Extravasation* occurs when medication or contrast medium is introduced into the tissues surrounding a vein rather than into the vein itself. It can occur when the patient's veins are particularly deep or small. The needle should be removed, pressure applied to prevent formation of a hematoma, and warm moist heat applied to relieve pain.

5. (C) The *antecubital* vein is the most commonly used injection site for contrast medium administration. It is not used for infusions that take longer than 1 hour due to its location at the bend of the elbow. The basilic vein, located on the dorsal surface of the hand, is used when the antecubital vein is inaccessible. The cephalic vein may also be used. Strict aseptic technique must be used for all intravenous injections.

6. (C) Patients who are seated or standing should be provided with a basin, tissues, and water for rinsing their mouth. It is essential that the recumbent patient have his or her head turned to the side to prevent choking from aspiration of vomitus. A patient who reports feeling nauseous is often apprehensive, as well, and may get some relief by breathing slowly and deeply through his or her mouth.

7. (A) *Orthostatic, or postural, hypotension* is a decrease in blood pressure that occurs on rising to the erect position. It can be severe enough to cause fainting in individuals who have been confined to bed for several days. A nosebleed (epistaxis) may be a result of any one of many causes, including hypertension, dry nasal mucous membranes, sinusitis, or trauma. The patient should be seated or placed in a Fowler's position. The radiographer should place cold cloths over the patient's nose and back of the neck. *Objective vertigo* is the sensation of having *objects* (or "the room") spinning about the person; *subjective vertigo* is the sensation of the *person* spinning about. It is usually associated with an inner-ear disturbance. Patients experiencing true vertigo (as opposed to dizziness or lightheadedness) are often very nauseous and must be protected from falls. A patient who reports feeling dizzy or faint should be immediately assisted to a chair. Bending forward and placing the head between the knees will often help relieve the lightheadedness as blood flow to the brain increases. In more severe cases, *a patient who cannot be assisted to a chair should be lowered to a recumbent position.* Elevation of the lower legs, or use of the Trendelenburg position, is helpful.

8. (C) Involuntary muscular contractions and relaxations, often associated with epilepsy, characterize a *convulsion.* No attempt must be made to restrain the patient's movements. The radiographer's responsibility here is to keep the patient from injury. Tight clothing may be loosened and objects that could harm the patient should be moved out of the way. A padded tongue blade or other suitable object should be placed between the patient's teeth to prevent biting the tongue.

9. (B) The inability of the lungs to perform ventilating functions is called *respiratory distress* and may be described as acute or chronic. *Acute* respiratory distress can be due to impaired gas exchange processes (requiring positive-pressure ventilation) or airway obstruction (requiring the *Heimlich maneuver*). Chronic respiratory failure is a result of a disease process that impairs breathing, such as emphysema, bronchitis, asthma, or cystic fibrosis. The radiographer should be able to distinguish between respiratory arrest (absence of chest movement and breathing sounds) and cardiopulmonary arrest (absence of pulse and respiration with loss of consciousness) and be able to initiate life-saving actions.

10. (B) Some intravenous medications are given at intervals through an established heparin lock. A *heparin lock* consists of a venous catheter established for a certain length of time to make a vein available for medications having to be administered at frequent intervals. This helps prevent the formation of scarred, sclerotic veins as a result of frequent injections at the same site.

It is essential that equipment used for urinary catheterization procedures be *sterile,* and that subsequent care of the catheterized patient prevent infection, as UTIs account for the greatest number of nosocomial infections.

Although oxygen is not a flammable substance, it does support combustion, so care must be taken to avoid spark or flame where oxygen is in use. There are various devices available to deliver oxygen to the patient; their use is determined by the amount of oxygen required by the patient. They are frequently classified as *low* or *high flow.*

part

II

Radiographic Procedures

3. Orbits, Optic Foramen, Orbital Fissures
4. Facial Bones, Nasal Bones, Zygomatic Arches
5. Mandible, Temporomandibular Joints (TMJs)
6. Paranasal Sinuses
7. Temporal Bone: Mastoids and Petrous Portions

III. Body Systems

A. Respiratory System
1. Introduction
2. Chest; PA, Lateral, Obliques
3. Chest; Axial and Decubitus
4. Airway
5. Terminology and Pathology

B. Biliary System
1. Introduction
2. Patient Preparation
3. Gallbladder
4. OR/T-Tube
5. ERCP
6. Terminology and Pathology

C. Digestive System
1. Introduction
2. Patient Preparation
3. Abdomen
4. Esophagus
5. Stomach and Small Intestine
6. Large Intestine
7. Terminology and Pathology

D. Urinary System
1. Introduction
2. Patient Preparation
3. Types of Examinations
4. KUB (Kidney, Ureter, and Bladder)
5. Bladder
6. Terminology and Pathology

E. Female Reproductive System
1. Introduction
2. Hysterosalpingogram
3. Terminology and Pathology

F. Central Nervous System
1. Introduction
2. Procedures
3. Myelogram
4. Terminology and Pathology

G. Circulatory System
1. Introduction
2. Venogram
3. Terminology and Pathology

An Overview of Positioning Principles and Terminology

KEY TERMS ◀

ARTIFACT	FRACTURE	PALPATION
ARTHRITIS	FRONTAL	POSITION
ARTICULATION	HYPERSTHENIC	PROJECTION
ASTHENIC	HYPOSTHENIC	RECUMBENT
AXIAL	IMMOBILIZATION	SAGITTAL PLANE
BODY HABITUS	LATERAL	STHENIC
BODY SURFACE LANDMARK	METASTATIC	TANGENTIAL
CORONAL PLANE	MIDCORONAL PLANE	TRANSVERSE PLANE
DECUBITUS	MIDSAGITTAL PLANE	VIEW
ERECT	OBLIQUE	

The development of positioning skills requires a thorough knowledge of anatomy and an awareness of possible pathologic conditions, including their impact on positioning limitations and technical factors.

A review of basic positioning principles and terminology is essential to an overview of radiographic procedures. Several tables and figures in this chapter summarize body planes (Fig. 6–2), body habitus and types (Fig. 6–3), the four quadrants and nine regions of the abdomen (Fig. 6–4), body surface landmarks and localization points (Fig. 6–5), and the ARRT standard terminology distinguishing among *position, projection,* and *view* (Fig. 6–6). The student ◀

should be thoroughly acquainted with these before approaching the study of specific positioning skills.

It must be emphasized that a patient's condition very often impacts his or her ability to cooperate. The descriptions of "Position of Part" in this section are most easily used on patients who are not severely injured or afflicted with debilitating pathology. One measure of a good radiographer is his or her ability to be cautious and resourceful when examining injured or debilitated patients. Patho-

▶ logic or traumatic conditions such as **metastatic** bone disease, vari-

▶ ous types of **arthritis,** and most bone **fractures** are examples of conditions such as these. The use of **body surface landmarks** and localization points (see Fig. 6–5) as external indicators of anatomic structures can increase the ease and accuracy of positioning. Thoughtful placement of a cushioning sponge, the use of a horizon-

▶ tal beam for **lateral** projections instead of moving the patient (see

▶ Fig. 6–1), performing the examination **erect** if the **recumbent** posi-

Figure 6–1. Lateral projection of knee performed in supine position on a patient with multiple injuries. A horizontal (cross-table) x-ray beam was used to reduce discomfort and the risk of further injury. Observe the sheet artifact from the mattress pad beneath the patient. Use this radiograph to review the skeletal anatomy of the knee and correctly identify the lettered parts. (Courtesy of The Stamford Hospital.)

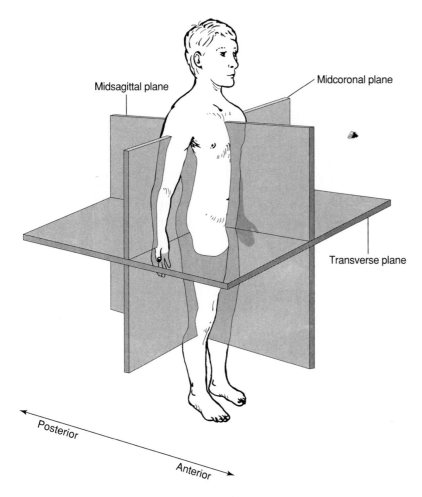

Figure 6–2. Body planes.

tion is uncomfortable, are examples of modifications that the considerate radiographer can make that will result in an appreciative patient, as well as a diagnostic exam. The radiographer must also be alert to the changes in technical factors that may be necessitated by various pathologic processes.

I. BODY PLANES (SEE FIG. 6–2)

- ***Midsagittal*** or *Median Sagittal Plane* (MSP): divides body ◀ into left and right halves.
- ***Sagittal Plane:*** any plane parallel to the MSP. ◀
- ***Midcoronal Plane*** (MCP): divides body into anterior and ◀ posterior halves.
- ***Coronal Plane:*** any plane parallel to the MCP. ◀
- ***Transverse***/*Horizontal* ***Plane:*** perpendicular to MSP and ◀ MCP, divides body axially into superior and inferior portions.

II. BODY TYPES AND HABITUS (SEE FIG. 6–3)

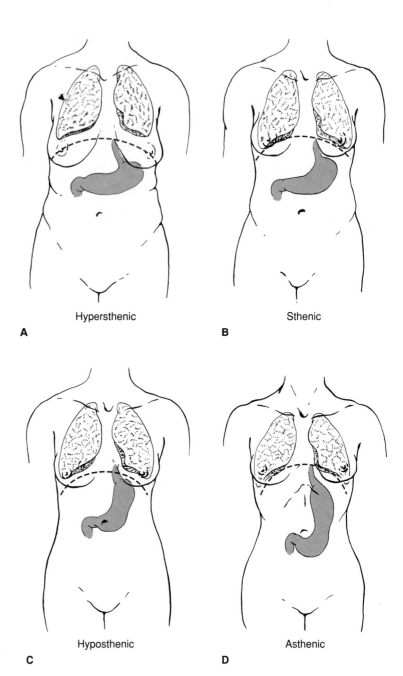

Hypersthenic

A

Sthenic

B

Hyposthenic

C

Asthenic

D

Body Types and Habitus

Hypersthenic and asthenic characterize the extremes in body types:

Hypersthenic
- Body is large and heavy
- Bony framework is thick, short and wide
- Lungs and heart are high
- Transverse stomach
- Gallbladder high and lateral
- Peripheral colon

Asthenic
- Body is slender and light
- Bony framework is delicate
- Long, narrow thorax
- Very low, long ("fish hook") stomach
- Gallbladder low and medial
- Low, medial, and redundant colon

Sthenic and hyposthenic types characterize the more average body
types:

Sthenic
- Average, athletic build
- Similar to hypersthenic, but modi-fied by elongation of abdomen and thorax

Hyposthenic
- Somewhat slighter, less robust
- Similar to asthenic, but stomach, intestines, and gallbladder situated higher in abdomen

Figure 6–3. The position, shape, and motility of various organs can differ greatly from one body habitus to another. Each of the body habitus types is shown and the characterstic variations in shape and position of the diaphragm, lungs, and stomach are illustrated. The radiographer must take these characterstic differences into considera-tion while performing radiographic examinations on individuals of various body habitus.

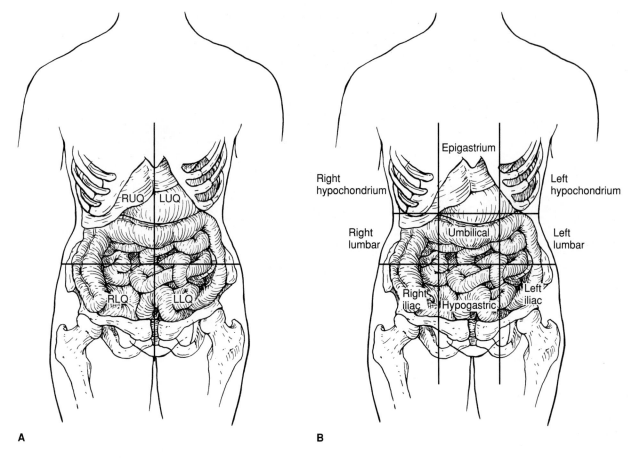

A   **B**

Figure 6–4. **A.** Four quadrants of the abdomen, illustrating position of major organs. **B.** Nine regions of the abdomen, illustrating position of major organs.

III. SURFACE LANDMARKS AND LOCALIZATION POINTS (SEE FIG. 6–5)

VERTEBRA(E)		LOCALIZATION POINT
Cervical region	C1	mastoid process
	C5	thyroid cartilage (Adam's Apple)
	C7	vertebra prominens
Thoracic region	T2–3	suprasternal (manubrial) notch
	T4–5	sternal angle
	T7–8	inferior angle of scapula
	T10	xyphoid (ensiform) process
Lumbar region	T12–L3	kidneys
	L1	transpyloric plane
	L3	inferior costal margin
	L4	iliac crest
Sacral and	S1–2	anterior superior iliac spine (ASIS)
coccygeal regions	Coccyx	symphysis pubis and greater trochanter

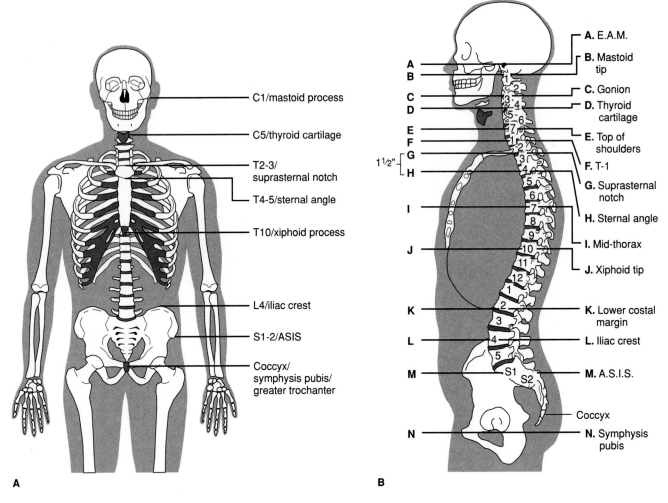

Figure 6–5. Body surface landmarks and localization points.

STANDARD TERMINOLOGY FOR POSITIONING AND PROJECTION

Radiographic view
Describes the body part as seen by an x-ray film or other recording media, such as a fluoroscopic screen. Restricted to the discussion of a *radiograph* or *image.*

Radiographic position
Refers to a specific body position, such as supine, prone, recumbent, erect, or Trendelenburg. Restricted to the discussion of the patient's *physical position.*

Radiographic projection
Restricted to the discussion of the *path of the central ray.*

Positioning terminology
   A. *Lying down*
   1. Supine: lying on the back
   2. Prone: lying face downward
   3. Recumbent: lying down in any position
   4. Decubitus: lying down with a horizontal x-ray beam

B. *Erect or Upright*
1. Anterior position: facing the film
2. Posterior position: facing the radiographic tube
3. Oblique positions

a. Anterior: facing the film
(1) *Left anterior oblique:* body rotated with left anterior portion closest to the film

(2) *Right anterior oblique:* body rotated with right anterior portion closest to the film

b. Posterior facing the radiographic tube
(1) *Left posterior oblique:* body rotated with left posterior portion closest to the film

(2) *Right posterior oblique:* body rotated with right posterior portion closest to the film

---

Figure 6–6. ARRT Standard Terminology for Positioning and Projection is used to clarify positioning terminology *(continued). (Standard Terminology.* © 1990 The American Registry of Radiologic Technologists. Reproduced with permission.)

Anteroposterior projection

Posteroanterior projection

Right lateral position

Left lateral position

Left posterior oblique position

Right posterior oblique position

Left anterior oblique position

Right anterior oblique position

Figure 6–6 *(Continued). (Standard Terminology.* © 1990 The American Registry of Radiologic Technologists. Reproduced with permission.)

IV. SKELETAL MOTION TERMINOLOGY

- **Supination:** turns the body or arm so that the palm faces forward, with thumb away from midline of body.
- **Pronation:** turns the body or arm so that the palm faces backward, with thumb toward midline of body.
- **Abduction:** movement of a part away from the body's MSP.
- **Adduction:** movement of a part toward the body's MSP.
- **Flexion:** bending motion of an articulation, decreasing the angle between associated bones.
- **Extension:** bending motion of an articulation, increasing the angle between associated bones.
- **Eversion:** a turning outward or lateral motion of an articulation, sometimes with external tension or stress applied.
- **Inversion:** a turning inward or medial motion of an articulation, sometimes with external tension or stress applied.
- **Rotation:** movement of a part about its central or long axis.
- **Circumduction:** movement of a limb that produces circular motion; circumscribes a small area at its proximal end and a wide area at the distal end.

V. PRELIMINARY STEPS AND PROCEDURAL GUIDELINES

The following are steps and procedures that help ensure high quality patient care and diagnostic radiographs.

1. Read the requisition carefully, noting the type of examination, patient condition, and mode of travel (make mental notes of any modifications or accessory equipment that may be required).
2. Prepare the radiographic room. Be certain the x-ray room is neat and orderly with a clean x-ray table and a fresh pillowcase. All accessories needed for the exam should be in the room before bringing the patient in.
3. Identify the correct patient, quickly evaluating any special needs; introduce yourself and establish rapport en route to the radiographic room—being careful not to discuss confidential or personal issues within earshot of others.
4. Instruct the patient to change into a dressing gown, as necessary, removing or moving appropriate clothing and objects (eg, jewelry, dentures, braided hair) that may cast *artifacts* within the area of interest (see Figs. 6–7 and 6–8).
5. Speak in a well-modulated voice, give a clear and succinct explanation of the procedure and address any patient questions or concerns. Obtain a short pertinent patient history of why the exam has been requested. The radiographer should explain that a number of different positions may be needed to evaluate the area of interest and may require *palpation* of bony landmarks and instructions to turn into various positions.

Figure 6–7. The PA chest film is accurately positioned and exposed, but observe the braids of hair that extend past the neck and superimpose on the pulmonary apices. Braided hair should be pinned up or otherwise removed from superimposition on thoracic structures. (Courtesy of The Stamford Hospital.)

Figure 6–8. LPO spot films of the esophagus are shown above with a jewelry artifact near the area of interest. The radiographer should instruct the patient to remove clothing and any other objects, such as jewelry, from the area to be examined before donning the dressing gown. (Courtesy of The Stamford Hospital.)

6. Radiography of most structures usually requires a minimum of two projections—most frequently at right angles to each other. A side-to-side (left/right) relationship is demonstrated in the *frontal* projection, while an anterior and posterior relationship is seen in the lateral projection. This is especially important in localizing foreign bodies and tumors, and demonstrating fracture displacement or alignment.

7. It is customary and economical to use the smallest size film that will include all necessary information. It follows, then, that the smallest possible anatomic area (consistent with a diagnostic examination) will be irradiated, and patient dose will therefore be kept to a minimum.

8. In radiography of the extremities, every effort should be made to include both **articulations** associated with the injured bone, but it is essential to include *at least* the articulation nearest the injury.

9. So that an accurate diagnosis can be made, supplemental radiographs of any anatomic part may be required, eg, *oblique, axial, tangential, erect,* or *decubitus.* Exposure factors must be correctly adjusted for each change of position.

10. Each radiograph *must* be accurately labeled with patient information such as name or identification number, institution name, date of examination, and side marker. Other information may be included according to institution policy.

VI. IMMOBILIZATION AND RESPIRATION

Motion obliterates recorded detail; it is therefore essential that the radiographer be able to reduce patient motion as much as possible. Even the slightest movement can cause severe degradation of the radiographic image. Several means can be employed to reduce motion unsharpness, but good patient communication is required for any to be effective.

Probably the single most important way to reduce *involuntary* motion is to use the shortest possible exposure time. Various types of *immobilization* devices can also be used to effectively reduce motion. Motion from muscular tremors as a result of anxiety or pain are involuntary and can be greatly minimized with good communication, a carefully placed positioning sponge or sandbag, and the use of the shortest exposure time possible.

Suspension of patient respiration for parts other than the extremities is an effective means of reducing *voluntary* motion; patient understanding and cooperation is required, thus making good *communication* the most effective means of reducing voluntary motion. The phase of respiration in which the exposure is made can be essential to the diagnostic quality of the radiographic image. Chest radiography, for example, normally requires that the exposure be made on inspiration (the second inspiration if the patient is of the hypersthenic type). Most abdominal examinations are exposed on expiration. The phase of respiration in which the exposure is made can make a significant difference in the resulting radiographic density as well (discussed in Part IV).

Chapter Exercises

 Congratulations! *You have completed this chapter. If you are able to answer the following group of very comprehensive questions, you should feel confident that you have really mastered this section. You are then ready to go on to "Registry-type" questions that follow. For greatest success, do not go to these multiple choice questions without first completing the short answer questions below.*

1. Discuss how knowledge of anatomy and pathologic conditions relates to positioning skills *(pp. 82, 84).*

2. Identify the sagittal and midsagittal, coronal and midcoronal, and transverse (horizontal) planes *(p. 77).*

3. List the four types of body habitus and provide physical characteristics of each *(p. 78).*

4. Name, identify, and describe the quadrants and nine regions of the abdomen *(p. 79).*

5. Identify anatomic localization points and their corresponding vertebrae *(p. 80).*

6. Define and identify various skeletal movement terms *(p. 82).*

7. Discuss the importance of establishing an orderly sequence of preparation for performing radiologic examinations *(pp. 82).*

8. Explain the importance of obtaining two views at right angles to each other for most radiologic examinations *(p. 84).*

9. Discuss the inclusion of articulations in radiography of the extremities *(p. 84).*

10. List the information that must be included on the radiographic image *(p. 84).*

A&U Chapter Review Questions

1. Prior to bringing the patient into the radiographic room, the radiographer should:
   1. be certain the x-ray room is clean and orderly
   2. check that all necessary accessories are available in room
   3. check for clean x-ray table and fresh pillowcases
   (A) 1 only
   (B) 1 and 2 only
   (C) 2 and 3 only
   (D) 1, 2, and 3

2. The position of the hypersthenic gallbladder compared to the position of the asthenic gallbladder is more:
   (A) superior and lateral
   (B) superior and medial
   (C) inferior and lateral
   (D) inferior and medial

3. What is the relationship between the midsagittal and coronal planes?
   (A) parallel
   (B) perpendicular
   (C) 45°
   (D) 70°

4. The best way to control involuntary motion is:
   (A) immobilization
   (B) careful explanation
   (C) short exposure time
   (D) physical restraint

5. X-ray examinations of the skull and cervical spine require that prior to the exam the patient remove which of the following?
   1. dentures
   2. earrings
   3. necklaces
   (A) 1 only
   (B) 1 and 2 only
   (C) 2 and 3 only
   (D) 1, 2, and 3

6. Film identification markers should include:
   1. patient's name and/or ID number
   2. date
   3. a right or left marker
   (A) 1 only
   (B) 1 and 2 only
   (C) 1 and 3 only
   (D) 1, 2, and 3

7. The radiographer should be able to:
    1. take a short patient history prior to the exam
    2. give a preliminary diagnosis for stat exams
    3. fluoroscope a GI in the absence of the radiologist
    (A) 1 only
    (B) 1 and 2 only
    (C) 1 and 3 only
    (D) 1, 2, and 3

8. With the patient recumbent and the central ray directed horizontally, the patient is said to be in the:
    (A) Trendelenburg position
    (B) Fowler's position
    (C) decubitus position
    (D) Sim's position

9. The plane that passes vertically through the body dividing it into equal left and right halves is termed the:
    (A) medial sagittal plane
    (B) midcoronal plane
    (C) sagittal plane
    (D) transverse plane

10. The uppermost portion of the iliac crest is approximately at the same level as the:
    (A) costal margin
    (B) umbilicus
    (C) xiphoid tip
    (D) fourth lumbar vertebra

Answers and Explanations

1. (D) A patient will naturally feel more comfortable and confident if brought into a clean, orderly x-ray room that has been prepared appropriately for the examination to be performed. A disorderly, untidy room and a disorganized radiographer hardly inspire confidence; more likely, they will increase anxiety and apprehension.

2. (A) The position, shape, and motility of various organs can differ greatly from one body habitus to another. The position of the diaphragm, lungs, stomach, gallbladder, and large and small intestines vary greatly with body habitus. The large extreme (hypersthenic) will have structures higher and more lateral, while these structures in individuals of the small extreme habitus (asthenic) have structures low and medial (see Fig. 6–3)

3. (B) The median sagittal, or midsagittal, plane (MSP) passes vertically through the midline of the body, dividing it into left and right halves. Any plane parallel to the MSP is termed a sagittal plane. *The midcoronal plane is perpendicular to the MSP* and divides the body into anterior and posterior halves. A transverse plane passes across the body, also perpendicular to a sagittal plane. These planes, especially the MSP, are very important reference points in radiographic positioning.

4. (C) Motion obliterates recorded detail; it is therefore essential that the radiographer be able to reduce patient motion as much as possible. Even the slightest movement can cause severe degradation of the radiographic image. Probably the single most important way to reduce *involuntary* motion is to use the shortest possible exposure time. Suspension of patient respiration for parts other than the extremities is an effective means of reducing *voluntary* motion; patient understanding and cooperation is required, thus making good *communication* the most effective means of reducing voluntary motion.

5. (D) The patient must remove any metallic objects if they are within the area(s) of interest. Dentures, earrings, and necklaces can obscure bony details in the skull or cervical spine. The radiographer must be certain the patient's belongings are cared for properly and returned following the examination (see Figs. 6–7 and 6–8).

6. (D) Correct and complete patient information on every radiograph is of paramount importance. Each radiograph must be accurately labeled with such patient information as name or identification number, institution name, date of examination, and side marker. Other information may be included according to institution policy.

7. (A) It is important that the radiologist receive a short, pertinent patient history of why an examination has been requested. Your information and any pertinent observations can be useful in making an accurate diagnosis. A radiographer does not have the training to deliver a diagnosis or perform fluoroscopy—this is strictly in the radiologist's realm.

8. (C) The decubitus position is used to describe the patient as recumbent (prone, supine, or lateral) with the central ray directed horizontally. When the patient is recumbent with his or her head lower than his or her feet, he or she is said to be in the Trendelenburg position. In the Fowler's position, the patient's head is positioned higher than his or her feet. The Sim's position is the (LAO) position assumed for enema tip insertion.

9. (A) The median sagittal, or midsagittal, plane (MSP) passes vertically through the midline of the body, dividing it into left and right halves. Any plane parallel to the MSP is termed a sagittal plane. The midcoronal plane is perpendicular to the MSP and divides the body into anterior and posterior halves. A transverse plane passes through the body at right angles to a sagittal plane. These planes, especially the MSP, are very important reference points in radiographic positioning.

10. (D) Surface landmarks, prominences, and depressions are very useful to the radiographer in locating anatomic structures not visible externally. The costal margin is about the same level as L3. The umbilicus is the same approximate level as the L3 to L4 interspace. The xiphoid tip is about the same level as T10. The fourth lumbar vertebra is at the same approximate level as the iliac crest.

Imaging Procedures, Including Anatomy, Positioning, and Pathology

I. THE APPENDICULAR SKELETON (FIG. 7–1)

KEY TERMS ◀

ANTEVERSION	ENDOSTEUM	PERIOSTEUM
AXIAL	EPIPHYSEAL PLATE	PROSTHESIS
BILATERAL	EPIPHYSIS	PROXIMAL
CANCELLOUS	FORESHORTENING	RADIOPAQUE
COMPACT	HYPEREXTEND	ROTATOR CUFF
CONTRAST AGENT	INTRAVENOUS UROGRAM	SPUR
DIAPHYSIS	MEDULLARY CAVITY	STRESS MANEUVER
DISPLACEMENT	MENISCI	SUPERIMPOSED
DISTAL	MORTISE	TANGENTIAL
DISTORTION	NONINVASIVE	

The appendicular skeleton is made of the extremities (appendages or limbs), the arms, shoulder girdle, legs, and pelvis. Most of these bones serve as levers for attachment of muscles, thereby making movement possible. Bones serve as a reservoir for minerals such as calcium and phosphorus, storing them until the body requires them. Bone tissue is osseous (*os* = bone), and there are two types of osseous tissue: ***cancellous*** (spongy) and ***compact*** (hard, cortical) ◀ (Fig. 7–2A).

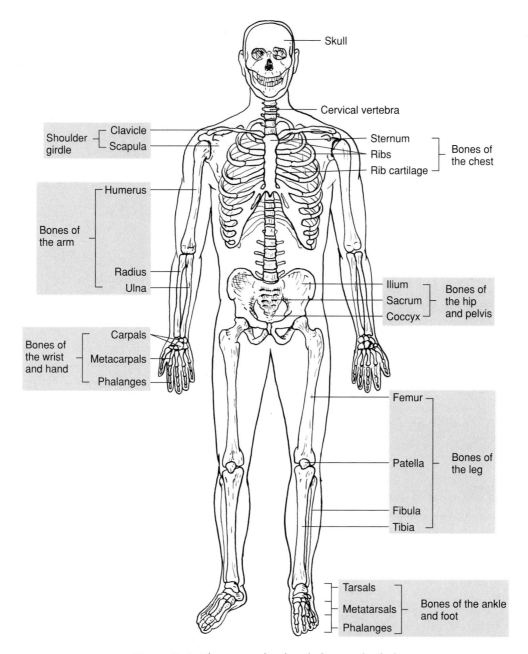

Figure 7–1. The appendicular skeleton (shaded).

Bones are classified as *long, short, flat,* and *irregular.* Many of the bones comprising the extremities are long bones. Long bones
▶ have a *shaft* and two extremities (ends). The shaft (or ***diaphysis***) (Fig. 7–2B) of long bones is the *primary ossification center* during bone development. It is composed of compact tissue and is covered
▶ with a membrane called ***periosteum.*** Within the shaft is the
▶ ***medullary cavity,*** which contains *bone marrow* and is lined by the
▶ membrane called ***endosteum.*** In the adult, yellow marrow occupies
▶ the shaft and red marrow is found within the ***proximal*** and ***distal***

extremities of long bones. The *secondary ossification center,* the ***epi-*** ◀
physis (Figure 7–2B), is separated from the diaphysis in early life by ◀
a layer of cartilage, the ***epiphyseal plate.*** As bone growth takes ◀
place, the epiphysis becomes part of the larger portion of bone, the
epiphyseal plate disappears but a characteristic line remains and is
thereafter recognizable as the *epiphyseal line.* The articular ends of
bones are covered with *articular (hyaline) cartilage.*

A. UPPER EXTREMITY AND SHOULDER GIRDLE

1. Hand, Fingers, and Thumb (Fig. 7–3). The hand is composed
of five *metacarpal* bones, which correspond to the palm of the hand,
and 14 *phalanges,* the fingers. The second through fifth fingers have
three phalanges each (proximal, middle, and distal rows) and the
first finger or thumb has two phalanges (proximal and distal). The
rows of phalanges articulate with each other forming proximal and
distal *interphalangeal joints* (hinge type joints), which permit flexion
and extension motion. The bases of the proximal row of phalanges
articulate with the heads of the metacarpals to form the (condyloid)
metacarpophalangeal joints (MPJ), which permit flexion and extension, abduction and adduction, and circumduction. The bases of the
metacarpals articulate with each other and the distal row of carpals
at the *carpometacarpal joints.* The first carpometacarpal joint (thumb)
is a saddle joint, permitting flexion and extension, abduction and
adduction, and circumduction. Traumatic **fractures** of the metacarpals and phalanges are common. Fractures of the distal (ungual)
phalangeal tufts usually occur from crushing injuries, such as being
closed in car doors or struck with a hammer.

2. Wrist. The wrist (Fig. 7–3) is composed of eight carpal bones
arranged in two rows (proximal and distal). The proximal row consists of, from lateral to medial, the *navicular/scaphoid,* the
lunate/semilunar, the *triangular/triquetrum,* and the *pisiform.* The
distal row, from lateral to medial, consists of the *greater multangu-
lar/trapezium,* the *lesser multangular/trapezoid,* the *capitate/os
magnum* (the largest carpal), and the *hamate/unciform* (which has
a hook-like process, the hamulus). The joints of the wrist include the
articulations between the carpals *(intercarpal joints),* which provide
a gliding motion, and the *radiocarpal joint* (between the distal radius
and navicular), which provides flexion and extension and abduction
and adduction. **Carpal tunnel syndrome** is a painful condition of
the wrist. If the anteroposterior (AP) diameter of the tunnel is diminished, the median nerve, which passes through the tunnel, is
impinged upon, causing severe pain and disability in the affected
hand and wrist. Surgical decompression of the carpal tunnel can provide significant relief.

3. Forearm. The bones of the forearm, or antebrachium (Fig. 7–4),
consist of the *radius* (laterally) and *ulna* (medially), which participate in formation of the elbow joint proximally and the wrist distally.
The distal ulna presents a head and *styloid process* and articulates
with the distal radius to form the *distal radioulnar joint.* The ulna is
slender distally but enlarges proximally and becomes the larger of
the two bones of the forearm. At its proximal end, the ulna presents
the *olecranon process* (posteriorly) and *coronoid process* (anteriorly)

A

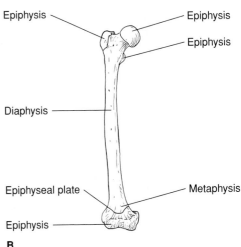

B

Figure 7–2. **(A)** and **(B)** Characteristics and ossification centers of long bones.

Articulations May Be Classified As

Diathrotic: freely movable
Amphiarthrotic: partially movable
Synarthrotic: immovable

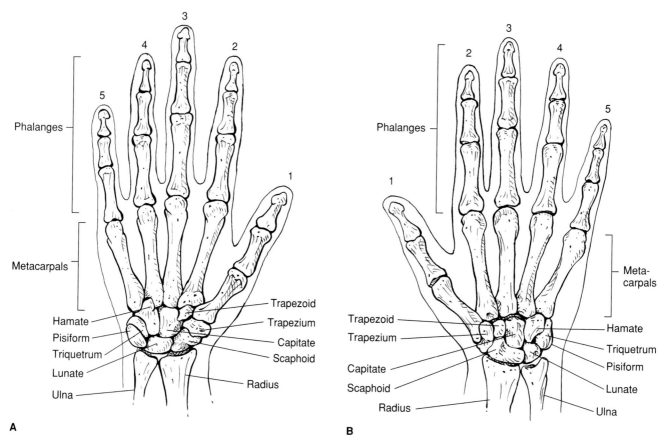

Figure 7–3. **(A)** AP (palmar) and **(B)** (PA) (dorsal) aspects of the right hand and wrist.

Carpal Bones

Proximal Row, Lateral to Medial
Navicular/Scaphoid
Lunate/Semilunar
Triangular/Triquetrum
Pisiform
Distal Row, Lateral to Medial
Greater Multangular/Trapezoid
Lesser Multangular/Trapezium
Capitate/Os Magnum
Hamate/Unciform

that are joined by a large articular cavity, the *semilunar,* or *trochlear, notch.* The coronoid process fits into the humeral *coronoid fossa* during flexion and the olecranon process fits into the humeral *olecranon fossa* during extension. Just distal and lateral to the semilunar notch is the *radial notch* (Fig. 7–4), which provides articulation for the radial head to form the *proximal radioulnar articulation.* Just as the ulna is the principal bone associated with the elbow joint, the radius is the principal bone associated with the wrist joint. Fracture of the distal radius is one of the most common skeletal fractures. The distal radius presents a *styloid process* laterally; the *ulnar notch* is located medially, helping to form the *distal radioulnar articulation.* The distal surface of the radius (carpal articular surface) is smooth for accommodating the navicular and lunate in the formation of the *radiocarpal joint.* The proximal radius has a cylindrical *head* with a medial surface that participates in the *proximal radioulnar joint;* its superior surface articulates with the capitulum of the humerus. **Fractures** of the radial head and neck frequently result from a fall onto an outstretched hand with the elbow *partially flexed.* Severe fractures are often accompanied by posterior dislocation of the elbow joint. **Colles' fractures** of the distal radius usually result from a fall onto an outstretched hand with the arm *extended.*

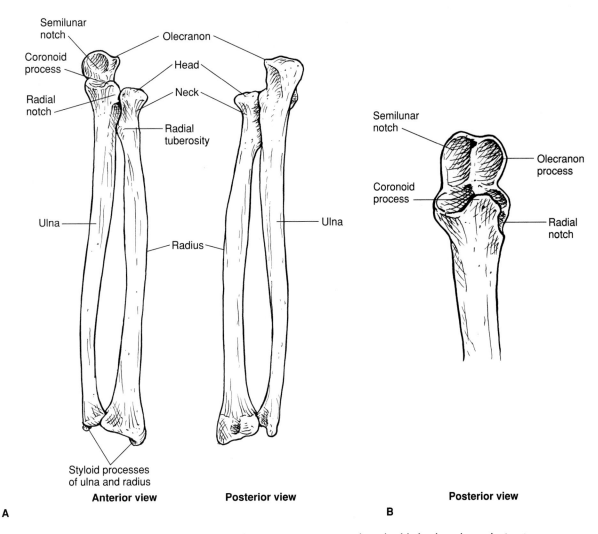

Figure 7–4. **(A)** Bones of the left forearm. **(B)** Proximal end of left ulna (lateral view).

4. Elbow. The distal *humerus* articulates with the radius and ulna to form the elbow joint (Figs. 7–5 and 7–6). The lateral aspect of the distal humerus presents a raised, smooth, rounded surface, the *capitulum,* which articulates with the superior surface of the *radial head* (Fig. 7–4). The *trochlea* is on the medial aspect of the distal humerus and articulates with the semilunar notch of the ulna. Just proximal to the capitulum and trochlea are the *lateral* and *medial epicondyles;* the medial is more prominent and palpable. **Lateral epicondylitis** (tennis elbow) is a painful condition caused by prolonged rotary motion of the forearm. The *olecranon fossa* is found on the posterior distal humerus and functions to accommodate the olecranon process with the elbow in extension (Fig. 7–7).

5. Humerus. The *deltoid tuberosity* is found on the anterolateral surface of the humeral shaft. The large, round *humeral head* is covered with hyaline cartilage and articulates with the scapula's glenoid

Figure 7–5. Anterior and posterior views of the bony articulation of the right elbow joint.

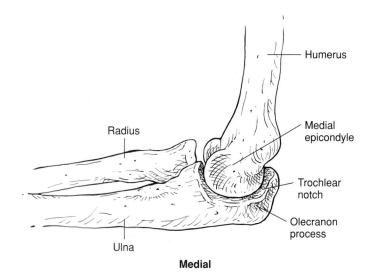

Figure 7–6. Medial and lateral views of the bony articulation of the right elbow joint.

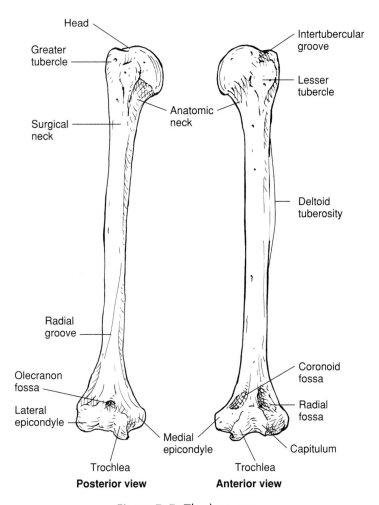

Figure 7–7. The humerus.

fossa. The *anatomical neck* marks the location of the fused epiphyseal plate in the adult and separates the head and metaphysis. The proximal humerus presents two protuberances on its anterior surface; the *greater tubercle* is lateral and the *lesser tubercle* is medial. Between the tubercles is the *bicipital,* or *intertubercular, groove.* The humeral shaft narrows just distal to the tubercles at the point of the *surgical neck.* Humeral **fractures** usually involve the surgical neck or its distal end.

6. Shoulder. The shoulder (pectoral) girdle consists of the scapulae (Fig. 7–8) and clavicles (Fig. 7–9). The S-shaped *clavicle* (collar bone) is the last bone to completely ossify, at about age 21, and is one of the most commonly fractured bones in young people. Its medial end articulates with the sternum to form the *sternoclavicular joint;* it articulates laterally with the scapula's acromion process, forming the *acromioclavicular joint.* Superior **dislocation** of the *acromioclavicular joint* is a common athletic injury. The *scapula* is a flat bone, shaped like an inverted triangle, with a *costal surface* that lies against the upper posterior rib cage. The scapula has a *superior*

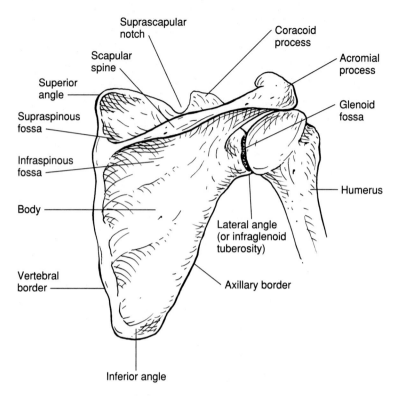

Figure 7–8. Posterior view of the right scapula.

Articulation Summary: Upper Extremity and Shoulder Girdle

- Acromioclavicular
- Sternoclavicular
- Shoulder (glenhumeral)
- Elbow: three articulations:
  1) b/w humeral trochlea and semi-lunar/trochlear notch
  2) b/w capitulum and radial head
  3) proximal radioulnar joint
- Distal radioulnar
- Radiocarpal (distal radius w/scaphoid and lunate)
- Intercarpal
- Carpometacarpal
- Metacarpophalangeal
- Interphalangeal

border, a *medial,* or *vertebral, border,* a *lateral,* or *axillary, border,* and an *inferior angle,* or *apex.* Its superior border presents a *scapular notch* and, projecting anteriorly just medial to the humeral head, the palpable *coracoid process.* The *scapular spine* divides the posterior surface into a *supraspinatus fossa* and *infraspinatus fossa;* the *acromion process* is the lateral extension of the scapular spine. The *glenoid fossa* is on the lateral aspect of the scapula and, with its articulation with the humeral head, forms the (ball and socket) ▶ *shoulder joint.* The **rotator cuff** is composed of a group of shoulder muscles. Rotator cuff injuries are a result of acute injury or chronic wear and tear. The articular capsule of the shoulder is loose, permitting a great range of movement but also making it susceptible to dislocation.

7. Positioning. Positioning of the upper extremity and shoulder girdle requires a thorough knowledge of the anatomy concerned and an awareness of possible pathologic conditions as well as their impact on positioning limitations and technical factors.

▶ **Radiopaque** objects such as watches, bracelets, and rings should be removed whenever possible, since they can obscure important information. The patient must be instructed regarding the importance of remaining still, and immobilization devices such as sandbags or tape should be used as required. The shortest possible exposure time should be employed, especially when involuntary

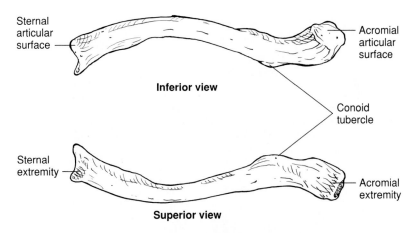

Figure 7–9. The right clavicle.

motion can be a problem, as with trauma, pediatric, or geriatric patients.

Most upper-extremity examinations are more comfortably and accurately positioned with the patient seated at the end of the x-ray table, with the forearm and elbow resting on the table. Most can be performed table-top (ie, without a Bucky grid); the humerus sometimes requires a grid, while the shoulder, clavicle, and scapula usually do. *Suspended respiration* is suggested for radiography of the proximal portion of the upper extremity and shoulder girdle. Patients should be adequately shielded.

The use of just a few important bony landmarks and their correct placement with respect to the film is the basis for accurate positioning. Rotation of the arm and placing the humeral epicondyles in correct relationship to the film is the foundation of forearm, elbow, and shoulder positioning. Positioning of the wrist and hand utilizes the radial and ulnar styloid processes, bending maneuvers (ie, radial and ulnar flexion), metacarpophalangeal joints (MPJ), and interphalangeal joints (IPJ).

The following tables provide a summary of routine and frequently performed special projections of the upper extremity and shoulder girdle.

HAND	POSITION OF PART	CENTRAL RAY DIRECTED	STRUCTURES INCLUDED/ BEST SEEN
PA	Pronated, elbow flexed 90°, fingers extended and slightly spread	$\perp$ 3rd MPJ	PA carpals, metacarpals, phalanges and their articulations; see Fig. 7–10. Provides obl proj of thumb

This position is often performed to include the wrist for *bone age* studies; 30″ SID is sometimes recommended, with the CR entering vertically at the head of the 3rd metacarpal.

(continued)

List of Abbreviations and Symbols Used in the Following Tables

$\angle$	angle
ASIS	anterior superior iliac spine
$\approx$	approximately (about)
b/w	between
CMC	carpometacarpal jt
dist	distal
fx	fracture
>	greater than
jt	joint
IPJ	interphalangeal jt
lat	lateral
LAO	left anterior oblique
LPO	left posterior oblique
<	less than
MPJ	metacarpophalangeal *or* metatarsophalangeal jt
MSP	midsagittal plane
OID	object-image distance
obl	oblique
$\parallel$	parallel to
$\perp$	perpendicular to
proj	projection
prox	proximal
RAO	right anterior oblique
RPO	right posterior oblique
SID	source-image distance
w/	with
w/o	without

Figure 7–10. PA projection of the hand; note that an oblique projection of the first metacarpal and phalange is obtained. Review the skeletal anatomy of the hand and correctly identify each of the lettered structures. (Courtesy of Bob Wong, RT.)

HAND (con't)	POSITION OF PART	CENTRAL RAY DIRECTED	STRUCTURES INCLUDED/ BEST SEEN
OBL	Prone, elbow flexed 90°, hand and forearm obliqued 45° on finger sponge	⊥ 3rd MPJ	Obl proj carpals, metacarpals, phalanges and their articulations; use of a "finger sponge" places jts ‖ to film and opens jt spaces

(continued)

HAND (con't)	POSITION OF PART	CENTRAL RAY DIRECTED	STRUCTURES INCLUDED/ BEST SEEN
LAT *in extension*	Elbow flexed 90°, fingers extended, wrist lateral, ulnar surface down	⊥ MPJs	***Superimposed*** carpals, metacarpals, phalanges and their articulations. Decrease 10 kV for foreign body ◄
LAT *in flexion*	Elbow flexed 90°, fingers slightly flexed and superimposed	⊥ MPJs	Superimposed carpals, metacarpals, phalanges and their articulations. *Shows anterior/ posterior fracture* ***displacement*** ◄

A "fan lateral" with the fingers separated is often performed to better visualize each phalange.
Routine: PA, obl, lat on (1) 11 × 14 or (1) 10 × 12 and (1) 8 × 10

FINGERS	POSITION OF PART	CENTRAL RAY DIRECTED	STRUCTURES INCLUDED/ BEST SEEN
PA	Hand pronated and fingers extended, elbow flexed 90°	⊥ proximal IPJ	PA proximal, middle, and distal phalanges
LAT	Elbow flexed 90°, forearm lateral, finger(s) extended and ‖ film	⊥ proximal IPJ	Lat of proximal, middle, and distal phalanges. 2nd and 3rd digits are done *radial side down;* 4th and 5th done *ulnar side down*

Routine: PA hand, obl, and lat of affected fingers on (1) 10 × 12

THUMB	POSITION OF PART	CENTRAL RAY DIRECTED	STRUCTURES INCLUDED/ BEST SEEN
AP	Dorsal surface adjacent and ‖ film	⊥ MPJ	
PA	Palmar surface ‖ film, *requires increase OID*	⊥ MPJ	
LAT	Lateral surface adjacent to film, fingers elevated and resting on sponge	⊥ MPJ	AP, PA, or lat projection of 1st digit. *3 articulations should be seen;* CMC, MPJ, and IPJ

Routine: PA hand, (obl thumb), lat and AP thumb on (1) 10 × 12

Figure 7–11. Lateral projection of wrist. Note large bone cyst on distal radius. (Courtesy of The Stamford Hospital.)

Figure 7–12. Radial flexion maneuver of left wrist. Radial flexion is used to better demonstrate the medial carpals (pisiform, triangular, hamate, and medial aspect of capitate and lunate). (Saia, DA. *Appleton & Lange's Review for the Radiography Examination,* 2nd ed. East Norwalk, CT: Appleton & Lange, 1993.)

WRIST	POSITION OF PART	CENTRAL RAY DIRECTED	STRUCTURES INCLUDED/ BEST SEEN
PA	Hand pronated w/MPJs slightly flexed, elbow flexed 90°	⊥ mid-carpal region	PA carpals, prox metacarpals, dist radius and ulna. *Flexion of MPJs reduces OID*
LAT	Elbow flexed 90°, ulnar surface down, radius and ulna superimposed	⊥ mid-carpal region	Lat carpals, superimposed prox metacarpals and dist radius and ulna; see Fig. 7–11
PA *semi-pronation* **OBL**	Elbow flexed 90°, wrist 45° w/film, ulnar surface down	⊥ mid-carpal region	Useful for navicular (scaphoid), and other *lat carpals* (greater and lesser multangular) *and their interspaces*
AP *semi-supination* **OBL**	Arm extended, 45° w/film, ulnar surface down	⊥ mid-carpal region	Useful for pisiform, triangular (triquetrum), and hamate (unciform); *medial carpals and their interspaces*
Ulnar Flexion	Position as PA wrist, evert hand (laterally) without moving forearm	⊥ navicular	Navicular and other *lat* carpal interspaces; *reduces foreshortening of navicular*
Radial Flexion	Position as PA wrist, move elbow toward body w/o moving hand/wrist	⊥ mid-carpal region	*Medial* carpal interspaces; see Fig. 7–12
▶ **Navicular** *(Stecher)*	Forearm a) Pronated *or* b) Pronated and elevated 20°	a) 20° toward elbow entering navicular *or* b) ⊥ navicular	Navicular w/o ***foreshortening*** and self-superimposition
▶ **Carpal Canal** *(Gaynor–Hart)*	*Hyperextend* wrist w/palm vertical	25°–30° into long axis of hand	Carpal canal *(tunnel);* greater multangular (trapezium), navicular, capitate, triangular, pisiform

Routine: PA, PA obl, lat on (1) 10 × 12 or 11 × 14, and special projections as requested

FOREARM	POSITION OF PART	CENTRAL RAY DIRECTED	STRUCTURES INCLUDED/ BEST SEEN
AP	Supinated and extended, epicondyles ∥ film; *shoulder and elbow on same plane*	⊥ mid-forearm	AP radius and ulna, including wrist and elbow joints; see Fig. 7–13, *arm must be supinated* to avoid overlap of radius and ulna
LAT	Elbow flexed 90°, epicondyles superimposed and ⊥ film, hand lateral; *shoulder and elbow on same plane*	⊥ mid-forearm	Radius and ulna superimposed distally, lat proj of radius and ulna, elbow and wrist joints

Routine: AP and lat on (1) 11 × 14

Figure 7–13. Lateral (external) oblique view of elbow. Note that the radial tuberosity is free of ulnar superimposition. The proximal radioulnar articulation is nicely shown at C. *Review the skeletal anatomy of the elbow by correctly identifying each of the labeled structures.* (Courtesy of Bob Wong, RT.)

ELBOW	POSITION OF PART	CENTRAL RAY DIRECTED	STRUCTURES INCLUDED/ BEST SEEN
AP	Extended, supinated; epicondyles ∥ film	⊥ elbow jt	AP elbow jt, proximal radius and ulna, distal humerus; radial head and tuberosity partially superimposed on ulna
LAT	Flexed 90°, epicondyles ⊥ film, forearm and wrist lateral	⊥ elbow jt	Lat elbow jt, prox radius and ulna and distal humerus; radial head partially superimposed on ulna
Medial (internal) OBL	Arm extended, palm down, epicondyles 45° to film	⊥ elbow jt midway b/w epicondyles	Obl elbow jt; *coronoid process in profile;* see Fig. 7–14
Lateral (external) OBL	Forearm extended and rotated laterally, radial surface down, epicondyles 45° to film	⊥ elbow jt midway b/w epicondyles	Obl elbow jt; radial head, neck, and tuberosity free from superimposition of ulna; see Fig. 7–15
AP *in partial flexion*	1) Prox forearm ∥ film, supinated 2) Distal humerus ∥ film, epicondyles ∥ film	to elbow jt: 1) ⊥ prox forearm 2) ⊥ distal humerus elbow	AP of prox forearm and distal humerus; components of elbow jt seen without **distortion** created ◄ by flexed

(continued)

Figure 7–14. Medial (internal) oblique view of elbow; notice that coronoid process is seen free of superimposition. (Saia, DA. *Appleton & Lange's Review for the Radiography Examination,* 2nd ed. East Norwalk, CT: Appleton & Lange, 1993.)

Figure 7–15. PA oblique projection, scapular Y view of the shoulder. Useful for demonstration of dislocations. Humeral head displaced inferior to coracoid process indicates *anterior dislocation,* while humeral head displaced inferior to acromion process indicates *posterior dislocation.* (From Cornuelle et al. *Radiographic Anatomy and Positioning.* Stamford, CT: Appleton & Lange, 1998.)

ELBOW (con't)	POSITION OF PART	CENTRAL RAY DIRECTED	STRUCTURES INCLUDED/ BEST SEEN
Radial Head	Lateral elbow w/hand: 1) externally rotated 2) lateral 3) pronated 4) internally rotated	⊥ elbow jt	Entire perimeter of radial head; used as supplemental examination when routine elbow is negative w/*elevated fat pad* and clinical point tenderness

Routine: AP, lat, both obl on (1) 11 × 14 or (2) 10 × 12 and additional projections as needed

HUMERUS	POSITION OF PART	CENTRAL RAY DIRECTED	STRUCTURES INCLUDED/ BEST SEEN
AP	Arm extended and supinated; epicondyles ‖ film	⊥ mid-humerus	AP humerus, includes shoulder and elbow jts; *greater tubercle in profile;* epicondyles ‖ film
LAT	Elbow flexed 90°, epicondyles ⊥ film	⊥ mid-humerus	Lat humerus including shoulder and elbow jts; *lesser tubercle in profile;* epicondyles superimposed

Routine: AP and lat on (2) 11 × 14

SHOULDER	POSITION OF PART	CENTRAL RAY DIRECTED	STRUCTURES INCLUDED/ BEST SEEN
AP *rotational projections*	Arm extended and 1) supinated, w/epicondyles ‖ film 2) palm against thigh, epicondyles 45° to film 3) elbow slightly flexed, back of hand against thigh	⊥ coracoid process	1) External rotation: true AP humerus, shows greater tubercle in profile 2) neutral position: good for calcific deposits, trauma 3) internal rotation: lateral of humerus, shows lesser tubercle in profile; see Fig. 7–16
Transthoracic Lateral	Patient erect lateral w/affected surgical neck centered to film; unaffected arm over head	⊥ affected surgical neck	Lateral shoulder and proximal humerus through thorax

(continued)

Figure 7–16. Shoulder in external rotation places humerus in a true AP position and places the greater tubercle (J) in profile. *Review the skeletal anatomy* of the shoulder by correctly identifying each of the labeled structures. (Courtesy of Bob Wong, RT.)

SHOULDER (con't)	POSITION OF PART	CENTRAL RAY DIRECTED	STRUCTURES INCLUDED/ BEST SEEN
Axial *superoinferior*	Seated at end of table with arm extended over cassette and shoulder centered to film	to shoulder joint, ∠5 to 15° to elbow	Superoinferior axial of shoulder, acromioclavicular jt and lesser tubercle
PA Obl *scapular Y*	Affected shoulder centered with MCP 60° to film	⊥ shoulder joint	Oblique shoulder; especially good for *demonstration of dislocations* (Fig. 7–15)

Routine: For fx: AP and transthoracic lat on (2) 10 × 12

CLAVICLE	POSITION OF PART	CENTRAL RAY DIRECTED	STRUCTURES INCLUDED/ BEST SEEN
PA or AP	Patient recumbent or erect; center affected clavicle to film; less OID in PA position	⊥ mid-shaft	Entire length of clavicle and articulations, best done PA erect or AP recumbent for patient comfort
PA Axial	Patient PA, affected clavicle centered to film	to supraclavicular fossa 25 to 30° caudad	*Axial* projection of clavicle; can demonstrate fractures not seen in direct PA or AP

Routine: PA and PA axial on (2) 10 × 12

ACROMIO-CLAVICULAR JOINTS	POSITION OF PART	CENTRAL RAY DIRECTED	STRUCTURES INCLUDED/ BEST SEEN
	Patient AP or PA *erect,* MSP to mid-film, arms at sides (always bilateral for comparison)	⊥ midline at level of AC jts	AP/PA projection of acromioclavicular jt and associated soft tissues; demonstrates *dislocation/ separation* when performed erect; it is often recommended that two exposures be made: one w/o and one w/weights (w/ films properly identified)

Routine: (1) 7 × 17 or (2) 8 × 10

SCAPULA	POSITION OF PART	CENTRAL RAY DIRECTED	STRUCTURES INCLUDED/ BEST SEEN
AP	AP upright or recumbent; scapula centered w/arm abducted and elbow flexed	⊥ mid-scapula, ≈ 2″ inferior to coracoid process	AP scapula with lateral portion drawn away from ribs; exposure may be made during quiet breathing to blur lung markings; see Fig. 7–17
LAT	Erect PA obl w/affected side toward film and arm across chest; palpate scapular borders and rotate body until superimposed	⊥ to mid-vertebral border	Lateral scapula, acromion and coracoid processes, superimposed vertebral and axillary borders free of rib cage

Routine: AP and lat on (2) 10 × 12

B. LOWER EXTREMITY AND PELVIS

1. Foot and Toes. The bones of the foot (Fig. 7–18) include the seven *tarsal bones,* five *metatarsal bones,* and 14 *phalanges.* The *calcaneus* (os calsis), or heel bone, is the largest tarsal. It serves as attachment for the Achilles tendon posteriorly, articulates anteriorly with the *cuboid bone,* presents three articular surfaces superiorly for its articulation with the *talus,* and has a prominent shelf on its anteromedial edge called the *sustentaculum tali.*

The inferior surface of the talus *(astragalus)* articulates with the superior calcaneus to form the 3-faceted *subtalar joint.* The talus also articulates anteriorly with the navicular *(scaphoid)* bone. Articulating anteriorly with the navicular are the three *cuneiform bones:*

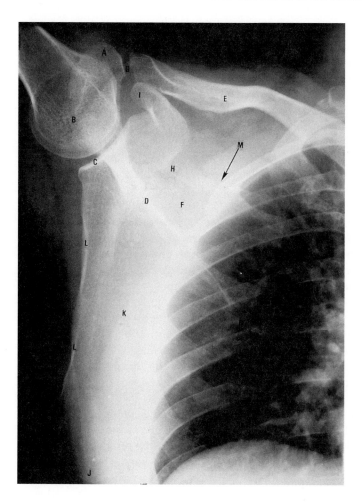

Figure 7–17. AP projection of scapula. Note that arm abduction moves scapula away from rib cage, revealing a greater portion of the scapular body. *Review the skeletal anatomy* of the scapula by correctly identifying each of the labeled structures. (Courtesy of Bob Wong, RT.)

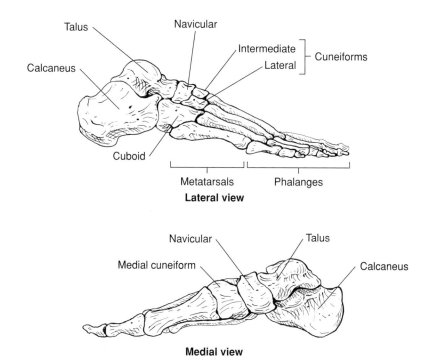

Figure 7–18. Bones of the foot.

Figure 7–19. Dorsoplantar projection of the foot demonstrates fractured shaft of the second metatarsal and dislocated third and fourth metatarsophalangeal joints. (From Way, LW, ed. *Current Surgical Diagnosis & Treatment* 10th ed. East Norwalk, CT: Appleton & Lange, 1994, Figure 43–51; p 1070.)

medial/first, intermediate/second, and lateral/third. The navicular articulates laterally with the cuboid.

Fractures of the calcaneus can occur, especially as a result of a fall from a height directly onto the heel. The calcaneus can also be ▶ associated with painful *spur* formation.

The metatarsals and phalanges of the foot are similar to the metacarpals and phalanges of the hand. The bases of the first three metatarsals articulate with the three cuneiforms. The bases of the fourth and fifth metatarsals articulate with the cuboid. The fifth (most lateral) metatarsal projects laterally and presents a large *tuberosity* at its base making it very susceptible to fracture. **Stress fractures** are common to the metatarsals (Fig. 7–19).

The first, or great, toe *(hallux)* has two phalanges; the second through fifth toes have three phalanges each. The phalanges of the toes are shorter than those of the fingers. Stubbing and crushing-type injuries are common causes of **fractured** phalanges. The articulations of the foot are named similarly to those of the hand.

2. Ankle. The ankle joint *(mortise)* is formed by the articulation of the talus and distal portions of the tibia and fibula (Fig. 7–20). The medial and lateral malleoli are the most frequently fractured components of the ankle joint; severe **fractures** can disrupt the integrity of the joint and lead to permanent instability and/or arthritis.

3. Lower Leg (Fig. 7–21). The *tibia* and *fibula* compose the bones of the lower leg. The tibia is the larger of the two and is situated medially. It articulates superiorly with the femur and inferiorly with the talus to form a portion of the ankle joint. The tibia consists

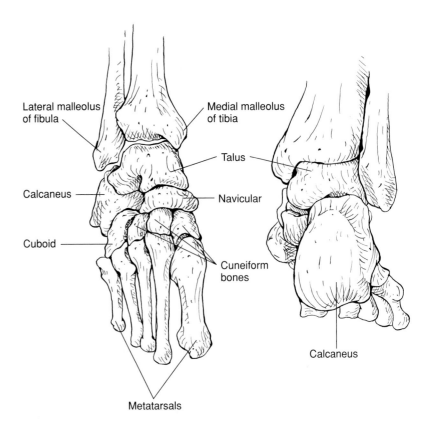

Figure 7–20. Ankle and foot: anterior and posterior views.

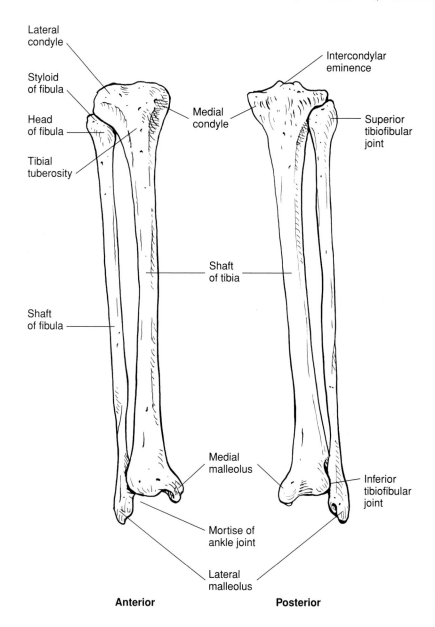

Figure 7–21. Right tibia and fibula.

of a shaft and two expanded extremities. Its distal extremity has a prominence, the *medial malleolus,* which also participates in the formation of the ankle ***mortise.*** The fibular notch provides articulation ◀ for the fibula to form the *distal tibiofibular joint.*

The proximal end of the tibia presents a *medial* and a *lateral condyle,* on whose superior surfaces there are facets for articulation with the femur. The articular facets form a smooth surface called the *tibial plateau,* which provides attachment for the cartilaginous *menisci* of the knee joint. Between the two articular surfaces is a raised prominence, the *intercondylar eminence (tibial spine).* The proximal anterior surface of the tibia presents the *tibial tuberosity,* which provides attachment for the patellar ligament. **Osgood–Schlatter's disease** is a chronic ***epiphysitis*** of the tibial tuberosity ◀ that occurs in some active young adults. Its symptoms include pain

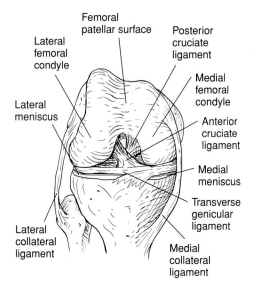

Figure 7–22. Ligaments of the knee joint.

and tenderness and it is manifested radiographically by separation at the epiphysis.

The fibula is the slender, lateral non–weight-bearing bone forming the lower leg; it also consists of a shaft and two expanded extremities. The bulbous distal end is the *lateral malleolus* (projects more distally than medially), which helps to form the ankle joint and has a facet for articulation with the tibia *(distal tibiofibular joint)*. The expanded proximal portion of the fibula is the *head,* which articulates with the lateral tibial condyle, forming the *proximal tibiofibular joint*. A *styloid process* extends superiorly from the head of the fibula. The *neck* is the constricted portion just distal to the fibular head. The fibula is most commonly fractured at the malleolus, just above the ankle joint.

4. Knee. The knee is formed by the proximal tibia, the patella, and the distal femur, which articulate to form the *femorotibial* and *femoropatellar* joints. The distal posterior femur presents two large *medial* and *lateral condyles* separated by the deep *intercondyloid fossa*. Two small prominences, the *medial* and *lateral epicondyles,* are just superior to the condyles. The femoral and tibial condyles articulate to form the *femorotibial joint*. Semilunar cartilages, the ▸ *menisci,* lie medially and laterally between the articulating bones and, together with the *cruciate* and *collateral ligaments,* help to form the *articular capsule* of the knee (Fig. 7–22). The *patella* is the largest *sesamoid* bone and, attached to the tibial tuberosity by the patellar ligament, glides over the patellar surface of the distal femur (femoropatellar joint) during flexion and extension of the knee. The congenital anomaly, **bipartite patella,** can be misinterpreted as a fracture. Just opposite the *patellar surface,* on the posterior distal femur, is the smooth *popliteal surface,* which accommodates the popliteal artery.

5. Femur. The *femur* (Fig. 7–23) is the longest and strongest bone in the body. The femoral *shaft* is bowed slightly anteriorly and presents a long, narrow ridge posteriorly, called the *linea aspera*. The proximal end of the femur consists of a *head* that is received by the *accetabulum* of the pelvis. The femoral head has a small notch, the *fovea capitis femoris,* for ligament attachment. The *femoral neck,* which joins the head and shaft, normally angles upward about 120° ▸ and forward (in **anteversion**) about 15°. The *greater* (lateral) and *lesser* (medial) *trochanters* are large processes on the posterior proximal femur. The greater trochanter is a prominent positioning landmark that lies in the same transverse plane as the pubic symphysis and coccyx. The *intertrochanteric crest* runs obliquely between the trochanters; the *intertrochanteric line* runs anteriorly parallel to the crest. The femoral neck is the most commonly fractured portion of the femur (Fig. 7–24). **Fractures** of the femoral shaft are usually the result of a direct blow; fracture *displacement* is dependent on muscular pull.

6. Pelvis. The pelvic girdle consists of two *innominate* (hip, or coxal) bones, one on each side of the sacrum. Each innominate bone consists of three fused bones, the *ilium, ischium,* and *pubis* (Fig. 7–25). Parts of these three bones contribute to the formation of the *acetabulum*—the socket articulation for the femoral head. The ilia are the large, superior bones whose medial *auricular* surfaces form the

---

Articulation Summary: Lower Extremity and Pelvic Girdle

- Sacroiliac
- Hip (femoral head w/acetabulum)
- Knee (femorotibial)
- Proximal tibiofibular
- Distal tibiofibular
- Ankle (distal tibia and fibula w/superior talus)
- Intertarsal
- Tarsometatarsal
- Metatarsophalangeal
- Interphalangeal

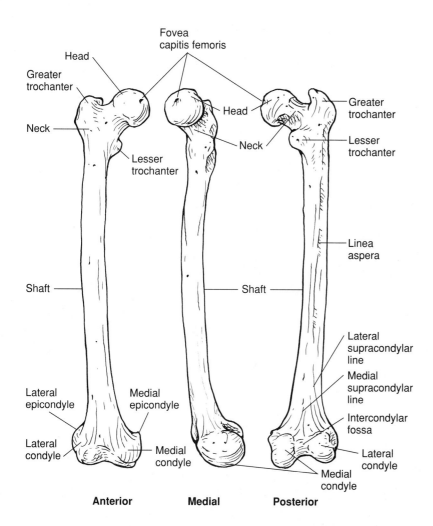

Figure 7–23. The right femur.

Anterior   Medial   Posterior

Labels on the figure: Greater trochanter, Head, Fovea capitis femoris, Neck, Lesser trochanter, Shaft, Lateral epicondyle, Medial epicondyle, Lateral condyle, Medial condyle, Head, Neck, Greater trochanter, Lesser trochanter, Linea aspera, Lateral supracondylar line, Medial supracondylar line, Intercondylar fossa, Lateral condyle, Medial condyle

Figure 7–24. AP projection of the hip demonstrating fracture of the femoral neck. (From Way, LW, ed. *Current Surgical Diagnosis & Treatment,* 10th ed. East Norwalk, CT: Appleton & Lange, 1994, Figure 43–34; p 1044.)

A

B

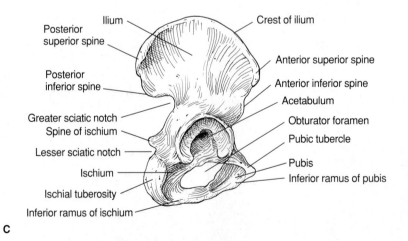

C

Figure 7–25. **(A)** The pelvis (anterior view). (Redrawn with permission from Martini, F. *Fundamentals of Anatomy and Physiology,* 2nd ed. Englewood Cliffs, NJ: Prentice-Hall, 1992.) **(B)** The pelvic girdle (posterior view). **(C)** The right hip bone (lateral view), showing the acetabulum.

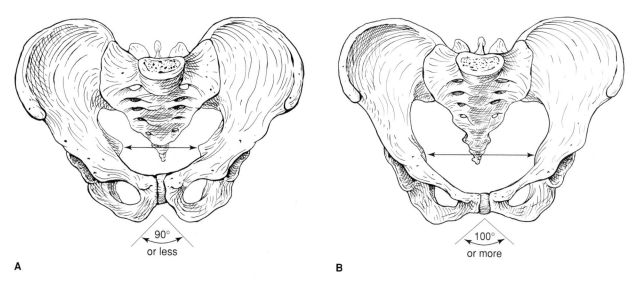

Figure 7–26. Architectural differences in the male (**A**) and female (**B**) pelves.

sacroiliac joints bilaterally. The broad, flat portion of each ilium is the *ala*, or wing; the upper part of the ala forms a ridge of bone called the *iliac crest,* which terminates in *anterior* and *posterior iliac spines.*

The ischium forms the posteroinferior portion of the pelvis. The posterior part of the ischium forms the major portion of the *greater* and *lesser sciatic notches* separated by the *ischial spine.* The most inferior portion is the *ischial tuberosity,* a large, rough prominence that provides attachment for posterior thigh muscles. The inferior *ramus* of the ischium extends medially from the tuberosities to unite with the inferior ramus of the pubis. The pubic bones form the anterior portion of the pelvis. Their bodies unite to form the *pubic symphysis.* The superior ramus fuses with the ilium and inferior ramus with the ischium to form the large *obturator foramen.*

Pelvic fractures frequently cause disturbance of the urinary bladder or urethra; an ***intravenous urogram*** (IVU, IVP) may be required to diagnose any urinary leakage. The **female pelvis** differs from the **male pelvis** in that it is shallower and its bones are generally more delicate. The pelvic outlet is wider and more circular in the female; the ischial tuberosities and acetabula are further apart; the angle formed by the pubic arch is also greater in the female; all these bony characteristics facilitate the birth process (Fig. 7–26).

7. Positioning.

Positioning of the lower extremity and pelvis requires a thorough knowledge of the skeletal anatomy and an awareness of possible pathologic conditions and their potential impact on positioning and technical factors.

Clothing with radiopaque objects such as buttons, snaps, or zippers should be removed whenever possible. Bulky or bunched clothing can produce undesirable radiographic artifacts and should therefore be removed whenever possible and replaced with a hospital dressing gown. Elastic-waisted garments can contribute to nonuniform density on abdominal radiographs.

The patient must be instructed about the importance of remaining still, and immobilization devices such as radioparent sponges, sandbags, or tape should be used as required. The shortest possible exposure time should be employed, especially when involuntary motion is a potential problem.

Many lower extremity examinations can be performed table-top (ie, non-Bucky); the knee frequently requires a grid; femur, hip, and pelvis almost always do. *Suspended respiration* is suggested for radiography of the proximal portion of the lower extremity and the pelvis. Patients must be appropriately shielded.

Some of the lower leg examinations can be performed either AP or PA, depending on the condition and comfort of the patient. Lateral projections can be easily obtained using a horizontal (cross-table lateral) beam when extremity or patient movement is contraindicated.

The following tables provide a summary of routine and frequently performed special projections of the lower extremity and pelvis.

Figure 7–27. Medial oblique view of left foot demonstrates the articulations of the cuboid with the calcaneus, fourth and fifth metatarsals, and lateral cuneiform. The talonavicular articulation and sinus tarsi are also demonstrated. Note the fractured shaft of the fifth metatarsal. (Courtesy of The Stamford Hospital.)

FOOT	POSITION OF PART	CENTRAL RAY DIRECTED	STRUCTURES INCLUDED/ BEST SEEN
Dorso-plantar	Knee flexed ≈45°, plantar surface on cassette	⊥ or 10° toward heel to base of 3rd metatarsal	Tarsals (except calcaneus and part of talus), metatarsals and phalanges with their articulations, in frontal projection
Medial Obl	Start as dorso-plantar, rotate medially 30°	⊥ base of 3rd metatarsal	Most tarsals and metatarsals (except the most medial) and their articulations, sinus tarsi, tuberosity of 5th metatarsal; see Fig. 7–27
Lateral Obl	Start as dorso-plantar, rotate laterally 30°	⊥ base of 3rd metatarsal	Articulations b/w 1st and 2nd metatarsals, 1st and 2nd cuneiforms; less foreshortened position of navicular
Lateral (medio-lateral)	Patient on affected side, patella ⊥ tabletop, foot slightly dorsiflexed with plantar surface ⊥ cassette	⊥ base of 3rd metatarsal	Lateral foot and ankle joint; distal tibia and fibula; superimposed tarsals, tibia and fibula; see Fig. 7–28

Routine: Dorsoplantar, obl, lat on (1) 11 × 14 or (1) 10 × 12 and (1) 8 × 10

Figure 7–28. Lateral projection of foot demonstrates superimposed tarsals, metatarsals, and phalanges; a little more of the distal tibia and fibula should be visualized. (Courtesy of The Stamford Hospital.)

TOES	POSITION OF PART	CENTRAL RAY DIRECTED	STRUCTURES INCLUDED/ BEST SEEN
Dorso-plantar	Knee flexed ≈45°, plantar surface on cassette	⊥ or 10° toward heel, to 2nd MPJ	Phalanges, their articulations and distal metatarsals in frontal projection
Medial Obl	Start as dorso-plantar, rotate medially 30 to 45°	⊥ 3rd MPJ	Oblique projection of phalanges, their articulations and distal metatarsals
LAT	Turn to side that brings affected toe(s) closest to film; unaffected toes may be taped back or occlusal film used for individual toes	⊥ proximal pip	Lateral projection of toe(s) and associated articulations

Routine: Dorsoplantar foot, obl and lat of affected toes on (1) 10 × 12 or 11 × 14

CALCANEUS	POSITION OF PART	CENTRAL RAY DIRECTED	STRUCTURES INCLUDED/ BEST SEEN
Planto-dorsal	Patient seated on table with leg extended, plantar surface ⊥ tabletop (immobilize w/strip of tape held by patient)	40° cephalad to base of 3rd metatarsal	Axial projection of calcaneus; trochlear process, sustentaculum tali, talocalcaneal jt; see Fig. 7–29
Dorso-plantar	Patient prone, plantar surface ⊥ tabletop; cassette placed against plantar surface	40° caudally to level of base of 2nd metatarsal	Axial proj of calcaneus; trochlear process, sustentaculum tali, talocalcaneal jt
LAT	Patient on affected side, patella ⊥ tabletop, foot and ankle lateral	⊥ mid-calcaneus	Lateral calcaneus, talus, navicular, ankle jt, and sinus tarsi; see Fig. 7–30

Routine: Plantodorsal axial and lat on (1) 8 × 10

Figure 7–29. Plantodorsal projection of calcaneus; sustentaculum tali, trochlear process, and calcaneal tuberosity are well visualized. (Courtesy of The Stamford Hospital.)

Figure 7–30. Lateral calcaneus; sinus tarsi is well visualized. (Courtesy of The Stamford Hospital.)

Figure 7–31. AP projection of the ankle joint. (Courtesy of The Stamford Hospital.)

ANKLE	POSITION OF PART	CENTRAL RAY DIRECTED	STRUCTURES INCLUDED/ BEST SEEN
AP	Leg extended AP, plantar surface vertical (⊥ film)	⊥ midway b/w malleoli thru tibiotalar jt	AP ankle jt, distal tibia/fibula, talus; see Fig. 7–31
LAT	Patient turned onto affected side, patella ⊥ table-top, foot dorsi-flexed (≈90°)	⊥ ankle jt	Lateral distal tibia/fibula, ankle jt, talus, calcaneus, navicular
Medial Obl *(mortise view)*	Leg extended, plantar surface vertical w/leg rotated 15–20° medially and malleoli parallel to cassette	⊥ ankle jt, midway between malleoli	Ankle mortise, oblique distal tibia/fibula and proximal talus, and their articular surfaces; see Fig. 7–32
Lateral Obl	Leg extended, plantar surface vertical w/leg rotated 45° laterally	⊥ ankle jt, midway between malleoli	Lateral oblique distal tibia/fibula and ankle jt

Routine: AP, lat, both obl on (1) 11 × 14 or (2) 10 × 12

LOWER LEG	POSITION OF PART	CENTRAL RAY DIRECTED	STRUCTURES INCLUDED/ BEST SEEN
AP	Leg extended AP, no pelvic rotation, foot dorsiflexed	⊥ mid-shaft tibia	AP lower leg, both jts should be included

(continued)

Figure 7–32. The 15 to 20° medial oblique projection of the ankle is used to demonstrate the ankle mortise. An oblique projection of the distal tibia/fibula, proximal talus, and their articular surfaces is also demonstrated. (Courtesy of The Stamford Hospital.)

LOWER LEG (con't)	POSITION OF PART	CENTRAL RAY DIRECTED	STRUCTURES INCLUDED/ BEST SEEN
LAT	Patient on affected side, patella ⊥ table-top, ankle and foot lateral	⊥ mid-shaft	Lateral tibia/fibula, both jts should be included

Routine: AP and Lat on (1) or (2/diagonally) 14 × 17

KNEE	POSITION OF PART	CENTRAL RAY DIRECTED	STRUCTURES INCLUDED/ BEST SEEN
AP	Leg extended AP, no pelvic rotation (leg may be rotated 3–5° internally)	5–7° cephalad to 1/2″ below patellar apex (knee jt)	AP knee jt, distal femur, and proximal tibia/ fibula, patella seen thru femur
LAT	Patient on affected side, patella ⊥ tabletop, knee flexed 20–30°	5° cephalad to knee jt	Lateral proj of knee and patellofemoral jts; superimposed femoral condyles; *knee should not be flexed >10° with known or suspected patellar fx;* see Fig. 7–33

(continued)

Figure 7–33. The knee should not be flexed more than 10° when transverse fracture of patella is known or suspected; flexion can cause pain, fragment separation, and fracture complication. CR angulation of 5° cephalad will superimpose the magnified medial femoral condyle on the lateral condyle and permit a better view of the joint space; angulation was not employed in this projection and the joint space is obscured by the magnified medial femoral condyle. (Courtesy of The Stamford Hospital.)

KNEE (con't)	POSITION OF PART	CENTRAL RAY DIRECTED	STRUCTURES INCLUDED/ BEST SEEN
AP *weight bearing (bilateral)*	Patient AP erect with back to upright Bucky, weight evenly shared on legs	⊥ CR midway b/w knees at level of patellar apices	AP weight bearing knee joints particularly useful for evaluation of *arthritic conditions*

Note: The *proximal tibiofibular articulation* is best demonstrated in a 45° internal/medial oblique knee position.

Intercondyloid Fossa *(Camp–Coventry)*	Patient PA recumbent, knee flexed so tibia forms 40°∠ w/ *tabletop and foot* rested on support	CR 40° caudad (⊥ long axis of tibia) to knee jt	*PA axial* (superoinferior) proj of intercondyloid fossa, tibial plateau, and eminences; *"tunnel view";* see Fig. 7–34
Intercondyloid Fossa *(Bêclerê)*	Patient AP w/knee flexed ≈20–30° resting on supported cassette	∠ed cephalad (⊥ long axis of tibia) to knee jt	*AP axial* (inferosuperior) proj of intercondyloid fossa, tibial plateau and eminences; "tunnel view"

Routine: AP and lat on (2) 8 × 10 . . . supplemental projections as necessary

Note: The *Holmblad* method of intercondyloid fossa is performed w/the patient in the kneeling position on the x-ray table. The affected knee is centered, CR forms a 20° angle w/femur (femur is 70° with table).

A

B

Figure 7–34. **(A)** Intercondyloid fossa, using the Camp–Coventry method. The tibial plateau and eminences are well visualized. (Courtesy of The Stamford Hospital.) **(B)** Patient and CR positioning for Camp–Coventry method. From Cornuelle et al. *Radiographic Anatomy and Positioning.* Stamford, CT: Appleton & Lange, 1998.)

PATELLA	POSITION OF PART	CENTRAL RAY DIRECTED	STRUCTURES INCLUDED/ BEST SEEN
PA	Patient prone, leg rotated ≈5–10° laterally to place patella ‖ tabletop	⊥ patella (enters popliteal region)	PA patella, usually including knee jt; better detail than that afforded by the AP position (less OID)
Tangential *(Hughston)*	Patient prone, knee flexed 50–60° with foot resting against tube head	45° cephalad through patellofemoral jt	Tangential proj of patella, patellofemoral articulation; particularly useful to r/o patellar *subluxation*
Tangential *(Settegast)*	Patient prone or seated on x-ray table; knee flexed to place patella nearly ⊥ tabletop	Directed to patellar apex, exiting at its base	***Tangential*** projection of the patella, patellofemoral articulation; especially useful for demonstrating *vertical* fx; *must not be attempted when there is known or suspected transverse fx of patella*

Routine: PA and tangential on (2) 8 × 10

FEMUR	POSITION OF PART	CENTRAL RAY DIRECTED	STRUCTURES INCLUDED/ BEST SEEN
AP	Patient supine, affected femur centered to midline of grid w/leg internally rotated 15°	⊥ mid-femoral shaft (to include hip and possibly knee jt	AP proj femur, including hip jt; leg rotation *overcomes anteversion* of femoral neck and places it ‖ film
LAT	Patient recumbent lateral w/affected leg centered to grid; patella ⊥ tabletop	⊥ mid-shaft	Lateral proj femur, from knee jt up; may be performed w/horizontal beam in case of known or suspected fracture or pathologic disease

Note: If an orthopedic appliance is present, the radiograph should include the entire appliance and the articulation closest to it. *Routine:* AP and lat on (2) 14 × 17 (two films are usually needed to demonstrate both joints in each position.)

HIP	POSITION OF PART	CENTRAL RAY DIRECTED	STRUCTURES INCLUDED/ BEST SEEN
AP	Patient supine, sagittal plane 2″ medial to ASIS centered to midline of grid, no pelvic rotation, leg rotated 15° internally	⊥ sagittal plane 2″ medial to ASIS at level of greater trochanter	AP hip jt, femoral neck and proximal femur; a portion of the pelvic bones is included. *The greater trochanter should be seen in profile.* Another method of hip localization is to bisect the ASIS and pubic symphysis: this locates the peak of the femoral head. A point ≈2–1/2″ distal and ⊥ is the mid-point of the femoral neck

Note: *Leg inversion must never be forced and is contraindicated in cases of known or suspected fx or destructive disease.*

(continued)

HIP (con't)	POSITION OF PART	CENTRAL RAY DIRECTED	STRUCTURES INCLUDED/ BEST SEEN
AP Oblique (*modified Cleaves*)	Patient supine, ASIS of affected side centered to grid, knee and hip acutely flexed, thigh(s) abducted 40°	⊥ the affected hip at a level 1″ above the pubic symphysis	AP oblique proj hip jt, femoral neck and associated structures; lesser trochanter should be seen on the medial aspect of the femur; see Fig.7–35; bilateral examination can be performed by positioning both hips and directing the CR to the MSP at a point 1″ above the pubic symphysis (Fig. 7–35)

Figure 7–35. AP oblique (modified Cleaves) view of hip. The femoral neck and greater and lesser trochanters are well defined; the lesser trochanter is seen medially. (Courtesy of The Stamford Hospital.)

Note: This position must not be attempted when fracture is suspected.

Axiolateral	Patient supine, unaffected leg elevated; leg rotated internally 15°, grid placed against thigh ‖ to femoral neck*	⊥ femoral neck* and grid	Lateral proj of proximal femur and its articulation with the acetabulum; *the lesser trochanter will be prominently seen on the posterior aspect of the femur*

*This position requires localization of the long axis of the femoral neck. First *mark* the midpoint between the ASIS and pubic symphysis of affected side; next *mark* a point 1″ distal to the prominence of the greater trochanter. A line between these 2 points parallels the long axis of the femoral neck.
Routine: For fracture and destructive disease: AP and axiolateral on (2) 10 × 12; for bursitis, etc: AP and AP axial on (2) 10 × 12

PELVIS	POSITION OF PART	CENTRAL RAY DIRECTED	STRUCTURES INCLUDED/ BEST SEEN
AP	Patient supine, MSP ⊥ tabletop, no pelvic rotation, legs rotated internally 15°	⊥ midline at a level 2″ above greater trochanter; top of cassette 1 to 2″ above iliac crest	AP proj pelvis and upper femora w/ femoral necks ‖ film and greater trochanters free of superimposition; see Fig. 7–36

Routine: (1) 14 × 17

Figure 7–36. AP projection of the pelvis. The femoral necks are seen in their entirety: internal rotation of the feet/legs places them parallel to the film. *Review the skeletal anatomy* of the pelvis by correctly identifying each of the lettered structures. (Courtesy of Bob Wong, RT.)

ILIUM	POSITION OF PART	CENTRAL RAY DIRECTED	STRUCTURES INCLUDED/ BEST SEEN
AP	Patient supine, sagittal plane passing through hip jt of affected side centered to grid, patient obliqued 40° toward affected side	⊥, enters the sagittal plane 2″ medial to ASIS at level mid-way between crest and greater trochanter	AP proj of ilium, patient obliquity "opens" the ilium by placing it ∥ to the film

Routine: (1) 10 × 12 ea

SACROILIAC JTS	POSITION OF PART	CENTRAL RAY DIRECTED	STRUCTURES INCLUDED/ BEST SEEN
AP Obl *(LPO and RPO)*	Patient supine and *obliqued 25–30°* affected side up with sagittal plane passing 1″ medial to ASIS centered to grid	⊥ a point 1″ *medial to* ASIS	Sacroiliac (SI) jt of the *elevated side;* the opposite obl is similarly obtained; the correct degree of obliquity "opens" the SI jt; axial projection may be made with CR 20 to 25° cephalad

Routine: (1) 8 × 10 ea

8. Long-Bone Measurement. Accurate measurement of long bones, usually lower extremities, is occasionally required to evaluate abnormal growth patterns in children or lower back disorders in adults.

LONG BONE MEASUREMENT	POSITION OF PART	CENTRAL RAY DIRECTED	STRUCTURES INCLUDED/ BEST SEEN
AP (leg)	Patient supine, leg extended and centered to grid w/metal ruler taped alongside; one exposure each at hip, knee, and ankle jts (on one film)	⊥ hip, knee, ankle jts	Tightly collimated AP projections of hip, knee, and ankle jts with metallic ruler alongside; if **bilaterally,** ruler ◄ is placed between legs, there must be no rotation, and if one knee is somewhat flexed, the other must be identically flexed for the exposure

Routine: (1) 14 × 17

> ### To Locate Joints
>
> **Hip:** Bisect the ASIS and pubic symphysis; center 1″ distal and lateral to that point
> **Knee:** Center immediately below the patellar apex
> **Ankle:** Center midway between the malleoli

9. Arthrography. *Arthrography* is a contrast examination performed to evaluate soft-tissue joint structures, such as articular cartilages, menisci, ligaments, and bursae. The examination is most often performed as *double* contrast, with a *positive* **contrast agent** (water- ◄ soluble iodinated) coating the structures and a *negative* contrast agent filling the joint cavity. Fluoroscopic spot films are made during the examination while applying various **stress maneuvers.** Over- ◄ head radiographs are frequently requested to follow. The knee is the most common joint to be examined in this way, although the hip, wrist, shoulder and temporomandibular joint (TMJ) can also be evaluated with contrast arthrography.

At the start of the procedure, any effusion is first aspirated from the joint. The contrast agent(s) are then introduced into the joint cavity and the joint is manipulated to distribute the contrast material throughout.

Knee arthrography requires the use of a stress device. Manipulation of the knee within the device serves to open the medial and lateral articulating surfaces to better advantage. Knee arthrography is useful in evaluating ligamentous and meniscal injuries.

Hip arthrography may be used to evaluate the condition or position of a **prosthesis** in the adult, and in children is used to assess ◄ congenital hip dislocation.

Wrist arthrography is useful in cases of restricted motion and continuous pain or weakness, eg, certain arthritic conditions.

Shoulder arthrography is commonly performed to evaluate soft-tissue injuries such as rotator cuff tears (Fig. 7–37A).

TMJ arthrography may be used to evaluate the clicking, severe pain, and tinnitis often associated with TMJ syndrome.

Many arthrographic procedures have been replaced by magnetic resonance imaging (MRI) studies, which have the advantage of being **noninvasive** and providing excellent soft-tissue diagnostic value ◄ (Fig. 7–37B).

A

B

Figure 7–37. **(A)** A normal shoulder arthrogram. (Way, LW, ed. *Current Surgical Diagnosis & Treatment,* 10th ed. East Norwalk, CT: Appleton & Lange, 1994, Figure 43–18A; p 1026.) **(B)** MR image of the shoulder is accomplished noninvasively and provides visualization of structures having subtle differences in tissue density. (Courtesy of The Stamford Hospital.)

10. Terminology and Pathology. Radiologically significant skeletal disorders or conditions of upper and lower extremities with which the student radiographer should be familiar are listed as follows.

Achondroplasia
Acromegaly
Battered child syndrome
Bone metastases
Bursitis
Carpal tunnel syndrome
Congenital hip dislocation
Enchondroma
Epicondylitis
Fracture
Gout
Osgood–Schlatter disease
Osteoarthritis
Osteochondroma

Osteogenesis imperfecta
Osteomalacia
Osteomyelitis
Osteopetrosis (see Fig. 7–38)
Osteoporosis
Paget's disease (see Fig. 7–39)
Rickets
Slipped femoral capital epiphysis
   (see Fig. 7–40)
Subluxation
Talipes
Tendinitis
Thalassemia
   (see Fig. 7–41)

Summary of Common Fracture Types

- **Simple: an undisplaced fx**
- **Compound: fractured end of bone has penetrated skin (open fx)**
- **Incomplete: fx does not traverse entire bone; little or no displacement**
- **Greenstick: break of cortex on one side of bone only; found in infants and children**

(continued, p. 125)

Some Conditions Requiring Adjustment in Exposure

Decrease In Exposure Factors	*Increase* In Exposure Factors
Arthritis	Acromegaly
Ewing's sarcoma	Chronic gout
Osteomalacia	Multiple myeloma
Osteoporosis	Osteochondroma
Rickets	Osteopetrosis
Thalassemia	Paget's disease (osteitis deformans)

Figure 7–38. Radiographic appearance of osteopetrosis (marble-bone disease). Osteopetrosis is a rare bone dysplasia characterized by bone that is dense throughout, lacking the softer medullary spongiosa. (From the American College of Radiology Learning File. Courtesy of the ACR).

Figure 7–39. Lateral projection of skull demonstrates Paget's disease. Early lytic changes are seen throughout the skull; observe the beginning of typical "cotton wool" appearance in the frontal region. (From the American College of Radiology Learning File. Courtesy of the ACR.)

Figure 7–40. AP pelvis demonstrating left slipped femoral capital epiphysis. The growth plate is displaced. The femoral head remains within the acetabulum and the femoral neck moves anteriorly. *Note* correct placement of gonadal shield. (Reproduced with permission from Way LW, ed. *Current Surgical Diagnosis & Treatment,* 10th ed. East Norwalk, CT: Appleton & Lange, 1994.)

Figure 7–41. Effect of thalassemia on bone density and example of pathologic fracture. Thalassemia is a congenital and hereditary disorder found in Mediterranean countries and descendants of their peoples. It is demonstrated radiographically by diminished bone density that often results in pathologic fractures as seen here in the distal tibia and fibula. (From the American College of Radiology Learning File. Courtesy of the ACR.)

Figure 7–42. Torus/buckle-type greenstick fracture. (From Simon, RS, Koenigsknecht, SJ. *Emergency Orthopedics: The Extremities*, 3rd ed. East Norwalk, CT: Appleton & Lange, 1995, Figure X-ray 32–X5, p 511.)

- **Torus/buckle (see Fig. 7–42): greenstick fx with one cortex buckled/compacted and the other intact**
- **Stress/Fatigue: response to repeated strong, powerful force (eg, jogging, marching)**
- **Avulsion: small bony fragment pulled from bony prominence as a result of forceful pull of the attached ligament or tendon (chip fracture)**
- **Hairline: faint undisplaced fx**
- **Comminuted: one fracture composed of several fragments**
- **Butterfly: comminuted fx with one or more wedge or butterfly-wing–shaped pieces**
- **Spiral: long fx encircling a shaft; result of torsion (twisting force); especially lower leg: distal tibia and proximal fibula**
- **Oblique: longitudinal fx forming an angle (about 45°) with the long axis of the shaft**
- **Transverse: fx occurring at right angles to long axis of bone**
- **Boxer's: fx just proximal to head of fifth metacarpal**
- **Monteggia: fx proximal third of ulnar shaft with anterior dislocation of radial head**
- **Colles' (see Fig. 7–43): transverse fracture of distal third of radius with posterior angulation and associated avulsion fx of ulnar styloid process**
- **Trimalleolar: fx lateral malleolus, fx medial malleolus on medial and posterior surfaces**
- **Jones': fx base of fifth metatarsal**
- **Potts: fx distal tibia and fibula with dislocation of ankle joint**
- **Pathologic: fx of bone weakened by pathologic condition, eg, metastatic bone disease**

Figure 7–43. Severely comminuted Colles' fracture. (Way, LW, ed. *Current Surgical Diagnosis & Treatment,* 10th ed. East Norwalk, CT: Appleton & Lange, 1994, Figure 43–30, p 1038.)

Chapter Review Questions

★ *Congratulations! You have completed a large portion of this chapter. You may go on to the "Registry-type" multiple-choice questions that follow. For greatest success, be sure to also complete the short answer questions found at the end of this chapter.*

1. A Colles' fracture involves the following:
   1. transverse fracture of the distal radius
   2. chip fracture of the ulnar styloid process
   3. posterior/backward displacement
   (A) 1 only
   (B) 1 and 2 only
   (C) 1 and 3 only
   (D) 1, 2, and 3

2. Which of the following projections will best demonstrate the carpal navicular?
   (A) lateral wrist
   (B) ulnar flexion
   (C) radial flexion
   (D) carpal tunnel

3. Which of the following projections requires that the humeral epicondyles be super-imposed?
   1. lateral elbow
   2. lateral forearm
   3. lateral humerus
   (A) 1 only
   (B) 1 and 2 only
   (C) 1 and 3 only
   (D) 1, 2, and 3

4. An axial projection of the clavicle is often helpful in demonstrating a fracture not visualized using a perpendicular central ray. When examining the clavicle in the PA position, how is the central ray directed for the axial projection?
   (A) cephalad
   (B) caudad
   (C) medially
   (D) laterally

5. Which of the following should not be performed until a transverse fracture of the patella has been ruled out?
   1. AP knee
   2. lateral knee
   3. axial/tangential patella
   (A) 1 only
   (B) 1 and 2 only
   (C) 2 and 3 only
   (D) 1, 2, and 3

6. The cuboid, sinus tarsi, and tuberosity of the fifth metatarsal are best demonstrated in which of the following?
   (A) lateral foot
   (B) lateral oblique foot
   (C) medial oblique foot
   (D) weight-bearing foot

7. In which of the following positions or projections will the subtalar joint be visualized?
   (A) dorsoplantar projection of the foot
   (B) plantodorsal projection of the os calsis
   (C) medial oblique position of the foot
   (D) lateral projection of the foot

8. The proximal tibiofibular articulation is best demonstrated in which of the following positions?
   (A) medial oblique
   (B) lateral oblique
   (C) AP
   (D) lateral

9. In the medial oblique projection of the ankle, the:
   1. talofibular joint is visualized
   2. talotibial joint is visualized
   3. plantar surface should be vertical
   (A) 1 only
   (B) 1 and 3 only
   (C) 2 and 3 only
   (D) 1, 2, and 3

10. The scapular Y projection of the shoulder demonstrates:
   1. an oblique projection of the shoulder
   2. anterior or posterior dislocation
   3. a lateral projection of the shoulder
   (A) 1 only
   (B) 1 and 2 only
   (C) 1 and 3 only
   (D) 1, 2, and 3

Answers and Explanations

1. (D) A Colles' fracture is usually caused by a fall onto an outstretched (extended) hand, in order to "brake" a fall. The wrist then suffers an impacted transverse fracture of the distal inch of the radius with accompanied chip fracture of the ulnar styloid process. Because of the hand position at the time of the fall, the fracture is usually displaced backward approximately 30°.

2. (B) The carpal navicular/scaphoid is somewhat curved, and consequently, is foreshortened radiographically in the PA projection. To better separate it from the adjacent carpals, the ulnar flexion maneuver is frequently employed. Radial flexion is used to better demonstrate the medial carpals. The navicular is superimposed on adjacent carpals in the lateral projection. The carpal tunnel/canal does not demonstrate the carpal navicular.

3. (D) The lateral elbow and lateral forearm must be flexed 90° to superimpose the distal radius and ulna and humeral epicondyles. The lateral humerus can also be performed with the elbow flexed 90°, but if the patient is unable to flex the arm, it may be left AP and a transthoracic lateral projection of the upper one-half to two-thirds of the humerus may be obtained. Since a coronal plane passing through the epicondyles is perpendicular to the film in this position, the epicondyles are superimposed.

4. (B) With the patient PA, the central ray is directed caudally. This serves to project the pulmonary apices away from the clavicle. The reverse is true when examining the clavicle in the AP position.

5. (C) If a transverse fracture of the patella is present and the knee is *flexed,* there is danger of *separation* of the fractured segments. Since both a lateral knee and axial patella require knee flexion, they should be avoided until a transverse fracture is ruled out. When present, a transverse fracture may be seen through the femur on the AP projection. The axial ("sunrise") projection of the patella is generally used for demonstration of vertical patellar fractures.

6. (C) To best demonstrate *most* of the tarsals and intertarsal spaces, including the cuboid, sinus tarsi, and tuberosity of the fifth metatarsal, a medial oblique is required (plantar surface and film form 30° angle). The lateral oblique demonstrates the navicular and first and second cuneiforms. Weight-bearing lateral feet are used to demonstrate the longitudinal arches.

7. (B) The subtalar, or talocalcaneal, joint is a three-faceted articulation formed by the talus and os calsis (calcaneus). The plantodorsal and dorsoplantar projections of the os calsis should exhibit density sufficient to visualize the subtalar joint. If evaluation of the subtalar joint is desired, special views (such as Broden and Isherwood methods) would be required.

8. (A) With the femoral condyles of the affected side rotated *medially/internally* to form a 45° angle with the film, the *proximal* tibiofibular articulation is placed parallel with the film and the fibula is free of superimposition with the tibia. The lateral oblique completely superimposes the tibia and fibula. The AP and lateral projections superimpose enough of the tibia and fibula so that the tibiofibular articulation is "closed."

9. (D) The medial oblique projection (15 to 20° mortise view) of the ankle is valuable because it demonstrates the tibiofibular joint as well as the talotibial joint, thereby visualizing all the major articulating surfaces of the ankle joint. To demonstrate maximum joint volume, it is recommended that the plantar surface be vertical.

10. (B) The scapular Y projection requires that the coronal plane be about 60° to the film, thus resulting in an oblique projection of the shoulder. The vertebral and axillary borders of the scapula are superimposed on the humeral shaft and the resulting relationship between the glenoid fossa and humeral head will demonstrate anterior or posterior dislocation. Lateral or medial dislocation is evaluated on the AP projection.

II. THE AXIAL SKELETON (FIG. 7–44)

KEY TERMS ◀

AMPHIARTHROTIC	HEEL EFFECT	LORDOTIC
BIFID	HYPEREXTENSION	MIDAXILLARY LINE
COMPENSATING FILTRATION	HYPERFLEXION	SCOLIOSIS
DIARTHROTIC	HYPERTROPHY	SYNARTHROTIC
FORAMEN	KYPHOTIC	

A. VERTEBRAL COLUMN

The vertebral column (Fig. 7–45) is composed of 33 bones divided into cervical, thoracic, lumbar, sacral, and coccygeal regions, with each region having its own characteristic shape. *Intervertebral disks* between the vertebral bodies form **amphiarthrotic** joints. The cer- ◀ vical and lumbar regions form **lordotic** curves; the thoracic and ◀ sacral regions form **kyphotic** curves (Fig. 7–45, lateral). An exagger- ◀ ated thoracic curve is called *kyphosis* ("hunchback"); an exaggerated lumbar curve is *lordosis* ("swayback"). Lateral curvature of the vertebral column is called **scoliosis.** ◀

The typical vertebra has a *body* and a *neural arch* surrounding the vertebral **foramen.** The neural arch is composed of two *pedicles,* ◀ one on each side supporting a *lamina.* The laminae extend posteriorly to the midline and join to form the *spinous process* (lack of union, or malunion, results in *spina bifida*). Each pedicle has notches superiorly and inferiorly *(superior* and *inferior vertebral notches)* that form the *intervertebral foramina,* through which the spinal nerves pass. The neural arch also has lateral *transverse processes* for muscle attachment and *superior* and *inferior articular processes* for the formation of *apophyseal joints.* The vertebral column permits flexion, extension, lateral, and rotary motions through its various articulations.

1. Cervical Spine. There are seven cervical vertebrae (Fig. 7–46). The *atlas* (C1) is a ring-shaped bone having no body and no spinous process; it is composed of an anterior and posterior arch, lateral masses, and transverse processes. Its superior articular processes articulate superiorly with the skull at the *atlantooccipital joint,* where flexion and extension motion occurs. The atlas articulates inferiorly with the *axis* (C2). The axis has a superior projection, the *dens,* or *odontoid process.* The axis articulates superiorly with the atlas at the *atlantoaxial joint,* a *pivot* joint where rotation takes place, and inferiorly with C3 at the apophyseal articulation. The typical cervical vertebra is small and has a *transverse foramen* in each transverse process for passage of the vertebral artery. Cervical spinous

---

Neural Arch

Composed of:
Two pedicles
Two laminae
Encloses:
Vertebral foramen
Supports 7 processes:
Two superior articular processes
Two inferior articular processes
Two transverse processes
One spinous process

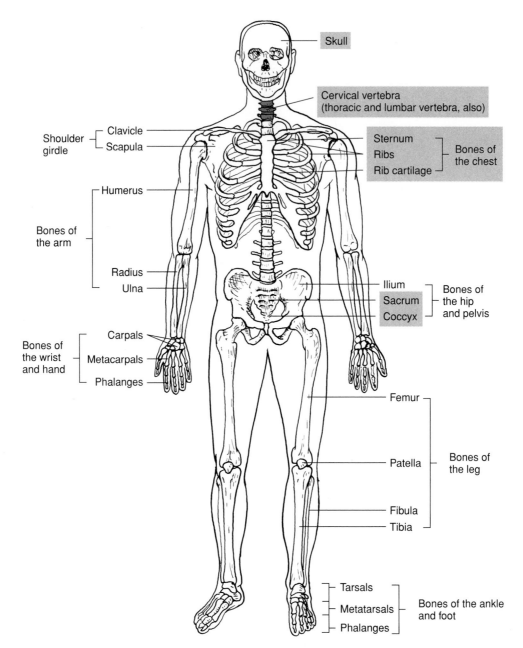

Figure 7–44. The axial skeleton. (Modified with permission from Rice, J. *Medical Terminology with Human Anatomy,* 3rd ed. East Norwalk, CT: Appleton & Lange, 1995.)

▶ processes angle downward and are usually **bifid.** The spinous process of C7 *(vertebra prominens)* is not bifid, is larger, horizontal, and is a useful positioning landmark. Fractures and/or dislocations of
▶ the cervical spine are usually due to acute **hyperflexion** or **hyper-**
▶ **extension** as a result of indirect trauma. Neurologic damage can occur on manipulation, hence the importance of immobilization. *Whiplash* injury is caused by a sudden, forced movement in one direction and then the opposite direction (as in rear-end automobile impacts). Whiplash symptoms frequently include neck pain and stiffness, headache, and pain and numbness of the upper extremities.

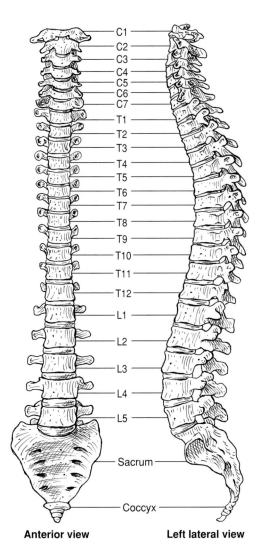

C1
C2
C3
C4
C5
C6
C7
T1
T2
T3
T4
T5
T6
T7
T8
T9
T10
T11
T12
L1
L2
L3
L4
L5
Sacrum
Coccyx

Anterior view   **Left lateral view**

Figure 7–45. AP and lateral views of the vertebral column.

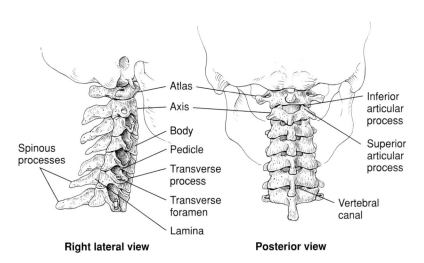

Atlas
Axis
Body
Pedicle
Transverse process
Transverse foramen
Lamina

Spinous processes

Inferior articular process
Superior articular process
Vertebral canal

Right lateral view   **Posterior view**

Figure 7–46. Right lateral and posterior views of the cervical spine.

Articulation Summary: Vertebral

- Occipitoatlantal
- Atlantoaxial
- Costovertebral
- Costotransverse
- Lumbosacral
- Sacroiliac
- Sacrococcygeal
- Intervertebral
- Apophyseal/interarticular

Whiplash is often evidenced radiographically by straightening or reversal of the normal lordotic curve. Osteoarthritis is characterized in the cervical and lumbar spine by chronic, progressive degeneration of cartilage and **hypertrophy** of bone along the articular margins, characterized radiographically by narrowed joint spaces, and *osteophytes*. It is also seen in the articulations of the fingers, toes, hips, and knees.

CERVICAL SPINE	POSITION OF PART	CENTRAL RAY DIRECTED	STRUCTURES INCLUDED/ BEST SEEN
AP	Patient supine, MSP ⊥ table; adjust flexion so mastoid tip and occlusal plane are aligned	15 to 20° cephalad to thyroid cartilage	AP of *lower five* cervical vertebrae and intervertebral disk spaces
AP *Atlas and Axis*	Patient supine, MSP ⊥ table, w/patient's mouth open, adjust flexion so mastoid tips and occlusal plane are aligned	⊥ center of opened mouth	AP proj of C1 and C2 (atlas and axis) and their articulations. *Too much flexion* superimposes teeth on odontoid; *too much extension* superimposes base of skull on odontoid
LAT	Patient erect w/L side adjacent to cassette, chin slightly elevated, shoulders depressed, MSP ∥ cassette centered, at level of C4	⊥ C4	Lat proj of all 7 vertebrae. Shows intervertebral jt spaces, apophyseal jts, spinous processes, bodies; due to the unavoidable OID, a 72″ SID should be used

Note: Flexion and extension views may be obtained in this position in cases of *whiplash* injury (Fig. 7–47). This proj is often performed recumbent w/a horizontal beam as the first radiograph in cases of suspected *subluxation*.

OBL *(LAO and RAO)*	Patient PA erect, MSP 45° to cassette centered to C5 (1″ inferior to thyroid cartilage), chin slightly raised	15 to 20° caudad to center of cassette	Oblique cervical spine; best view of intervertebral foramina *closest* to cassette; a similar view can be obtained w/the patient *LPO* and *RPO,* CR ∠ed cephalad, and showing the foramina *farthest* from the film (see Fig. 7–48)

Note: Oblique cervical spine may be performed in the *recumbent position* on patients whose trauma prohibits moving them. The CR is directed 45° medially for one oblique and 45° laterally for the other.

(continued)

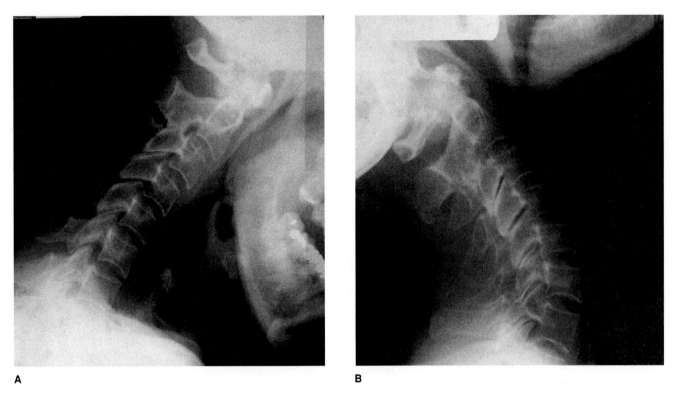

A   B

Figure 7–47. Flexion **(A)** and extension **(B)** lateral views are often performed in whiplash injuries to demonstrate degree of anterior/posterior motion. (Courtesy of The Stamford Hospital.)

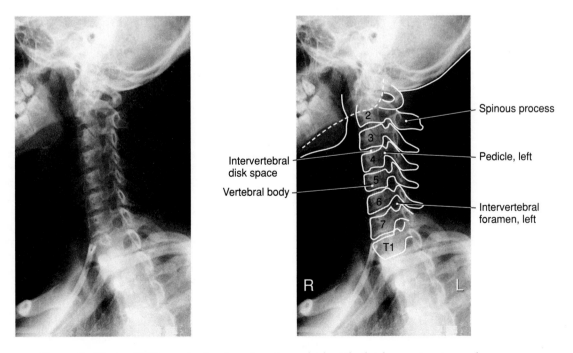

Figure 7–48. An RPO cervical spine. Locate and identify the bony structures shown particularly well in the oblique. (From Cornuelle et al. *Radiographic Anatomy and Positioning.* Stamford, CT: Appleton & Lange, 1998.)

CERVICAL SPINE (con't)	POSITION OF PART	CENTRAL RAY DIRECTED	STRUCTURES INCLUDED/ BEST SEEN
LAT *cervico-* ▶ *thoracic ("swimmer's position")*	Patient erect (or recumbent) lat w/**midaxillary line** centered to grid, MSP ‖, adjacent arm over head, depress shoulder farthest from grid	⊥ T2	Lateral proj of lower cervical and upper thoracic vertebrae; particularly useful for lower cervical and upper thoracic vertebrae of broad-shouldered individuals

Routine: AP, open mouth, lat, both obl on (5) 8 × 10

2. Thoracic Spine.

There are 12 thoracic vertebrae, which are larger in size than cervical vertebrae and which increase in size as they progress inferiorly toward the lumbar region. Thoracic spinous processes are fairly long and are sharply angled caudally. The bodies ▶ and transverse processes have *articular facets* for the **diarthrotic** rib articulations. A common metabolic bone disorder frequently noted in radiographic examinations of the thoracic spine is osteoporosis. **Osteoporosis** is characterized by bone demineralization and can result in compression fractures of the vertebrae. The condition is most common in sedentary and postmenopausal women.

THORACIC SPINE	POSITION OF PART	CENTRAL RAY DIRECTED	STRUCTURES INCLUDED/ BEST SEEN
AP ▶ ▶	Patient supine, MSP ⊥ tabletop, top of cassette 1″ above shoulders	⊥ T7	AP proj of thoracic vertebrae and intervertebral spaces; it is helpful to use the **heel effect** and/or **compensating filtration** to provide more uniform density
Note: To demonstrate *apophyseal joints, 70° obliques* are performed.			
LAT	Patient L lat recumbent, midaxillary line centered to table, arms ⊥ long axis of body, top of cassette 1″ above shoulders	5 to 15° cephalad (⊥ long axis of spine)	Lateral proj of thoracic vertebrae, especially bodies, intervertebral spaces and foramina; a vertical beam may be used if the patient's MSP is adjusted to ‖ the tabletop

Routine: AP and lat on (2) 14 × 17; some institutions include a "swimmer's" position routinely in order to better demonstrate the upper thoracic vertebrae in lateral projection.

3. Lumbar Spine.

The five lumbar vertebrae are the largest of the vertebral column and increase in size toward the sacral region. The spinous processes are short, horizontal and serve as attachment for

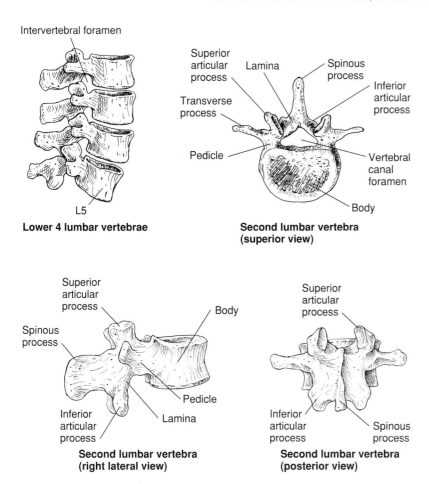

Figure 7–49. Lateral view of the lower lumbar vertebrae. Superior, right lateral, and posterior views of L2.

strong muscles (see Fig. 7–49). The causes of lumbar pain are numerous. Trauma, fracture, spasm of the paralumbar muscles, herniated intervertebral disk, and osteoarthritis are a few causes of low back pain. Disorders that may be detected radiographically include **osteoarthritis, spondylolysis, spondylolisthesis,** and **ankylosing spondylitis.** Myelography and MRI are used to evaluate **herniated intervertebral disks.**

LUMBAR SPINE	POSITION OF PART	CENTRAL RAY DIRECTED	STRUCTURES INCLUDED/ BEST SEEN
AP	Patient supine, MSP ⊥ tabletop, knees flexed	⊥ to L3	AP proj of lumbar vertebrae, intervertebral spaces (except L5–S1), transverse processes; *flexion of the knees reduces lumbar curve and OID (see Fig. 7–50)*

Figure 7–50. AP projection of the lumbar spine. Flexion of the knees reduces lumbar curve and OID; relieves strain on lower back muscles; patients are most comfortable with sponge or pillow support placed under knees. (From Cornuelle et al. *Radiographic Anatomy and Positioning.* Stamford, CT: Appleton & Lange, 1998.)

Figure 7–51. Lateral projection of the lumbar spine. If MSP is adjusted parallel to tabletop CR angulation is unnecessary. (From Cornuelle et al. *Radiographic Anatomy and Positioning.* Stamford, CT: Appleton & Lange, 1998.)

LUMBAR SPINE *(con't)*	POSITION OF PART	CENTRAL RAY DIRECTED	STRUCTURES INCLUDED/ BEST SEEN
AP (L5–S1)	Patient supine, MSP ⊥ tabletop, legs extended	To MSP at 30 to 35° cephalad to a point midway b/w ASIS and pubic symph	AP of lumbosacral articulation not seen on AP lumbar; the CR parallels the angle formed by L5–S1, thus "opening" it
OBL *(RPO and LPO)*	Patient AP recumbent, obliqued 45° w/spine centered to grid	⊥ L3	Obl proj of lumbar vertebrae, especially for apophyseal articulations (L1–L4) of side *adjacent* to table; opposite obl is done to show opposite articulations. L5–S1 apophyseal articulations shown in 35° obl (see Fig. 7–52 A and B).

Note: *This proj demonstrates the characteristic "scotty dogs"* (see Fig. 7–52 A and B). Obl lumbar spine may also be performed in the PA position and demonstrates the apophyseal articulations *away* from the film.

LAT	Patient L lateral recumbent, midaxillary line centered to grid	5 to 8° caudad L3	Lat proj of lumbar vertebrae, especially for vertebral bodies, interspaces, intervertebral foramina, spinous processes; if MSP adjusted ‖ tabletop, CR is vertical (see Fig. 7–51)
LAT (L5–S1)	Patient L lat recumbent, centerplane 1-1/2″ posterior to midaxillary line to grid, adjust MSP ‖ tabletop	⊥ coronal plane at level midway b/w crest and ASIS	Lat proj L5–S1; if MSP not adjusted ‖ tabletop CR is ∠ed 5 to 8° caudad

Routine: AP, lat, coned L5–S1 on (2) 11 × 14 and (1) 8 × 10; additional projections as required

4. Sacrum. There are five fused sacral vertebrae (Fig. 7–53); the fused *transverse processes* form the *alae.* The anterior and posterior *sacral foramina* transmit spinal nerves. The *sacrum* articulates superiorly with the fifth lumbar vertebra, forming the L5–S1 articulation and inferiorly with the *coccyx* to form the *sacrococcygeal joint.*

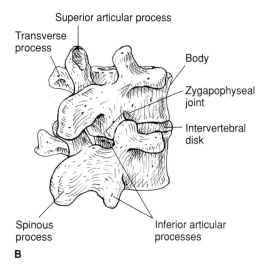

Figure 7–52. **(A)** Oblique lumbar spine, illustrating the lumbar apophyseal joints. Note "scotty dog" images. The scotty's "ear" corresponds to the *superior articular process,* his "nose" to the *transverse process,* his "eye" is the *pedicle,* his "neck" the *pars interarticularis,* his "body" is the *lamina,* and his "front foot" is the *inferior articular process.* (Courtesy of The Stamford Hospital.) **(B)** Forty-five degree posterolateral view of lumbar vertebrae. Note structures that form the classic "scotty dog." (From Cornuelle et al. *Radiographic Anatomy and Positioning.* Stamford, CT: Appleton & Lange, 1998.)

SACRUM	POSITION OF PART	CENTRAL RAY DIRECTED	STRUCTURES INCLUDED/ BEST SEEN
AP	Patient AP supine, MSP ⊥ tabletop	15° cephalad to midline, to point midway b/w pubic symphysis and ASIS	AP proj of sacrum; CR ∠ parallels sacral curve and provides less distorted visualization
LAT	Patient L lat recumbent, coronal plane 3″ posterior to midaxillary line centered to grid	⊥ specified coronal plane at level of ASIS	Lat proj of sacrum (see Fig. 7–54)

Routine: AP and lat on (2) 10 × 12

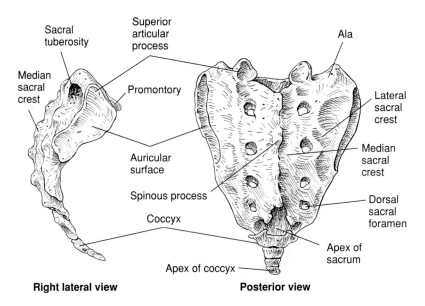

Right lateral view   **Posterior view**

Figure 7–53. Sacrum and coccyx. (Reproduced with permission from Chusid, JG. *Correlative Neuroanatomy & Functional Neurology,* 19th ed. East Norwalk, CT: Appleton & Lange, 1985.)

Figure 7–54. Lateral projection of the sacrum and coccyx. A little more of the L5–S1 articulation should have been included; otherwise, both structures are well visualized on the single radiograph. (Courtesy of The Stamford Hospital.)

5. Coccyx. There are four or five fused coccygeal vertebrae (Fig. 7–53). Fracture of the coccyx usually results from a fall onto it, landing in a seated position. Fracture displacement is fairly common and occasionally requires removal of the fractured fragment to relieve the painful symptoms.

COCCYX	POSITION OF PART	CENTRAL RAY DIRECTED	STRUCTURES INCLUDED/ BEST SEEN
AP	Patient AP supine, MSP ⊥ tabletop	10° caudad to midline to point 2″ above pubic symphysis	AP proj of coccyx; CR ∠ parallels coccygeal curve and provides less distorted visualization
Lat	Patient L lat recumbent, coronal plane 5″ posterior to midaxillary line centered to grid	⊥ specified coronal plane at level of mid coccyx	Lat proj of coccyx and its articulation with the sacrum; (see Fig. 7–54)

Routine: AP and lat on (2) 8 × 10

6. Scoliosis Series

SCOLIOSIS SERIES	POSITION OF PART	CENTRAL RAY DIRECTED	STRUCTURES INCLUDED/ BEST SEEN
	14″ × 17″ film of vertebrae to include 1 in of iliac crest/L5–S1	⊥ center of cassette	4 exposures made in this way: PA recumbent, PA erect, PA/bending L and R; *radiation dose is reduced when breast and thyroid shields are used and when examination is performed PA rather than AP*

Routine: (4) 14 × 17

B. THORAX

1. Sternum and Sternoclavicular Joints. The bones of the *thorax* (sternum, ribs, thoracic vertebrae; Fig. 7–55) function to protect the vital organs within (heart, lungs, major blood vessels). The *sternum* forms the anterior central portion of the thorax and is composed of three major divisions: the *manubrium, body,* and *xiphoid process.* Sternal **fractures** are uncommon, and when they do occur fracture displacement is rare, but the possibility of traumatic injury to the heart must still be considered.

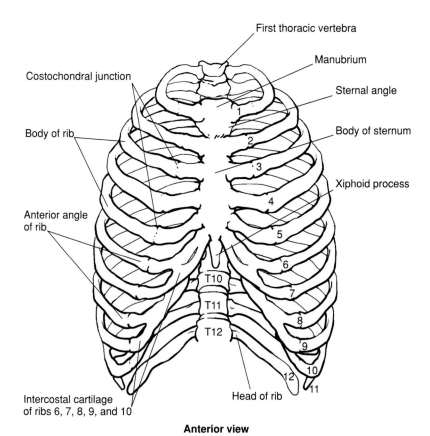

Anterior view

Articulation Summary: Thorax

- Sternoclavicular
- Sternochondral
- Costochondral
- Costovertebral
- Costotransverse

Figure 7–55. The thoracic cage: anterior, posterior, and lateral views.

2. Ribs. The *rib* cage (Fig. 7–55) consists of 12 pair of ribs. Ribs 1 to 7 articulate with thoracic vertebrae and the sternum, and are called "true ribs." Ribs 8 to 10 articulate with thoracic vertebrae and the superjacent costal cartilage to form the anterior costal margin, and are called *"false ribs."* The last two pairs of false ribs articulate only with thoracic vertebrae and are referred to as *"floating ribs."* **Rib fractures** are a common injury in thoracic trauma because of their relative thinness and exposed position. Their fracture may be complicated by **pneumothorax, hemothorax,** liver laceration (right lower ribs), or spleen laceration (left lower ribs).

STERNUM	POSITION OF PART	CENTRAL RAY DIRECTED	STRUCTURES INCLUDED/ BEST SEEN
PA OBL (RAO)	Patient 15 to 20° RAO; greater obliquity for thin patients, sternum centered to midline of table	⊥ mid-sternum	Obl-frontal proj of sternum, obliquity removes sternum from superimposition on vertebrae; *R obl proj sternum into heart shadow for uniform density;* long exposure can be made during quiet breathing to blur pulmonary vascular markings
LAT	Patient erect L lat, shoulders rolled back, MSP vertical, cassette 1-1/2″ above manubrial notch	⊥ mid-sternum	Lat proj of sternum free of superimposition of ribs; exposure made on deep inspiration to move sternum away from ribs

Routine: RAO and L Lat on (2) 10 × 12

STERNO-CLAVICULAR JOINTS	POSITION OF PART	CENTRAL RAY DIRECTED	STRUCTURES INCLUDED/ BEST SEEN
PA	Patient prone, MSP centered to grid, cassette centered at T3 (suprasternal notch)	⊥ T3	Bilateral PA proj of sternoclavicular jts visualized through superimposed vertebrae and ribs; for a unilateral examination, turn patient's head toward *affected* side to better "open" that jt—both sides done for comparison

Routine: (1) 8 × 10

Radiographically Significant Skeletal Disorders and Conditions of the Axial Skeleton

Achondroplasia
Ankylosing spondylitis
Cervical rib
Degenerative disk disease
Herniated disk
Hydrocephalus
Kyphosis
Lordosis
Osteophyte
Osteoporosis
Pectus excavatum
Scoliosis
Spina bifida
Spondylolisthesis
Spondylolysis
Transitional vertebra
Whiplash

PA OBL *(LAO and RAO)*	Patient prone, MSP centered to grid, rotate body ≈15° *affected side down*	⊥ affected joint	obl proj of sterno-clavicular jt closest to film; similar results can be obtained w/a ⊥ MSP and w/CR 15° toward midline from the affected side

Routine: (2) 8 × 10

RIBS	POSITION OF PART	CENTRAL RAY DIRECTED	STRUCTURES INCLUDED/ BEST SEEN
AP	Patient supine or AP recumbent, MSP ⊥ midline of table, top of cassette 1″ above shoulder	⊥ center of cassette, about level of T7	AP proj, upper posterior or ribs best delineated; do PA for better detail of anterior ribs
PA OBL *(LAO, RAO)*	Patient prone or erect PA, rotate 45°, *affected side down*	⊥ center of cassette, about level of T7 (at T10 to T12 for below diaphragm)	Right obl shows right ribs and their *axillary* portions, L obl shows left ribs and their axillary portions, especially useful for *posterior ribs* (because of less OID)
AP OBL *(LPO, RPO)*	Patient supine or erect AP, rotate to 45° affected side away from film	⊥ center of cassette, about level of T7 (at T10 to T12 for below diaphragm)	Right obl shows *left* ribs and their axillary portions, L obl shows *right* ribs and their axillary portions; sometimes preferred for *anterior ribs*

Note: *Above-diaphragm* ribs are exposed on deep *inspiration* or during quiet breathing (long exposure). *Below-diaphragm* ribs are exposed on forced *expiration*.

Routine: AP or PA, obl above and below diaphragm of affected side on (2) 14 × 17 and (1) 10 × 12. A PA and L lat chest are often performed to r/o perforated lung and/or air/fluid levels.

C. HEAD AND NECK

1. Skull. The *skull* (Figs. 7–56 to 7–58) has 2 major parts: the *cranium*, which is composed of eight bones and houses the brain; and the 14 irregularly shaped *facial bones*. The eight cranial bones are the paired *parietal* and *temporal* bones and the unpaired *frontal, occipital, ethmoid* and *sphenoid* bones. The 14 facial bones include the paired *nasal, lacrimal, palatine, inferior nasal conchae, maxillae,* and *zygomatic* bones and the unpaired *vomer* and *mandible.*

The average shaped skull is termed *mesocephalic* (petrous pyramids and MSP form ≈47°), the broad skull is termed *brachycephalic* (petrous pyramids and MSP form ≈54°), and the elongated

---

Cranial Bones (8)

(1) Frontal
(2) Parietal
(2) Temporal
(1) Occipital
(1) Ethmoid
(1) Sphenoid

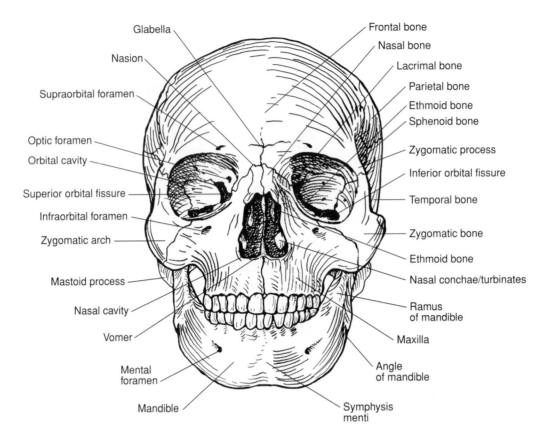

Figure 7–56. Anterior view of the skull, labeled.

skull is termed *dolichocephalic* (petrous pyramids and MSP form ≈40°). These deviations are readily observable in axial CT and MR images. The inner and outer compact tables of the skull are separated by cancellous tissue called *diploë*. The internal table has a number of branching *meningeal grooves* and larger *sulci* that house blood vessels.

▶   The bones of the skull are separated by immovable **(synar-throtic)** joints called *sutures*. The major sutures of the cranium are the *sagittal,* which separates the parietal bones; the *coronal,* which separates the frontal and parietal bones; the *lambdoidal,* which separates the parietal and occipital bones; and the *squammosal,* which separates the temporal and parietal bones (Figs. 7–56 and 7–58). The articular surfaces of these bones have serrated-like edges with small projecting bones called *wormian* bones that fit together to form the articular sutures. The sagittal and coronal sutures meet at the *bregma,* which corresponds to the fetal anterior fontanel. The sagittal and lambdoidal sutures meet posteriorly at the *lambda,* which corresponds to the fetal posterior fontanel. The parietal, frontal, and sphenoid bones meet at the *pterion,* the location of the anterolateral fontanel. The highest point of the skull is called the *vertex.*

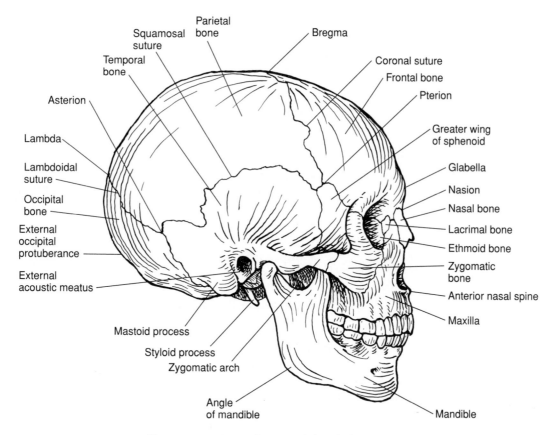

Figure 7–57. Lateral view of the skull, labeled.

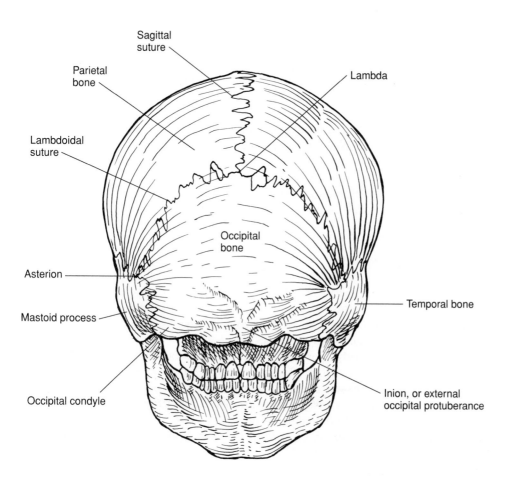

Figure 7–58. Posterior view of the skull.

a. Cranial Bones
Frontal Bone

- The frontal bone corresponds to the forehead region.
- **Orbital plates (2):** horizontal part of frontal bone; forms much of superior aspect of bony orbit.
- **Frontal eminences (2):** on anterior surface of frontal bone, lateral to MSP.
- **Glabella:** smooth prominence between eyebrows.
- **Frontal sinuses (2):** directly behind glabella, between the tables of the skull.
- **Superciliary arches/ridges (2):** ridge of bone under eyebrow region.
- **Supraorbital margins (2):** upper border/rim of bony orbit.
- **Supraorbital notches/foramina (2):** mid-portion of supraorbital margin; passage for artery and nerve to forehead.
- **Frontonasal suture:** where frontal bone articulates with nasal bones (corresponds exteriorly with *nasion*).

Parietal Bone

- Paired; form the vertex and part of lateral portions of cranium.
- Meet at midline to form sagittal suture; other borders help form coronal, squamosal, and lambdoidal sutures.
- **Parietal eminences:** rounded prominence on lateral surface of each parietal bone.

Ethmoid Bone (Figs. 7–57 and 7–60)

- Located between orbits; helps form parts of nasal and orbital walls.
- **Cribriform plate:** porous, passage for olfactory nerves; horizontal portion between orbital plates of frontal bone.
- **Crista galli:** extends superiorly from mid-portion of cribriform plate.
- **Perpendicular plate:** extends downward from crista galli to form major portion of nasal septum.
- **Superior and middle nasal turbinates/conchae:** cartilaginous; within nasal cavity, attached to perpendicular plate.
- **Ethmoidal labyrinths/lateral masses:** help form medial wall of orbit; ethmoidal sinuses within.

Sphenoid Bone (see Figs. 7–59 and 7–60)

- Wedge or bat-shaped bone located between frontal and occipital bones.
- Anchor for eight cranial bones.
- Forms small part of lateral cranial wall and part of skull base.
- Consists of: body, two lesser wings, two greater wings, two pterygoid processes and hamuli.
- **Body:** central portion; midline of skull base; anterior part joins ethmoid bone; contains the two sphenoid sinuses.
- **Lesser (minor) wings:** anterior portion, articulates with orbital plates; contain optic canals for passage of optic nerves and ophthalmic arteries.
- **Anterior clinoid processes:** formed by medial aspect of lesser wings.

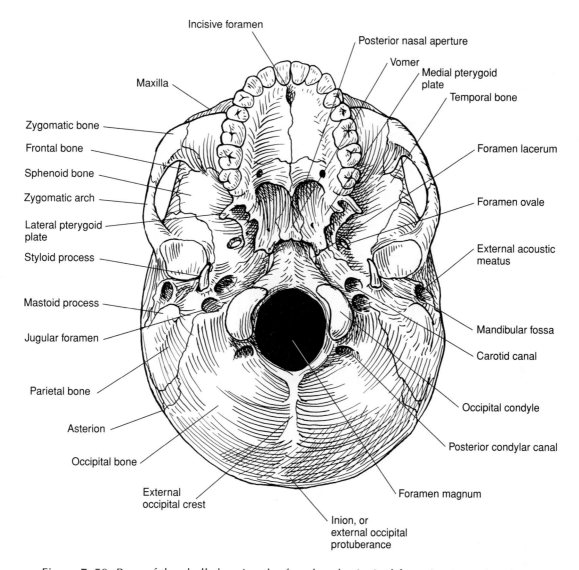

Figure 7–59. Base of the skull showing the fossal and principal foramina (superior view).

- **Tuberculum sellae:** ridge of bone between anterior clinoid processes; anterior boundary of sella turcica.
- **Optic (chiasmic) groove:** horizontal depression crossing body of bone in front of sella turcica; where optic nerves cross.
- **Optic foramen and canal:** passage for optic nerve and ophthalmic artery at the orbit's apex.
- **Sella turcica:** deep depression in sphenoid bone; houses pituitary gland.
- **Dorsum sellae:** posterior boundary/wall of sella turcica.
- **Posterior clinoid processes:** extend laterally from dorsum sellae.
- **Clivus:** basilar portion; slopes down and posteriorly from dorsum sellae; articulates with basilar portion of occipital bone.

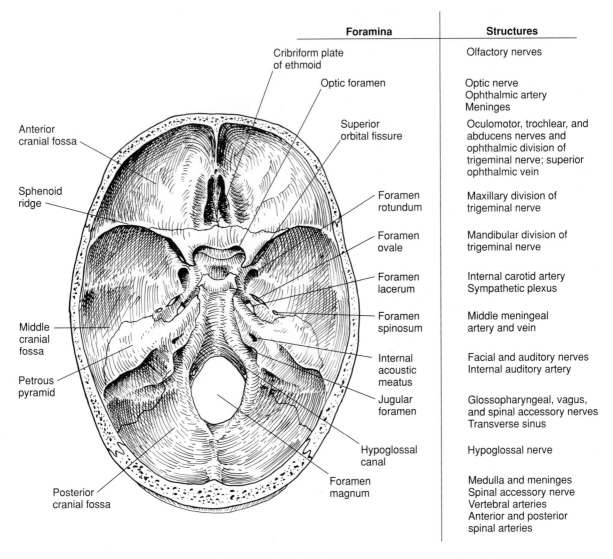

Foramina	Structures
Cribriform plate of ethmoid	Olfactory nerves
Optic foramen	Optic nerve Ophthalmic artery Meninges
Superior orbital fissure	Oculomotor, trochlear, and abducens nerves and ophthalmic division of trigeminal nerve; superior ophthalmic vein
Foramen rotundum	Maxillary division of trigeminal nerve
Foramen ovale	Mandibular division of trigeminal nerve
Foramen lacerum	Internal carotid artery Sympathetic plexus
Foramen spinosum	Middle meningeal artery and vein
Internal acoustic meatus	Facial and auditory nerves Internal auditory artery
Jugular foramen	Glossopharyngeal, vagus, and spinal accessory nerves Transverse sinus
Hypoglossal canal	Hypoglossal nerve
Foramen magnum	Medulla and meninges Spinal accessory nerve Vertebral arteries Anterior and posterior spinal arteries

Anterior cranial fossa

Sphenoid ridge

Middle cranial fossa

Petrous pyramid

Posterior cranial fossa

Figure 7–60. Basal view of the skull (external aspect, inferior view).

- **Superior orbital fissures:** large spaces between greater and lesser wings; for passage of four cranial nerves.
- **Greater (major) wings:** larger, posterior portion of sphenoid bone; contains the foramina rotundum, ovale, and spinosum for transmission of cranial nerves.
- **Pterygoid processes:** extend inferiorly from junction of body with great wing; each has a medial and lateral plate that articulates with posterior part of adjacent maxillae.
- **Inferior orbital fissures:** large openings, lie between the greater wings and the maxilla.

Occipital Bone

- Forms part of posterior wall and inferior part of cranium.
- Upper portion of each side articulates with parietal bones to form lambdoidal suture.

- **Basilar portion:** articulates anteriorly with basilar portion (clivus) of sphenoid bone.
- **Lateral portions (2):** bilateral to foramen magnum; **occipital condyles, hypoglossal canals,** and **jugular foramina** located here.
- **Foramen magnum:** large opening; transmits inferior portion of brain (medulla oblongata), which is continuous with spinal cord.
- **Squamosal portion:** posterior, superior portion; presents the **external occipital protuberance** (inion, occiput).

Temporal Bone (Figs. 7–57 and 7–59)

- Irregularly shaped bone forming lateral aspects of cranium.
- Located between greater wings of sphenoid bone and occipital bone.
- Dense, **petrous portions** form ridges and contain the organs of hearing.
- Contain internal auditory meati and carotid canals.
- **Zygomatic processes:** extend from flat, squamous portion; articulate with zygomatic (facial) bones.
- **Mandibular fossae:** articulate with mandibular condyles to form temporomandibular joints (TMJs).
- **Temporal styloid processes:** sharp, slender processes extending anteriorly and inferiorly to mastoid processes.
- **External auditory meatus (EAM):** external openings of the ear canal.
- **Mastoid processes:** inferior to EAM; contain numerous air cells; communicate with tympanic cavity (middle ear) at mastoid antrum

b. Facial Bones (Fig. 7–56)
Nasal Bone

- Small, rectangular.
- Form bridge of nose.
- Movable part of nose is composed of cartilage.
- Articulate with each other at midline to form **nasal suture.**
- **Frontonasal suture:** formed by articulation with frontal bone; corresponds to nasion externally.

Lacrimal Bones (Fig. 7–56)

- Smallest of facial bones.
- Form part of medial orbital wall.
- **Lacrimal groove:** accommodates lacrimal (tear) duct.

Zygomatic (Malar) Bones (Fig. 7–56)

- Inferior and lateral to outer canthus of eye; cheek bone.
- Have four **processes:** frontosphenoidal, orbital, temporal, and maxillary.

Maxillae (Figs. 7–56 and 7–57)

- Second largest of facial bones.
- Articulate with each other to form most of upper jaw (hard palate).

Types of Fractures

Linear fx
A skull fx, straight and sharply defined.

Depressed fx
A comminuted skull fx, with one or more portions pushed inward.

Hangman's fx
Fx of C2 with anterior subluxation of C2 on C3; result of forceful hyperextension.

Compression fx
Especially of spongy (cancellous) bone; diminished thickness or width as a result of compression-type force (eg, vertebral body).

Blowout fx
Fx of orbital floor as a result of a direct blow.

Facial Bones (14)

(2) Nasal
(2) Lacrimal (smallest)
(2) Palatine
(2) Inferior nasal conchae
(2) Zygomatic
(2) Maxillae
(1) Vomer
(1) Mandible (largest; only movable)

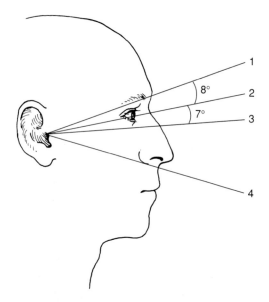

Figure 7–61. Four fundamental baselines are used in skull radiography: (1) the glabellomeatal (GML), (2) the orbitomeatal (OML, also known as canthomeatal or radiographic baseline), (3) the infraorbito-meatal (IOML), (4) the acanthiomeatal line. There is approximately a 7° difference between the OML and IOML and 8° between the OML and GML.

- **Palatine processes:** plates of bone that articulate at midline to form two-thirds of the hard palate.
- Form most of roof of mouth **(hard palate)** and floor of nasal cavity.
- Contain the **maxillary sinuses** (maxillary antra; antra of Highmore) just superior to bicuspid teeth; the thin floor of the maxillary sinus is formed by the alveolar process.
- **Alveolar ridge/process:** contains sockets for teeth; spongy ridge of bone.
- **Anterior nasal spine:** corresponds to *acanthion* externally.
- **Infraorbital foramen:** located below orbit, lateral to nasal cavity.

Palatine Bones (Fig. 7–61)

- Small bones; form posterior one-third of hard palate.
- L-shaped; have vertical and horizontal processes.
- **Horizontal parts:** articulate with palatine processes of maxillae to complete the hard palate.
- **Vertical parts:** project superiorly from horizontal part to articulate with the sphenoid bones.

Inferior Conchae (nasal turbinates; Fig. 7–56)

- Completely osseous.
- Placed inferiorly on each lateral wall of nasal cavity.

Vomer (Fig. 7–56)

- Inferior to perpendicular plate of ethmoid bone.
- Forms posterior bony septum.
- **Choanae:** posterior opening into nasopharynx; separated by posterior portion of vomer.

Mandible (Figs. 7–56 and 7–57)

- U-shaped bone; largest facial bone.
- Only movable facial bone.
- **Mandibular symphysis:** where two halves fuse after birth.
- **Mental tubercles:** prominences at inferolateral margin of symphysis.
- **Mental protuberance:** protuberance at lower portion of symphysis.
- **Alveolar process/ridge:** spongy ridge of bone with sockets for teeth.
- **Body:** horizontal position.
- **Ramus:** posterior vertical portion.
- **Angle:** junction of vertical and horizontal parts; corresponds to external landmark: *gonion*.
- **Condyloid process (capitulum/head):** extends posterior and superior from ramus.
- **TMJ:** articulation of head of condyle with mandibular fossa of temporal bone; only movable articulation in skull.
- **Coronoid process:** extends anterior and superior from ramus and has no articulation; serves as muscle attachment.
- **Mandibular notch:** deep notch between condyloid and coronoid processes.

- **Mental foramen:** small opening on outer surface of body, approximately below second premolar; passage for mandibular nerve.
- **Mandibular foramen:** opening on inner side of ramus for mandibular nerve.

SKULL (FIG. 7–62)	POSITION OF PART	CENTRAL RAY DIRECTED	STRUCTURES INCLUDED/ BEST SEEN
PA	Patient prone, MSP ⊥ mid-table, OMI (see Fig. 7–61) vertical (⊥ film)	⊥ nasion	PA proj of skull, *petrous pyramids should fill the orbits;* demonstrates frontal bone, lateral cranial walls, frontal sinuses, crista galli; see Fig. 7–62

The following variations of the basic true PA skull proj are used to demonstrate:

a) General survey cranium   CR ∠ed 15° caudad to nasion (ridges fill lower 1/3 orbits)

b) Superior orbital fissures   20 to 25° caudad to mid-orbits

c) Foramina rotundum   25 to 30° caudad to nasion (ridges below orbits)

d) Sella turcica   25° cephalad to a point 1-1/2″ above nasion (PA axial) *or* 10° cephalad to the glabella (PA proj)

Note: Similar projections of the same structures may be obtained in the AP position with the OML vertical if the CR is directed in the opposite direction. Anterior structures will be somewhat magnified and eye dose will be greater.

AP	Patient supine, MSP ⊥ mid-table, OML vertical (⊥ film)	⊥ nasion	AP proj of skull, *petrous pyramids should fill the orbits*
AP Axial *(Towne/ Grashey)*	Patient supine, MSP ⊥ mid-table, OML vertical, top of cassette 1-1/2″ below vertex	30° caudad to a point ≈ 1-1/2″ above glabella (or 37° to IOML)	AP axial of skull, especially for *occipital bone,* symmetrical proj of petrous pyramids, projects dorsum sella and posterior clinoid processes within the foramen magnum (see Fig. 7–63) (excessive tube ∠ or neck flexion will project posterior arch of C1 in foramen magnum)

Note: A collimated proj of the *sella turcica* can be obtained in this proj; an AP axial of the *zygomatic arches* can be obtained by directing the CR to the glabella and decreasing the technical factors. Similar results can be obtained in the prone position (PA axial, Haas method) with the CR ∠ed 25° cephalad to the OML. Particularly useful for hypersthenic or kyphotic patients although some magnification of the occipital bone must be expected.

Figure 7–62. PA skull radiograph; the correct amount of flexion places the petrous pyramids within the orbits.

Figure 7–63. AP axial (Grashey position) projection of the skull; demonstrates the dorsum sella and posterior clinoid processes within the foramen magnum; useful for demonstration of the occipital bone. (Courtesy of the Stamford Hospital.)

Figure 7–64. Submentovertical (SMV) skull. The success of this projection rests with positioning the CR ⊥ the IOML and cassette.

SKULL (con't)	POSITION OF PART	CENTRAL RAY DIRECTED	STRUCTURES INCLUDED/ BEST SEEN
LAT	Patient PA oblique w/skull MSP ‖ grid, interpupillary line vertical, IOML ‖ transverse axis of cassette	⊥ a point 2″ superior to EAM	Lateral proj of skull demonstrating superimposed cranial and facial structures; anterior and posterior clinoid processes and supraorbital margins should be superimposed
Basal Proj Submento-vertical (SMV)	Patient supine or seated AP, neck hyperextended to place IOML ‖ film and ⊥ CR, MSP ⊥ cassette	⊥ IOML and film, enters MSP at level of sella	Full basal proj of skull, useful for many foramina (spinosum, ovale, carotid canals), sphenoid and maxillary sinuses, odontoid process seen through foramen magnum, symmetrical proj of petrous pyramids w/ mandibular condyles projected anterior to petrosae and symphysis superimposed on frontal bone (see Fig. 7–64)

Note: A decrease in 10 kVp will demonstrate a bilateral axial projection of the zygomatic arches.

Vertico-submental (VSM)	Patient recumbent prone MSP ⊥ table, chin extended	Caudad and ⊥ IOML, pass through the sella	Similar to SMV with some magnification and distortion as a result of increased OID and direction of CR

Routine: AP axial, PA and/or PA general survey, both lat on (5) 10 × 12; supplemental views as required

2. Sella Turcica

LAT	Patient PA oblique w/skull MSP ‖ grid, interpupillary line vertical, IOML ‖ transverse axis of cassette	⊥ a point 3/4″ anterior and superior to EAM	Lat proj of sella turcica, sphenoid sinus, superimposed supraorbital margins
AP Axial	See AP axial skull		
PA and PA Axial	See PA skull variations		

Routine: both lat, PA on (3) 8 × 10

3. Orbits, Optic Foramen, Orbital Fissures

ORBIT

The orbital cavities are formed by seven bones (frontal, sphenoid, ethmoid, maxilla, palatine, zygoma/malar, and lacrimal). The orbital walls are fragile and the orbital floor is subject to traumatic **"blow-out" fractures.** Orbital floor fractures can be demonstrated using the *parietoacanthial (Waters)* projection; conventional tomography and CT may be indicated for further evaluation.

OPTIC FORAMEN	POSITION OF PART	CENTRAL RAY DIRECTED	STRUCTURES INCLUDED/ BEST SEEN
Parieto-orbital *(Rhese)*	Patient prone centered to table; skull resting on forehead, zygoma, chin w/MSP 53° to cassette and 37° to CR, acanthiomeatal line ⊥ cassette	⊥ through orbit adjacent to table	Parietoorbital proj of optic foramen (canal) in cross-section should be seen in lower outer quadrant of orbit: *longitudinal* displacement indicates incorrect baseline adjustment, *lateral* displacement indicates incorrect rotation

Note: This can be performed AP as the orbitoparietal projection with the MSP 53° to table and acanthiomeatal line vertical. CR passes through orbit farthest from film.

SUPERIOR ORBITAL FISSURES

See PA skull variations

INFERIOR ORBITAL FISSURES	POSITION OF PART	CENTRAL RAY DIRECTED	STRUCTURES INCLUDED/ BEST SEEN
PA Axial *(Bertel)*	Patient PA, MSP centered to grid, IOML ⊥ tabletop	20–25° cephalad through nasion	PA axial proj of inferior orbital fissures within the orbits and projected between the pterygoid processes

Figure 7–65. Parietoacanthial (Water's position) is the single best projection for the facial bones. (Courtesy of The Stamford Hospital.)

4. Facial Bones, Nasal Bones, Zygomatic Arches

FACIAL BONES	POSITION OF PART	CENTRAL RAY DIRECTED	STRUCTURES INCLUDED/ BEST SEEN
Parieto-acanthial *(Waters)*	Patient PA, MSP ⊥ centered to grid, chin extended so OML is 37° to table	⊥ to parietal region, exiting at acanthion	Axial proj of facial bones, especially orbits, zygomas, and maxillae; best single proj for *facial bones;* see Fig. 7–65

Note: Patient should be upright to demonstrate air/fluid levels.

FACIAL BONES	POSITION OF PART	CENTRAL RAY DIRECTED	STRUCTURES INCLUDED/ BEST SEEN
AP AXIAL *(Reverse Waters)*	Patient supine, MSP ⊥ mid-table, IOML ⊥ table, center cassette ≈3″ above inion	30° cephalad to lips	Axial, but *magnified,* proj of facial bones
LAT	Patient PA obl, MSP of skull ∥ table, inter-pupillary line ⊥, IOML ∥ to transverse axis of film	⊥ zygoma	Lat proj of super-imposed facial bones

Routine: (2) 8 × 19; additional proj as requested

NASAL BONES	POSITION OF PART	CENTRAL RAY DIRECTED	STRUCTURES INCLUDED/ BEST SEEN
LAT	Patient recum-bent prone, MSP of skull ∥ table, interpu-pillary line ⊥, IOML parallel to transverse axis of film	⊥ a point 3/4″ distal to nasion	Lat proj of superim-posed nasal bones and their associat-ed soft tissue; see Fig. 7–66

NASAL BONES (con't)	POSITION OF PART	CENTRAL RAY DIRECTED	STRUCTURES INCLUDED/ BEST SEEN
Tangential	Skull aligned so that glabella is in same plane as superior border of alveolar ridge of maxilla	∥ glabelloalveolar line, passing through nasal bone	Axial proj of that portion of nasal bones projecting anterior to glabelloalveolar line, *shows medial or lateral fx displacement;* may be done intraorally (occlusal film) or extraorally w/ chin resting on cassette

Routine: both lat on (1) 8 × 10; tangential on request

ZYGOMATIC ARCHES	POSITION OF PART	CENTRAL RAY DIRECTED	STRUCTURES INCLUDED/ BEST SEEN
Tangential (SMV) (Full Basal)	See Skull: basal proj/SMV		

Note: In this projection, the skull may be rotated *15° toward the affected side* to better "open up" the zygomatic arches in individuals having flat cheekbones or a depressed fracture.

AP Axial   See Skull: AP axial (Towne/Grashey)

Routine: AP axial, SMV on (2) 8 × 10

Figure 7–66. Lateral nasal bones demonstrating fracture. (Courtesy of The Stamford Hospital.)

5. Mandible, Temporomandibular Joints (TMJs)

MANDIBLE	POSITION OF PART	CENTRAL RAY DIRECTED	STRUCTURES INCLUDED/ BEST SEEN
PA	Patient PA, nose and forehead on table, MSP ⊥, cassette centered to tip of nose	⊥ the lips	PA proj of mandible, especially body and rami
PA Axial	Patient PA, nose and forehead on table, MSP ⊥, cassette centered to glabella	20 to 25° cephalad to center of film	PA axial mandible, especially for rami and condyles
Axiolateral	Patient PA, MSP of skull ∥ cassette centered 1/2″ anterior and 1″ inferior to the EAM	25° cephalad, enters at angle of unaffected side	Axiolateral mandible, especially for body and ramus; rotate MSP 15° forward to better demonstrate body (see Fig. 7–67)

Routine: PA axial, both axiolateral on (3) 8 × 10

Figure 7–67. Axiolateral mandible, opening body and ramus for visualization.

Figure 7–68. **(A)** Radiograph demonstrates the oblique lateral projection of the TMJ in the closed-mouth position. **(B)** The open-mouth position. (Courtesy of The Stamford Hospital.)

TMJ	POSITION OF PART	CENTRAL RAY DIRECTED	STRUCTURES INCLUDED/ BEST SEEN
AP Axial	Patient AP, MSP ⊥ midcassette, OML ⊥ table	30° caudad, enters ≈3″ above nasion	AP axial proj of condyloid proc- esses and their articulations; unless contrain- dicated by suspected or known fracture or destructive disease another exposure is made with the *mouth open*
Infero- superior Trans- facial	Patient PA obl, skull MSP ≈ horizontal, inter- pupillary line ≈15° to verti- cal, cassette centered 1/2″ anterior and 1″ inferior to EAM	30° cephalad, exits TMJ adjacent to film	Obl lat TMJ; *both sides* examined in the open and closed-mouth po- sitions unless con- traindicated; see Fig. 7–68A and B
Obl Trans- facial *(Zanelli)*	Patient nearly lateral, MSP 30° (w/ chin away from table), cassette center- ed 1/2″ anterior to EAM	⊥; enters just distal to upper mandibular angle	Axiolateral proj of TMJs without superimposition; both sides examined in the open and closed- mouth positions unless contrain- dicated

Routine: AP axial, L and R transfacial on (3) 8 × 10

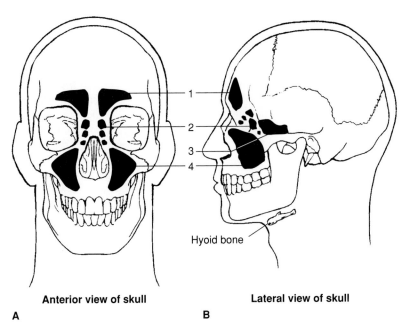

Figure 7–69. The paranasal sinuses, AP and lateral views.

6. Paranasal Sinuses. There are four paired *paranasal sinuses: frontal, ethmoidal, maxillary,* and *sphenoidal* (Fig. 7–69). The left and right frontal sinuses are usually asymmetrical. They are located behind the glabella and superciliary arches of the frontal bone. The frontal sinuses are not present in young children and reach their adult size in the 15th or 16th year. The ethmoidal sinuses are composed of 6 to 18 thin-walled air cells that occupy the bony labyrinth of the ethmoid bone. The ethmoidal sinuses of children are very small and do not fully develop until after the 14th year. The maxillary sinuses (antra of Highmore) are the largest of the paranasal sinuses and are located in the body of the maxillae. The *maxillary* sinuses are particularly prone to infection and collections of stagnant mucus. The maxillary sinuses reach their adult size around the 12th year. The sphenoidal sinuses are located in the body of the sphenoid bone and are usually asymmetrical. They generally reach adult size by the 14th year.

Radiography of the paranasal sinuses must be performed in the erect position so that any *fluid levels* may be demonstrated and to distinguish between fluid and other pathology such as *polyps*.

It is essential to remember that to demonstrate air and fluid levels the CR must always be directed parallel to the floor, even if the patient is not completely erect (just as in chest radiography). If the CR is angled to parallel the plane of the body, any fluid levels will be distorted or actually obliterated.

PARANASAL SINUSES	POSITION OF PART	CENTRAL RAY DIRECTED	STRUCTURES INCLUDED/ BEST SEEN
PA Axial *(Caldwell)*	Patient PA, skull MSP centered to grid, OML ⊥, grid, cassette centered to nasion	15° caudad to nasion	PA axial of *frontal* and *anterior ethmoid* sinuses, petrous pyramids are seen in the *lower one-third of the orbits;* see Fig. 7–70
Parieto-acanthial *(Waters)*	Patient PA, skull MSP centered to grid, OML 37° to cassette centered to acanthion	⊥, enters parietal region and exits acanthion	Parietoacanthial proj of *maxillary* sinuses projected *above petrous pyramids* (insufficient neck extension results in petrosa super-imposed on floor of maxillary sinus); distorted projec-tion of frontal and ethmoid; see Fig. 7–71

Figure 7–70. PA axial projection (Caldwell position) of the frontal and anterior ethmoid sinuses. The caudal angulation is somewhat excessive because the petrous pyramids are seen at the lowermost portion of the orbits. Correct angulation places the petrous pyramids in the lower one-third of the orbits. (Courtesy of The Stamford Hospital.)

Note: A modification of this projection made with the *mouth open* will demonstrate the *sphenoid sinuses* through the open mouth.

Figure 7–71. Parietoacanthial projection (Water's position) clearly demonstrates an air-fluid level in the left maxillary sinus. The radiograph is well collimated and the maxillary sinuses exactly centered to the film. The neck is adequately extended, projecting the petrous pyramids below the floor of the maxillary sinuses (too much extension projects teeth into maxillary sinuses). (Courtesy of The Stamford Hospital.)

Figure 7–72. Lateral projection of the sinuses (same patient as Figure 7–66) also demonstrates the importance of the erect position in paranasal sinus examinations. The air-fluid level is again observed within the maxillary sinus. CR is positioned too low, frontal sinus is cut off. Note also the fingerprint artifacts (around sphenoid sinus and on mandible) from careless film handling techniques. (Courtesy of The Stamford Hospital.)

PARANASAL SINUSES *(con't)*	POSITION OF PART	CENTRAL RAY DIRECTED	STRUCTURES INCLUDED/ BEST SEEN
LAT	Patient PA obl, skull MSP ∥ to cassette centered 1″ posterior to outer canthus, interpupillary line vertical	⊥ mid-cassette, enters 1″ posterior to outer canthus	Lat proj of all paranasal sinuses; see Fig. 7–72
SMV *(Basal)*	Patient AP erect, neck hyperextended to place IOML ∥ film and ⊥ CR, MSP ⊥ cassette	⊥ IOML and film, enters MSP at level of sella	Basal proj of sphenoid and ethmoid sinuses; mandibular symphysis should be superimposed on frontal bone

Routine: Caldwell, Waters, lat, SMV on (4) 8 × 10

7. Temporal Bones: Mastoids and Petrous Portions

TEMPORAL BONE: MASTOIDS AND PETROUS PORTION (see Fig. 7–73)

	POSITION OF PART	CENTRAL RAY DIRECTED	STRUCTURES INCLUDED/ BEST SEEN
PA Transorbital	Patient PA, MSP centered to grid, OML ⊥ table, tightly collimated beam centered to nasion	⊥ nasion	PA internal auditory canals projected through the orbits

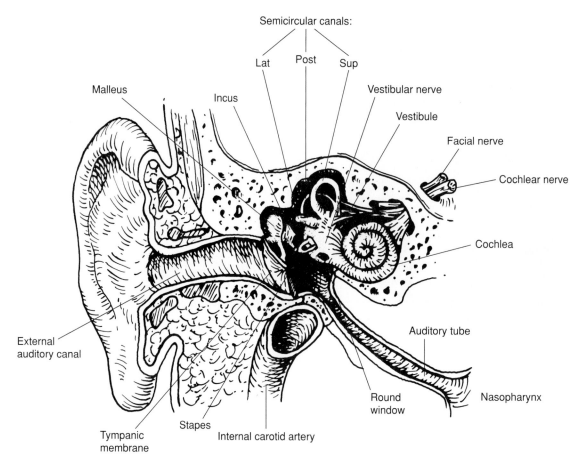

Figure 7–73. Temporal bone, demonstrating organs of hearing.

Figure 7–74. Axiolateral (Laws position) projection of right mastoid. (Courtesy of The Stamford Hospital.)

	POSITION OF PART	CENTRAL RAY DIRECTED	STRUCTURES INCLUDED/ BEST SEEN
AP Axial	See Skull: AP axial (Towne/Grashey) and center to MSP so that CR passes through level of EAMs		
Axio-lateral (Laws)	Patient prone obl, interpupillary line ⊥ table, IOML ∥ cassette, MSP rotated forward to form 15° ∠ w/table, mastoid centered to table	15° caudad, entering ≈ 2″ posterior to and 2″ above upper EAM	Axiolateral proj of mastoid air cells, superimposed internal and external auditory meatus of side closest to film (see Fig. 7–74)

Note: This projection can be duplicated with the patient in a true lateral position, using a double *tube* angulation of 15° caudad and 15° anteriorly and entering the same point. It can also be obtained by using double-angulation of the *part,* ie, skull rotated 15° anteriorly (toward the table) and 15° caudad so that the interpupillary line forms a 15° angle with the tabletop.

	POSITION OF PART	CENTRAL RAY DIRECTED	STRUCTURES INCLUDED/ BEST SEEN
SMV *(subbasal)*	Patient AP erect or supine, neck hyperextended to place OML ∥ film and ⊥ XP, MSP ⊥ cassette	⊥ OML and film, enters MSP at level 1″ anterior to EAMs	Axial projection of symmetrical petrous pyramids, external auditory meati, auditory ossicles and middle ears

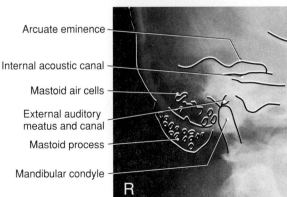

Arcuate eminence —

Internal acoustic canal —

Mastoid air cells —

External auditory meatus and canal —

Mastoid process —

Mandibular condyle —

R

Figure 7–75. Posterior profile projection, Stenvers method of petrous portions. The mastoid process is demonstrated in profile away from the bony structures of the skull and cervical spine. (From Cornuelle et al. *Radiographic Anatomy and Positioning.* Stamford, CT: Appleton & Lange, 1998.)

	POSITION OF PART	CENTRAL RAY DIRECTED	STRUCTURES INCLUDED/ BEST SEEN
Posterior Profile *(Stenvers)*	Patient PA, MSP 45°, head resting on forehead, zygoma, and nose, IOML ‖ transverse axis of film	12° cephalad exiting 1″ anterior to EAM closest to film	Pars petrosa projected in profile and parallel to film, mastoid process seen next to C1 and C2; middle ear, internal auditory canal, and bony labyrinth also demonstrated (see Fig. 7–75)
Anterior Profile *(Arcelin)*	Patient AP obl, MSP 45°, IOML ‖ transverse axis of film	10° caudad, entering 1″ anterior and 3/4″ above EAM away from film	Pars petrosa away from film projected in profile and parallel to film; internal auditory canal and bony labyrinth also demonstrated but somewhat magnified

Routine: AP axial, Laws, Stenvers; supplemental proj as required

  Chapter Review Questions

⭐ *Congratulations!* *You have completed a large portion of this chapter. You may go on to the "Registry-type" multiple-choice questions that follow. For greatest success, be sure also to complete the short answer questions found at the end of this chapter.*

1. Which of the following is/are part of the bony thorax?
    1. 24 ribs
    2. clavicles
    3. 12 thoracic vertebrae
   (A) 1 only
   (B) 1 and 2 only
   (C) 1 and 3 only
   (D) 1, 2, and 3

2. All of the following statements regarding a PA projection of the skull, with central ray perpendicular to the film are true, EXCEPT:
   (A) orbitomeatal line is perpendicular to the film
   (B) petrous pyramids fill the lower third of the orbits
   (C) midsagittal plane (MSP) is perpendicular to the film
   (D) central ray exits at the nasion

3. Which of the following is demonstrated in a 25° RPO position and the central ray entering 1 inch medial to the elevated anterior superior iliac spine (ASIS)?
   (A) left sacroiliac joint
   (B) right sacroiliac joint
   (C) left ilium
   (D) right ilium

4. Which of the following is (are) demonstrated in the lateral projection of the cervical spine?
   1. intervertebral joints
   2. apophyseal joints
   3. intervertebral foramina
   (A) 1 only
   (B) 1 and 2 only
   (C) 2 and 3 only
   (D) 1, 2, and 3

5. To best visualize the lower ribs, the exposure should be made:
   (A) on normal inspiration
   (B) on inspiration, second breath
   (C) on expiration
   (D) during shallow breathing

6. With the body in the erect position, the diaphragm moves:
   (A) 2 to 4 inches higher than when recumbent
   (B) 2 to 4 inches lower than when recumbent
   (C) 2 to 4 inches superiorly
   (D) spasmodically

7. Which of the following is a functional study used to demonstrate the degree of AP motion present in the cervical spine?
   (A) open-mount projection
   (B) moving mandible AP
   (C) flexion and extension laterals
   (D) right and left bending

8. Which of the following statements is (are) correct regarding the parietoacanthial projection (Water's method) of the skull?
   1. patient should be examined erect
   2. OML is perpendicular to the film
   3. petrosa should be projected below the maxillary antra
   (A) 1 only
   (B) 1 and 2 only
   (C) 1 and 3 only
   (D) 1, 2, and 3

9. The apophyseal articulations of the thoracic spine are demonstrated with the:
   (A) coronal plane 45° to the film
   (B) midsagittal plane 45° to the film
   (C) coronal plane 70° to the film
   (D) midsagittal plane 70° to the film

10. To better demonstrate the mandibular rami in the PA position, the:
    (A) skull is obliqued toward the affected side
    (B) skull is obliqued away from the affected side
    (C) central ray is angled cephalad
    (D) central ray is angled caudad

Answers and Explanations

1. (C) The thorax consists of 12 pairs of ribs and the structures to which they are attached anteriorly and posteriorly: the sternum and thoracic vertebrae. The clavicles are part of the shoulder girdle. They articulate with the sternum to form the sternoclavicular joints, the only bony articulation between the upper extremities and thorax.

2. (B) In the "true" PA projection of the skull with perpendicular central ray exiting the nasion, the petrous pyramids should *fill* the orbits. As the central ray (CR) is angled caudally, the petrous pyramids are projected lower in the orbits and at about 25 to 30° they are below the orbits. The orbitomeatal line (OML) must be perpendicular to the film, or the petrous pyramids will not be projected into the expected location in the angled projection. The MSP must be perpendicular to the film or the skull will be rotated.

3. (A) The sacroiliac joints angle posteriorly and medially 25° to the MSP. Therefore, to demonstrate them with the patient in the AP position (RPO, LPO), the *affected* side must be elevated 25°. This places the joint space perpendicular to the film and parallel to the central ray. When performed with the patient PA position (RAO, LAO), the *unaffected* side will be elevated 25°.

4. (B) Intervertebral joints are well visualized in the lateral projection of all the vertebral groups. Cervical articular facets (forming apophyseal joints) are 90° to the MSP and are therefore well demonstrated in the lateral projection. The cervical intervertebral foramina lie 45° to the MSP (and 15 to 20° to a transverse plane) and are therefore demonstrated in the oblique position.

5. (C) *Full or forced expiration* is used to elevate the diaphragm and demonstrate ribs *below* the diaphragm to best advantage (with exposure adjustment). *Deep inspiration* is used to depress the diaphragm and demonstrate as many ribs *above the diaphragm* as possible. Shallow breathing technique is occasionally used to visualize above diaphragm ribs, while obliterating pulmonary vascular markings.

6. (B) When the body is erect the diaphragm is more easily moved to a lower position during inspiration. For this reason, chest radiography is performed erect to allow maximum lung expansion. With the body in the supine position, the abdominal viscera exert greater pressure on the diaphragm and it usually assumes a position 2 to 4 inches higher than when erect.

7. (C) The degree of anterior and posterior motion is occasionally diminished with a "whiplash"-type injury. Anterior (forward, flexion) and posterior (backward, extension) motion is evaluated in the lateral position with the patient assuming flexion and extension as best as possible. Left and right bending films of the vertebral column are frequently obtained to evaluate scoliosis.

8. (C) The parietoacanthial projection (Water's method) of the skull is valuable for the demonstration of facial bones or maxillary sinuses. The head is rested on extended chin so that the OML forms a 37° angle with the film. This projects the petrous pyramids below the floor of the maxillary sinuses and provides an oblique frontal view of the facial bones.

9. (C) The thoracic apophyseal joints are demonstrated by placing the patient in an oblique position with the coronal plane 70° to the film (MSP 20° to the film) This can be accomplished by first placing the patient lateral, then obliqueing him or her 20° "off lateral." The apophyseal joints closest to the film are demonstrated in the PA (RAO, LAO) oblique and those remote from the film in the AP (LPO, RPO) oblique. Comparable detail is obtained using either method since OID is about the same.

10. (C) The straight PA (0°) projection effectively demonstrates the mandibular body but the rami and condyles are superimposed on the occipital bone and petrous portion of the temporal bone. To better visualize the rami and condyles, the central ray is directed cephalad 20 to 30°. This projects the temporal and occipital bones above the area of interest.

III. BODY SYSTEMS

KEY TERMS ◄

ANAPHYLAXIS	ISCHEMIA	RETROPERITONEAL
ANTIHISTAMINE	JAUNDICE	SEROUS
CANALIZATION	LUMEN	SPHINCTER
CHOLECYSTECTOMY	MUCOSA	TORTUOUS
CYSTOSCOPY	OPACIFICATION	URTICARIA
ENDOSCOPE	PARENCHYMA	VARICES
FISSURE	PERISTALTIC	VENTILATION
HEMIDIAPHRAGM	REFLUX	
INFARCT	RETROGRADE	

A. RESPIRATORY SYSTEM

1. Introduction. The principle structures of the respiratory system are the lungs, which function to supply oxygen to the blood and relieve the body of carbon dioxide (Fig. 7–76). Pulmonary function depends upon the processes of *ventilation* and alveolar gas ◄ exchange. The right lung is shorter because the liver is below it; the left lung is narrower because the heart occupies a portion of the left

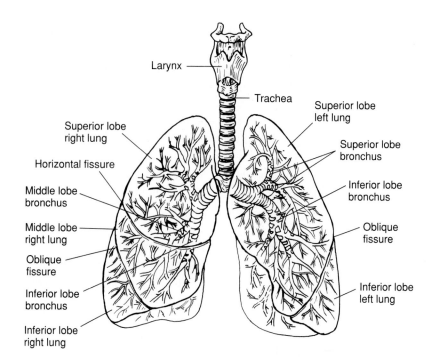

Figure 7–76. Trachea and bronchi (anterior view).

side. The lungs have a somewhat conical shape; their narrow upper portion is called the *apex,* their wide *base* is defined by the *diaphragmatic surface.* Structures such as the mainstem bronchi and pulmonary artery and veins enter and leave the lungs at the *hilum.* The *right lung* has three lobes; the upper and middle lobes are separated

▶ by the horizontal *fissure,* the middle and lower lobes are separated by the oblique fissure. The *left lung* has two lobes; the upper and lower lobes are separated by the oblique fissure (Fig. 7–76).

▶   The lungs are enclosed in a **serous** membrane, the *parietal pleura.* The *visceral pleura* lines the inner thoracic wall and covers the superior surface of the diaphragm; the potential space between the two layers of pleura is the *pleural cavity.*

Pneumothorax is the presence of air in the pleural cavity. A large pneumothorax is usually accompanied by a partial or complete collapse of the lung **(atelectasis).** Radiographic indications of atelec-

▶ tasis include elevation of the **hemidiaphragm** of the affected side and an increase in (tissue) density of the collapsed lung. **Thoracentesis** is the procedure required to remove significant amounts of air, blood, or other fluids in the pleural cavity.

One of the most diagnostically useful and frequently performed radiographic examinations is the chest x-ray examination. During the course of their illness and recovery, patients often need successive chest examinations to monitor their progress, and reproduction of quality images is an important part of quality control. Accurate positioning and selection of technical factors is critical to the diagnostic value of the radiographic images. *Even slight rotation or leaning can*

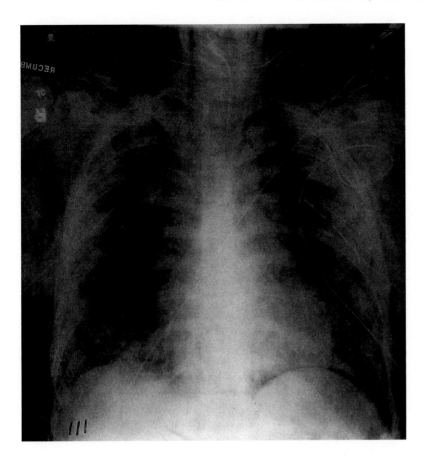

Figure 7–77. Mobile AP chest radiograph. Observe an endotracheal tube, ECG leads, one chest tube on the right and two on the left. The patient has extensive soft-tissue emphysema. Radiographers must exercise particular care when working around various patient tubes. (From the American College of Radiology Learning File. Courtesy of the ACR.)

cause significant distortion of the size and shape of the heart. Consistent and accurate positioning is essential to radiographic quality.

The radiographer must take careful note of each patient's apparel, body type, and clinical information. Important considerations include removal of any radiopaque clothing and accessories, placing the cassette transversely for broad-chested individuals (in order to include the *costophrenic angles*—blunting of the costophrenic angles is often due to pleural effusion), instructing female patients with large breasts to move them up and laterally for the PA projection, exposing on the second inspiration for hypersthenic individuals, and adjusting exposure factors for various pathologic conditions. Appropriate radiation protection measures must always be provided.

Mobile chest radiography often brings the radiographer into contact with seriously ill patients. The radiographer must be very cautious when positioning these patients for there are often numerous tubes (eg, chest tubes, endotracheal tubes, electrocardiographic (ECG) leads, Swan–Ganz lines, urinary catheters) associated with maintaining the patient's airway or reinflating a collapsed lung, removing fluid or air from the pleural cavity, administering medications, measuring central venous pressure, or measuring urine output (Fig. 7–77).

The following tables provide a summary of routine projections and frequently performed special projections.

2. Chest; PA, Lateral, Obliques

CHEST	POSITION OF PART	CENTRAL RAY DIRECTED	STRUCTURES INCLUDED/ BEST SEEN
PA	Patient erect PA, MSP exactly ⊥ cassette, shoulders depressed and rolled forward w/back of hands on hips, top of cassette 1-1/2–2″ above shoulders	⊥ T7	PA proj of thoracic viscera and skeletal anatomy; when exposed on *inspiration* demonstrates air filled trachea and lungs, 10 posterior ribs, on *expiration* shows pulmonary vascular markings; *inspiration and expiration* are done for pneumothorax, foreign body, diaphragm excursion, and atelectasis.

Note: Chest radiography is performed *erect* whenever possible to demonstrate air/fluid levels. The MSP must be exactly vertical (perpendicular); any *rotation can cause significant distortion* and misrepresentation of the visceral structures. *Rotation is detected on the PA radiograph by asymmetrical distance between the sternal ends of the clavicles and the lateral border of the thoracic vertebrae.* The shoulders are rolled forward to remove the scapulae from superimposition on the lung fields. Superiorly, the *pulmonary apices* must be seen; inferiorly the *costophrenic angles* must be seen in their entirety. *Inspiration must be adequate to demonstrate 10 posterior ribs.* A 72″ SID is recommended to decrease *magnification* of the heart. See Fig. 7–78.

LAT	Patient erect L lat, MSP vertical, midaxillary line 2″ posterior to center of cassette, arms over head, top of cassette 1-1/2 to 2″ above shoulders	Enters ⊥, 2″ posterior to midaxillary line at level of T7	L lat proj of chest particularly useful for heart, aorta, L lung and its fissures, and other left-sided structures/pathology; L lat usually done to place heart closer to film

Note: The MSP must be *exactly vertical;* any lateral leaning can cause significant distortion and misrepresentation of the visceral structures. *Rotation* is detected on the lateral radiograph by superimposition of ribs on sternum or vertebrae. Pulmonary apices and angles must be visualized. See Fig. 7–79.
Routine: (2) 14 × 17

OBL *(LAO and RAO)* *(For Lungs)*	Patient erect, PA obl, 45° to film, hand next to film on hip, other raised and supported	⊥ T7	L and R 45° obls for lungs; PA obls demonstrate lung closest to film, AP obls show lung away from film; to better see the aorta, the LAO should be 55 to 60°

Routine: (2) 14 × 17

(continued)

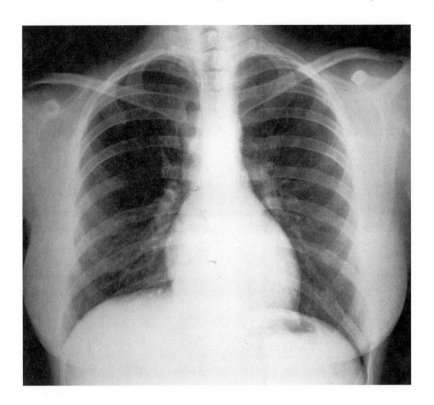

Figure 7–78. PA projection of the chest of a normal, healthy adult demonstrating the importance of positioning accuracy. Slight rotation has made the manubrium visible at the site of the right sternoclavicular joint, providing a density very similar to that created by a paraspinous or mediastinal mass. (From the American College of Radiology Learning File. Courtesy of the ACR.)

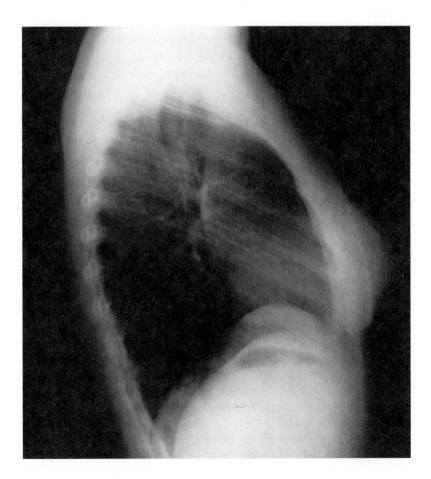

Figure 7–79. Lateral projection of the same chest as Figure 7–72 and without rotation. The sternum is seen free of superimposed ribs, the thoracic and lumbar vertebral spinous processes are seen. (From the American College of Radiology Learning File. Courtesy of the ACR.)

CHEST (con't)	POSITION OF PART	CENTRAL RAY DIRECTED	STRUCTURES INCLUDED/ BEST SEEN
OBL (LAO and RAO) (For Heart Size)	Patient erect, PA obl, 55 to 60° for L obl, and 45° for R obl	⊥ T7	LAO demonstrates L lung, heart, and aorta anterior to vertebrae; RAO demonstrates R lung, L atrium of the heart

Routine: (2) 14 × 17

3. Chest; Axial and Decubitus

	POSITION OF PART	CENTRAL RAY DIRECTED	STRUCTURES INCLUDED/ BEST SEEN
AP Axial (lordotic)	Patient erect AP, MSP ⊥ mid-cassette at level of T2	15 to 20° cephalad to T2	AP axial (lordotic) proj of pulmonary apices projected below clavicles (this position can also be done with patient leaning back and CR ⊥ film)

Routine: (1) 10 × 12 or 11 × 14

	POSITION OF PART	CENTRAL RAY DIRECTED	STRUCTURES INCLUDED/ BEST SEEN
Decubitus (L and R Lat)	Patient recumbent lat on affected or un-affected side as indicated by diagnosis; an-terior or pos-terior surface adjacent to cassette. MSP ⊥ mid-cassette w/ top 1-1/2″ above shoulders	⊥ mid-cassette	Frontal (AP or PA) proj of the chest useful for demon-stration of air or fluid levels; note: if free *air* is suspected, the affected side must be *up;* if *fluid* is suspected, the affected side must be placed *down*

Routine: (2) 14 × 17

4. Airway. AP and lateral projections of the airway and larynx are occasionally required to rule out *foreign body, polyps, tumors,* or any other condition suspected of causing some airway obstruction.

The AP is positioned as for an AP cervical spine with the CR perpendicular to the *laryngeal prominence.* The lateral is positioned as for a lateral cervical spine and centered to the coronal plane passing through the trachea (anterior to the cervical spine) at the level of the laryngeal prominence. *Exposures are made on slow inspiration* to visualize air-filled structures.

Depending on the structure(s) of interest being examined, these positions may be performed with barium and/or during performance of the *Valsalva/modified Valsalva maneuver.* Tomograms may be performed during phonation of vowel sounds to demonstrate more superior structures such as the larynx and/or vocal cords.

Figure 7–80. PA chest radiograph demonstrates the characteristic irreversible trapping of air found in emphysema, which gradually increases and overexpands the lungs, thus producing the characteristic flattening of the diaphragm and widening of the intercostal spaces. The increased air content of the lungs requires a compensating decrease in technical factors. (From the American College of Radiology Learning File. Courtesy of the ACR.)

5. Terminology and Pathology. The following is a list of radiographically significant conditions and devices with which the student radiographer should be familiar.

Asthma
Atelectasis
Bronchiectasis
Bronchitis
Central venous pressure line
Chest tube (see Fig. 7–77)
Chronic obstructive
   pulmonary disease
Cystic fibrosis
Emphysema (see Fig. 7–80)
Empyema

Endotracheal tube (see Fig. 7–77)
Hemothorax
Hickman catheter
Pleural effusion (see Fig. 7–81)
Pneumoconiosis
Pneumonia
Pneumothorax
Swan–Ganz catheter
Thoracentesis
Tuberculosis

Figure 7–81. PA chest demonstrating pleural effusion secondary to heart failure. (Reproduced with permission from Way, LW, ed. *Current Surgical Diagnosis & Treatment,* 10th ed. East Norwalk, CT: Appleton & Lange, 1994.)

Chapter Review Questions

☆ *Congratulations! You have completed your review of a large portion of this chapter. You may go on to the "Registry-type" multiple-choice questions that follow. For greatest success, be sure also to complete the short answer questions found at the end of this chapter.*

1. With the body in the erect position, the diaphragm moves:
   (A) 2 to 4 inches higher than when recumbent
   (B) 2 to 4 inches lower than when recumbent
   (C) cyclically
   (D) intermittently

2. Which of the following is (are) important when positioning the patient for a PA projection of the chest?
   1. the patient should be examined erect
   2. shoulders should be depressed
   3. shoulders should be rolled forward
   (A) 1 only
   (B) 1 and 2 only
   (C) 1 and 3 only
   (D) 1, 2, and 3

3. Which of the following criteria are used to evaluate a good PA projection of the chest?
   1. ten posterior ribs should be visualized
   2. sternoclavicular joints should be symmetrical
   3. scapulae should be outside the lung fields
   (A) 1 and 2 only
   (B) 1 and 3 only
   (C) 2 and 3 only
   (D) 1, 2, and 3

4. Blunting of the costophrenic angles seen on a PA projection of the chest may be indicative of:
   (A) pleural effusion
   (B) ascites
   (C) bronchitis
   (D) emphysema

5. To demonstrate the pulmonary apices below the level of the clavicles in the AP supine position, the CR should be directed:
   (A) perpendicularly
   (B) 15 to 20° caudad
   (C) 15 to 20° cephalad
   (D) 40° cephalad

6. Inspiration and expiration projections of the chest may be performed to demonstrate:
   1. pneumothorax
   2. diaphragm excursion
   3. bronchitis
   (A) 1 only
   (B) 1 and 2 only
   (C) 1 and 3 only
   (D) 1, 2, and 3

7. Chest radiography should be performed using 72 inches SID whenever possible in order to:
   1. minimize magnification of the heart
   2. obtain better lung detail
   3. blur out vascular markings
   (A) 1 only
   (B) 1 and 2 only
   (C) 1 and 3 only
   (D) 1, 2, and 3

8. All of the following statements regarding respiratory structures are true, EXCEPT:
   (A) the right lung has two lobes
   (B) the uppermost portion of the lung is the apex
   (C) each lung is enclosed in pleura
   (D) the trachea bifurcates into mainstem bronchi

9. All of the following statement completions regarding the oblique positions of the chest are correct, EXCEPT:
   (A) for lungs, the patient is obliqued 45°
   (B) for heart size, the right oblique is 45° and the left oblique is 60°
   (C) the RAO demonstrates the right atrium
   (D) the RAO may be used with barium to demonstrate the esophagus

10. Aspirated foreign bodies in older children and adults are most likely to lodge in the:
    (A) right main bronchus
    (B) left main bronchus
    (C) esophagus
    (D) proximal stomach

Answers and Explanations

1. (B) When the body is erect the diaphragm is more easily moved to a lower position during inspiration. For this reason, chest radiography is performed erect to allow maximum lung expansion. With the body in the supine position, the abdominal viscera exert greater pressure on the diaphragm and it usually assumes a position 2 to 4 inches higher than when erect.

2. (D) The chest should be examined in the erect position whenever possible to demonstrate any air or fluid levels. The shoulders should be relaxed and depressed to move the clavicles below the lung apices. The shoulders should be rolled forward to move the scapulae out of the lung fields.

3. (D) To evaluate sufficient inspiration and lung expansion, ten posterior ribs should be visualized. Sternoclavicular joints should be symmetrical; any loss of symmetry indicates rotation. Accurate positioning and selection of technical factors is critical to the diagnostic value of the radiographic images. Even slight rotation or leaning can cause significant distortion of the heart size and shape. To visualize maximum lung area, the shoulders are rolled forward to remove the scapulae from the lung fields.

4. (A) Fluid in the thoracic cavity between the visceral and parietal pleura is called *pleural effusion.* In the erect position, fluid gravitates to the lowest point, settling in, and "blunting," the costophrenic angles. *Ascites* is an accumulation of serous fluid in the peritoneal cavity. *Bronchitis* is an inflammation of the bronchial tubes. Pulmonary *emphysema* is a chronic pulmonary disease characterized by increase beyond the normal in the size of air spaces distal to the terminal bronchiole, and with destructive changes in the walls of the bronchioles.

5. (C) When the shoulders are relaxed, the clavicles are usually carried below the pulmonary apices. In order to examine the portions of the lungs lying behind the clavicles, the central ray is directed cephalad 15 to 20° to project the clavicles above the apices, when the patient is examined in the AP position.

6. (B) Phase of respiration is exceedingly important in thoracic radiography; lung expansion and the position of the diaphragm strongly influence the appearance of the finished radiograph. Inspiration and expiration radiographs of the chest are taken to demonstrate air in the pleural cavity (pneumothorax), to demonstrate degree of diaphragm excursion, or to detect the presence of foreign body. The expiration film will require a somewhat greater exposure (6 to 8 kVp more) to compensate for the diminished quantity of air in the lungs.

7. (B) Chest radiographs are performed in the erect position at 72 inches SID whenever possible. The long source-image-distance is easily achieved with a minimum patient exposure due to the low tissue densities being examined (ribs and lungs). The longer source-image-distance minimizes magnification of the heart and provides better lung detail (also because of less magnification). Rather than blurring the pulmonary vascular markings, their details are also improved.

8. (A) The trachea (windpipe) bifurcates into left and right mainstem bronchi, each entering its respective lung hilum. The left bronchus divides into two portions, one for each lobe of the left lung. *The right bronchus divides into three portions, one for each lobe of the right lung.* The lungs are conical in shape, consisting of upper pointed portions, termed the *apices* (singular = apex), and the broad lower portions (or *bases*). The lungs are enclosed in a double-walled serous membrane called the pleura.

9. (C) The RAO position demonstrates the left atrium of the heart. This position provides good visualization of the esophagus when it is full of barium because the esophagus is projected between the vertebrae and heart. The 45° obliques are used to demonstrate the lungs; the LAO for the right lung and the RAO for the left lung. For heart size, the left oblique must be increased to 55 to 60° to separate superimposed aorta and vertebrae.

10. (A) Because the right main bronchus is wider and more vertical, aspirated foreign bodies are more likely to enter it than the left main bronchus, which is narrower and angles more sharply from the trachea. An aspirated foreign body does not enter the esophagus or stomach, as they are not respiratory structures, but rather, digestive.

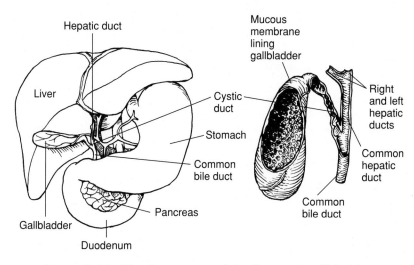

Figure 7–82. Bile duct system of the liver and gallbladder.

B. BILIARY SYSTEM

1. Introduction. The biliary tree consists of the left and right hepatic ducts, common hepatic duct, cystic duct, common bile duct, and the gallbladder (Fig. 7–82). The hepatic ducts leave the liver and join to form the *common hepatic duct*. The short *cystic duct* continues to the gallbladder. The common hepatic and cystic ducts unite to form the long *common bile duct,* which usually joins with the pancreatic duct to form the short *hepatopancreatic ampulla (of Vater).* The ampulla opens into the descending duodenum through the *duodenal papilla,* which is surrounded by the *hepatopancreatic sphincter (of Oddi).*

The *gallbladder* is located in a shallow fossa on the inferior surface of the liver between its right and quadrate lobes. Small gallstones are able to pass out the gallbladder through the cystic duct; those that are too large irritate the gallbladder mucosa, resulting in **cholecystitis.** *Gallstones* can also lodge in ducts. If a stone lodges in the cystic duct, cholecystitis without ***jaundice*** is the result, because bile can still drain into the duodenum. A stone lodged in the common bile duct will result in jaundice as well as cholecystitis. A "gallbladder attack" is the painful result of fatty chyme stimulating the release of *cholecystokinin,* which elevates pressure within the stone-laden gallbladder.

Radiographic examinations of the biliary system include *oral cholecystography, operative cholangiography, T-tube cholangiography,* and *endoscopic retrograde cholangiopancreatography (ERCP).* Each of these examinations requires the use of a contrast agent. With the exception of the ERCP, few of these exams are performed today, but rather are imaged via *sonography* (Fig. 7–83).

2. Patient Preparation. For *oral cholecystograms* (OCG), iodinated tablets are taken the evening before the examination. The gallbladder stores and concentrates the contrast-laden bile, rendering the

Figure 7–83. A sonogram of the gallbladder demonstrating the presence of gallstones.

gallbladder radiopaque. The evening meal must be fat-free to prevent gallbladder contraction and subsequent release of the radiopaque bile. Oral cholecystography is used to evaluate the function of the biliary system as well as demonstrate the structure and contents of the gallbladder.

▶ Operative cholangiography is used to examine the bile ducts and frequently follows a **cholecystectomy.** An iodinated contrast agent is introduced into the common bile duct to evaluate biliary patency and that of the hepatopancreatic ampulla. Any calculi can be detected and removed before completion of surgery.

Occasionally, a T-shaped tube is left in the common bile duct for postsurgical drainage. T-tube cholangiography is performed by injecting a contrast agent through the tube to detect any remaining calculi and evaluate the biliary tree patency.

▶ *ERCP* is a specialized procedure used to evaluate suspected biliary and/or pancreatic conditions. An **endoscope** is passed through the mouth, esophagus, stomach, and into the descending duodenum to the orifice of the hepatopancreatic ampulla. Contrast material is injected into the common bile duct for evaluation of the biliary system.

2. Gallbladder.
An oral cholecystogram frequently begins with a
▶ prone 14 × 17 film of the abdomen to check **opacification** and location of the gallbladder as well as patient preparation and technical factors. Collimated recumbent PA and oblique, and erect or decubitus radiographs follow. In the absence of gallstones, a fatty meal may then be given the patient and another similar series of films taken 20 to 30 minutes later. Fluoroscopic spot films may be taken in addition to, or in place of, these radiographs. *The gallbladder of the average build patient is located between the 10th and 12th ribs on the right,* midway between the vertebral column and lateral border of the body. *Hypersthenic* individuals usually require centering about 2″ higher and more laterally, while centering for *asthenic* individuals is usually 2″ lower and more midline. In the *erect* position, the gallbladder of an asthenic patient can be as low as the iliac fossa.

OCG	POSITION OF PART	CENTRAL RAY DIRECTED	STRUCTURES INCLUDED/ BEST SEEN
PA	Patient prone or PA erect, sagittal plane passing midway b/w spine and R lat border of body, at level of 9th rib centered to grid (CR lower when done erect)	⊥ center of cassette	PA recumbent or erect proj of GB. *The erect position will demonstrate layering of any gallstones* (see Fig. 7–84)

(continued)

A

B

C

Figure 7–84. **(A)** Note the position of the gallbladder (GB) in the PA erect projection with respect to the vertebrae and iliac crest. In the erect position, the GB moves inferiorly. Its medial location is characteristic of the asthenic/hyposthenic body type. (Courtesy of The Stamford Hospital.) **(B)** LAO view of gallbladder; no evidence of gallstones. **(C)** The same patient as **B** in the erect position, showing layering of gallstones. (From the American College of Radiology Learning File. Courtesy of the ACR.)

OCG (con't)	POSITION OF PART	CENTRAL RAY DIRECTED	STRUCTURES INCLUDED/ BEST SEEN
OBL (*LAO*)	Patient in recumbent LAO, sagittal plane passing midway b/w spine and R lat border of body centered to grid at level of 9th rib	⊥ center of cassette	Obl proj of GB, with somewhat less foreshortening and self-superimposition than in PA proj. *Greater obliquity* (40°) is *required for asthenic patients* than for hypersthenic (15°)
R Lat Decubitus	Patient recumbent R lat, posterior surface adjacent to upright grid and centered to level of gallbladder	⊥ center of cassette	R lat decubitus of gallbladder is useful for demonstration of *stratification* (layering) of gallstones (see Fig. 7–84) and demonstrating the GB free of superimposition of gassy bowel loops

4. OR/T-Tube

	POSITION OF PART	CENTRAL RAY DIRECTED	STRUCTURES INCLUDED/ BEST SEEN
RPO	Patient supine with L side elevated 15 to 20°, R upper quadrant centered to grid	⊥ center of cassette	RPO of biliary tree and gallbladder area; used to evaluate the hepatopancreatic ampulla and biliary tree for evidence of calculi or other pathology (following injection of contrast into common bile duct)

▶ **5. ERCP.** Following ***canalization*** of the hepatopancreatic ampulla, fluoroscopic spot films are taken in the AP (RPO) or PA (LAO) position. Filming procedure should immediately follow injection since, under normal conditions, contrast will empty from the biliary ducts in about 5 minutes (Fig. 7–85).

6. Terminology and Pathology. The following is a list of radiographically significant conditions with which the student radiographer should be familiar.

Cholecystitis   Hepatitis
Cholelithiasis   Jaundice
Cirrhosis   Pancreatitis

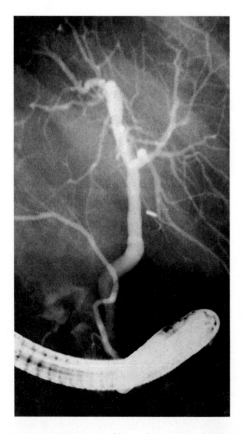

Figure 7–85. Spot film of a normal ERCP. The pancreatic and common bile ducts are clearly delineated. (Courtesy of The Stamford Hospital.)

C. DIGESTIVE SYSTEM

1. Introduction. The digestive system (Fig. 7–86) consists of the *gastrointestinal tract* and accessory organs. The *gastrointestinal tract,* or *alimentary canal,* is a continuous tube of varying dimensions consisting of the esophagus, stomach, and small and large intestines. The teeth, tongue, salivary glands, liver, gallbladder, and pancreas are accessory organs that aid in the mechanical and chemical breakdown of food. The major portion of the GI tract lies within the abdominopelvic cavity. Its principle functions are the chemical breakdown and absorption of nutrients.

The *esophagus* functions to propel a bolus of food toward the stomach through **peristaltic** motion. The *cardiac sphincter* is ◄

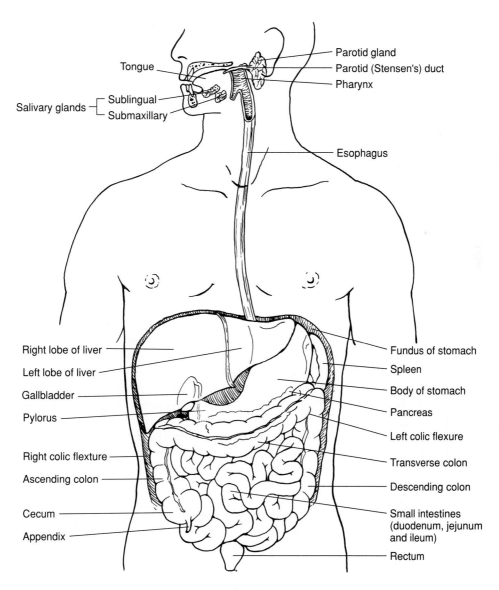

Figure 7–86. The digestive system.

Figure 7–87. **(A)** Normal position of the stomach. **(B)** Note protrusion of stomach through esophageal hiatus (hiatal hernia).

located at the distal end of the esophagus. **"Heartburn"** is an
▶ inflammation of the esophageal ***mucosa*** as a result of gastric ***reflux***
▶ of acidic material into the esophagus. ***Esophageal varices*** are
▶ dilated, ***tortuous*** veins directly beneath the esophageal mucosa. A
hiatal hernia is a herniation of the stomach through the esophageal
hiatus of the diaphragm, producing a sac-like dilatation above the
diaphragm (Fig. 7–87). The presence of varices or herniation can be
detected radiographically with the use of barium sulfate.

The *stomach* is the dilated, sac-like portion of the GI tract. When
the stomach is empty, its mucosal lining forms soft folds called *rugae*
(Fig. 7–88). Exteriorly, it presents a *greater curvature* on its lateral
surface and a *lesser curvature* on its medial surface. The proximal
opening of the stomach is the *cardiac sphincter;* the *pyloric sphincter* is located at its distal end. The portion of the stomach around
the distal esophagus is called the *cardia;* that portion superior to
the esophageal juncture is the *fundus.* The sharp angle (incisura)
between the esophagus and fundus is the *cardiac notch.* The major
portion of the stomach is the *body;* the distal portion is the *pylorus.*
The *incisura angularis* is located on the lesser curvature and marks
the beginning of the pylorus. The distal portion of the pylorus is
▶ marked by the pyloric ***sphincter.*** *Gastritis* is an inflammation of the
gastric mucosa that can be caused by excessive secretion of acids or
by ingestion of irritants such as aspirin or corticosteroids.

The *small intestine* is composed of the duodenum, jejunum, and
ileum. The *duodenum* is the shortest portion. It begins just beyond
the pyloric sphincter and is divided into four portions: the duodenal
cap or bulb, descending duodenum, transverse duodenum, and
ascending duodenum. These portions form a C-shaped loop *(duodenal loop)* that is occupied by the head of the pancreas. The descending portion receives the hepatopancreatic ampulla and duodenal
papilla (see biliary section). The ascending portion terminates at the
duodenojejunal flexure (angle of Treitz). While the position of the
short (9 in) duodenum is fixed, the *jejunum* (9 ft) and *ileum* (13 ft)
are very mobile. Their relative position may be seen radiographically
to change from day to day. Excessive twisting of the small intestine
is called **volvulus,** and can cause compression of blood vessels,
▶ leading to loss of blood supply, ***ischemia,*** and ***infarct*** of the
affected area. The small intestine terminates at the *ileocecal valve.*

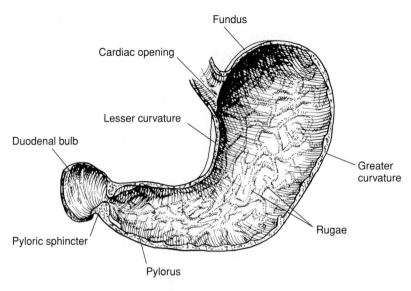

Figure 7–88. Stomach (internal aspect).

Figure 7–89. The colon.

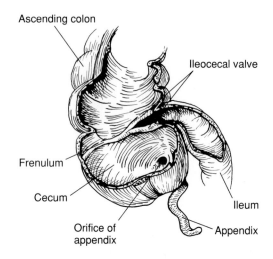

Figure 7–90. The ileocecal valve.

The approximately 5-ft-long *large intestine (colon)* (Fig. 7–89) functions in the formation, transport, and evacuation of feces. The colon begins at the terminus of the small intestine; its first portion is the dilated sac-like *cecum,* located inferior to the ileocecal valve (Fig. 7–90). Projecting posteromedially from the cecum is the short (about 3.5 in) *vermiform appendix.* Its lumen is particularly narrow in adolescents and young adults and may become occluded by a **fecalith** and result in inflammation **(appendicitis).**

The *ascending colon* is continuous with the cecum and is located along the right side of the abdominal cavity. It bends medially and anteriorly in the right hypochondrium, forming the *right colic (hepatic) flexure.* The colon traverses the abdomen as the *transverse colon* and bends posteriorly and inferiorly in the left hypochondrium, forming the *left colic (splenic) flexure.* The *descending colon* continues down the left side of the abdominal cavity and, at about the level of the pelvic brim, the colon moves medially to form the S-shaped *sigmoid colon.* The *rectum* is that part of the large intestine, about 5″ in length, between the sigmoid and the anal canal.

Diverticula are small saccular protrusions of intestinal mucosa through the intestinal wall (Fig. 7–91). They are most commonly associated with the sigmoid colon and can become occluded by fecaliths and subsequently inflamed **(diverticulitis).** If an inflamed diverticulum perforates, it can result in severe bleeding and **peritonitis.**

2. Patient Preparation. Preliminary patient preparation is generally required of patients undergoing radiographic examinations of various portions of the digestive system. The upper GI tract (stomach and small intestine) must be empty and the lower tract (large intestine) must be cleansed of any gas and fecal material. Patients should be questioned about their preparation and a preliminary "scout" film taken to check abdominal contents and for any radiopaque (eg, gallstones, residual barium) material.

Figure 7–91. Barium enema roentgenogram showing multiple diverticula of the colon. (From Way, LW, ed. *Current Surgical Diagnosis Treatment,* 10th ed. East Norwalk, CT: Appleton & Lange, 1994.)

In order to make up for the lack of subject contrast, radiography of the digestive system most often requires the use of artificial contrast media in the form of barium sulfate suspension or water-soluble iodine and, frequently, air. *Double-contrast studies* of the stomach and large intestine are frequently performed. Barium sulfate functions to coat the organ with radiopaque material, while air inflates the structure. This permits visualization of the shape of the structure as well as visualization of pathology within its lumen. Thus, conditions such as **polyps** can be seen projecting within the air-filled lumen, whereas a barium-filled *lumen* would make visualization of ◀ anything but the organ shape virtually impossible.

The speed with which barium sulfate passes through the alimentary canal depends on patient habitus (hypersthenic usually fastest) and the concentration of the barium suspension.

When performing examinations on patients suspected or known to have stomach or **intestinal perforation,** *water-soluble* iodinated contrast media should be used instead of barium sulfate. If the water-soluble medium leaks through a perforation into the peritoneal cavity, it will simply be absorbed and excreted by the kidneys. Water soluble contrast media are excreted more rapidly than barium sulfate preparations.

These studies are far from pleasant for patients and the radiographer should make every effort to fully explain the procedure while endeavoring to expedite the examination and make the patient as comfortable as possible.

With the increased use of digital fluoroscopy and 100-mm and 105-mm spot films, fewer "overhead" radiographs are done today. However, a summary of the most frequently performed examinations and projections follows.

3. Abdomen

	POSITION OF PART	CENTRAL RAY DIRECTED	STRUCTURES INCLUDED/ BEST SEEN
AP	Patient supine, MSP centered to grid, hands at sides, cassette center-ed to iliac crest; see Fig. 7–92	⊥ to midline at level of crest	AP proj of abdomen frequently used as "scout" film preliminary to con-trast studies of the abdomen; shows size and shape of kidneys, liver, and spleen, psoas mus-cles, as well as any calcifications or masses
Erect	Patient AP erect, MSP centered to grid, cassette centered ≈2″ above iliac crest	⊥ to mid-cassette	AP erect proj of abdomen used to demonstrate air/ fluid levels; both hemidiaphragms should be included; see Fig. 7–93

(continued)

Figure 7–92. When positioning the abdomen, it is important to position the patient's hands at his or her side or resting high on the chest. Note the position of the patient's right hand in this retrograde urogram. (From the American College of Radiology Learning File. Courtesy of the ACR.)

(con't)	POSITION OF PART	CENTRAL RAY DIRECTED	STRUCTURES INCLUDED/ BEST SEEN
LAT Decubitus	Patient lat recumbent, (AP or PA) MSP ⊥ and centered to upright grid, cassette centered ≈2″ above iliac crest	Horizontal and ⊥ mid-cassette	Usually *left* lat decubitus (PA or AP proj) of abdomen performed to demonstrate air/fluid levels in patients unable to assume the erect position; both hemidiaphragms should be included

Note: A "three-way abdomen" study is often performed to evaluate possible obstruction or free air and fluid within the abdomen and usually consists of AP recumbent, AP erect, and L lat decubitus projections of the abdomen (Fig. 7–94).

Routine: (3) 14 × 17

B

A

Figure 7–93. Observe the difference between these two radiographs. **(A)** Part of an intravenous urogram (IVU) examination taken in the recumbent position. **(B)** Part of an abdominal survey taken in the erect position. Observe the change in appearance and radiographic density, especially of the lower abdomen, as the patient is moved erect and the abdominal viscera assume a lower position; the lower abdomen essentially becomes "thicker" and radiographic density increases. Both hemidiaphragms must be observed on the erect abdomen. (**(A)** from the American College of Radiology Learning File. Courtesy of the ACR. **(B)** courtesy of Bob Wong, RT.)

Figure 7–94. Small-bowel obstruction indicated by the dilated bowel loops having a ladder-like pattern. Patient is recumbent; therefore air/fluid levels are not demonstrated. (From Way, LW, ed. *Current Surgical Diagnosis & Treatment,* 10th ed. East Norwalk, CT: Appleton & Lange, 1994.)

4. Esophagus

	POSITION OF PART	CENTRAL RAY DIRECTED	STRUCTURES INCLUDED/ BEST SEEN
AP	Patient supine, MSP centered and ⊥ table, top of cassette 1–2″ above shoulders, patient swallowing barium during (<0.1 sec) exposure	⊥ mid-cassette, ≈T6–T7	Barium-filled esophagus in AP proj
RAO	Patient prone obl, 35–40° RAO, top of cassette 1–2″ above shoulders, patient swallowing barium during exposure	⊥ mid-cassette, ≈T6–T7	Barium-filled esophagus in RAO proj, demonstrated between vertebrae and heart; best single proj of esophagus; see Fig. 7–95
LAT (L or R)	Patient recumbent lat, coronal plane 2″ posterior to midaxillary line, centered to grid, top of cassette just above shoulders, patient swallowing during exposure	⊥ mid-cassette	Barium-filled esophagus in lat proj

▶ **Note:** Esophagus for demonstration of *varices* must be performed in the *recumbent* position; table slightly Trendelenburg and/or performance of the Valsalva maneuver is also helpful. Exposure times of 0.1 sec or less should be used in order to avoid motion; however, respiration normally stops during and shortly after the act of swallowing, so that patients need not be instructed to stop breathing.

5. Stomach and Small Intestine. Radiologic examination of the stomach and/or small bowel generally begins with fluoroscopic examination. The fluoroscopist observes the swallowing mechanism, mucosal lining (rugae) of the stomach, and the filling and emptying mechanisms of the stomach and proximal small bowel in various positions. The patient is turned and rotated in various positions so that all aspects of the stomach and any abnormalities such as hiatal hernia (Fig. 7–101) can be visualized. Double-contrast examinations of the upper GI system are performed frequently. Occasionally glucagon or another similar drug will be given the patient (IV or IM) prior to the examination to relax the GI tract and permit more complete filling. Various spot films will be taken by the fluoroscopist and the radiographer may be required to take supplemental "overhead" projections. *Small-bowel series* examinations require that successive films be made of the abdomen at specified intervals;

Figure 7–95. RAO film of a barium-filled esophagus. The esophagus has three normal constrictions at the levels of the cricoid cartilage, the left bronchus, and the esophageal hiatus of the diaphragm. (Courtesy of The Stamford Hospital.)

an additional spot film is taken when barium reaches the *ileocecal valve*.

Contrast material (usually water soluble) may occasionally be instilled through a gastrointestinal (GI) tube for visualization of the GI tract. GI tubes can be used therapeutically to siphon gas and fluid from the GI tract or diagnostically, using contrast agent, to locate the site of obstruction or pathology.

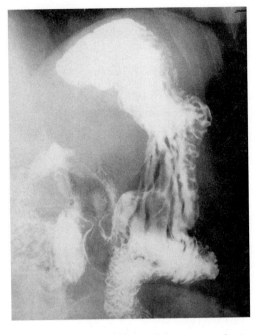

Figure 7–96. LPO view of the stomach. In this position, air replaces the barium that drains from the duodenal bulb and pylorus, thus providing double-contrast visualization of these structures. (Courtesy of The Stamford Hospital.)

	POSITION OF PART	CENTRAL RAY DIRECTED	STRUCTURES INCLUDED/ BEST SEEN
LPO	Patient supine, obliqued ≈40° to left, centered midway b/w vertebrae and L abdominal wall at level of L1	⊥ mid-cassette (at level of L1)	Barium-filled fundus (the fundus is most posterior portion of stomach, thus, it readily fills w/ barium in AP position and moves more superiorly); good position for *double contrast* of body, pylorus, and duodenal bulb; see Fig. 7–96
Routine: (1) 10 × 12			
LAT	Patient recumbent lat (usually R), center coronal plane b/w midaxillary line and anterior abdominal wall to cassette at level of L2 (b/w umbilicus and xiphoid)	⊥ mid-cassette (at level of L2)	Lat proj of stomach and proximal small bowel demonstrating anterior and posterior aspects of stomach, retrogastric space, pyloric canal, duodenal loop; this proj provides the best visualization of the pyloric canal and duodenal bulb in the hypersthenic patient; see Fig. 7–97
Routine: (1) 10 × 12			
RAO	Patient recumbent PA obliqued 40 to 70°, centered midway b/w vertebrae and lat abdominal wall at level of L2	⊥ mid-cassette (at level of L2)	Right PA obl proj of stomach particularly useful for barium-filled pyloric canal and duodenal loop; this position is helpful in studying the stomach's emptying mechanism, since *peristaltic activity is greatest in this position*
Routine: (1) 10 × 12			

Figure 7–97. Lateral projection demonstrates the anterior and posterior stomach surfaces and the retrogastric space. (Courtesy of The Stamford Hospital.)

(continued)

	POSITION OF PART	CENTRAL RAY DIRECTED	STRUCTURES INCLUDED/ BEST SEEN
PA	Patient prone, MSP centered to grid, cassette centered to level of L2	⊥ mid-cassette (at level of L2)	PA proj of somewhat transversely spread stomach, demonstrating its contours, greater and lesser curvatures

Note: Hypersthenic patients frequently have high, transverse stomachs with indistinguishable curvatures. The adult hypersthenic stomach can be "opened" and its contours made readily visible by angling the CR 35 to 45° cephalad. The top edge of a lengthwise 14 × 17 cassette is placed level with the patient's chin and the CR directed to mid-cassette.
Routine: (1) 14 × 17

	POSITION OF PART	CENTRAL RAY DIRECTED	STRUCTURES INCLUDED/ BEST SEEN
AP/ Small Bowel	Patient supine, MSP centered to grid, cassette centered to level of L2	⊥ mid-cassette (at level of L2)	AP proj of distal esophagus area, stomach, and proximal small bowel; demonstrates hiatal hernias w/ patient in Trendelenburg position

Note: This position is used to record progress of the barium column in *small bowel* examinations. The first radiograph is usually made 15 min after ingestion of the barium drink and centered at level of L2. Subsequent radiographs are made at 15 to 30-min intervals (and centered at level of crest), according to the individual patient and how quickly/slowly the barium progresses. Spot films are usually taken when the barium column reaches the ileocecal valve.

6. Large Intestine. The lower GI tract is most often examined by ▶ *retrograde* filling with barium sulfate and, frequently, air. The fluoroscopist observes filling of the large bowel in various positions and takes spot films as indicated. Much of the barium is then drained from the intestine, and air is introduced. The objective is to coat the bowel with barium, then distend its lumen with air. The double-contrast method is ideal for demonstration of intraluminal lesions, such as **polyps.**

The success of the barium enema examination depends on several factors, but without proper patient preparation a diagnostic examination is often impossible. *Poor preparation resulting in retained fecal material in the colon can mimic or conceal pathologic conditions.*

The barium enema is most easily tolerated and retained by the patient if it is cool or actually cold (≈40 to 45°F). There is probably no radiographic examination that causes more embarrassment and anxiety than the barium-enema and air-contrast procedure. The radiographer must be sensitive to the concerns and needs of the patient by providing a complete explanation of the procedure and by providing for the patient's modesty as much as possible.

The following table is a summary of frequently performed projections taken following the fluoroscopic procedure.

	POSITION OF PART	CENTRAL RAY DIRECTED	STRUCTURES INCLUDED/ BEST SEEN
AP	Patient supine, MSP centered to cassette at level of iliac crest	⊥ mid-cassette	AP proj of entire contrast-filled large intestine

Note: The large intestine of *hypersthenic* patients is high and around the periphery of the abdomen, hence they may require that the AP and PA be done on (2) 14 × 17s placed crosswise in the Bucky tray. In contrast, the colon of the *asthenic* patient is low, redundant, and more midline.

	POSITION OF PART	CENTRAL RAY DIRECTED	STRUCTURES INCLUDED/ BEST SEEN
PA	Patient prone, MSP centered to cassette at level of iliac crest	⊥ mid-cassette	PA proj of entire contrast-filled large intestine; AP or PA *erect* may be used to demonstrate double-contrast *flexures*

Routine: (1) 14 × 17

	POSITION OF PART	CENTRAL RAY DIRECTED	STRUCTURES INCLUDED/ BEST SEEN
PA Axial	Patient prone, MSP centered to cassette at level of pubic symphysis	35° caudad to midline at level of ASIS	PA axial proj of *sigmoid colon;* angulation opens the length of the S-shaped colon; see Fig. 7–98

Note: AP axial may be performed to show similar structures; CR is directed 35° cephalad.
Routine: (1) 10 × 12

(continued)

Figure 7–98. Double-contrast PA axial projection of the rectum and sigmoid. The caudal tube angulation serves to "open" the redundant S-shaped sigmoid colon. Similar results may be obtained in the AP position with a cephalad tube angle. (Courtesy of The Stamford Hospital.)

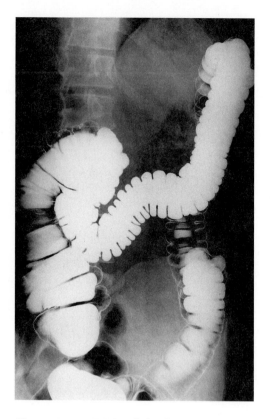

Figure 7–99. RAO of the barium and air-filled large bowel. Note that the hepatic flexure is "opened" for better visualization. An LPO would provide similar results. The opposite obliques (LAO, RPO) are used to demonstrate the splenic flexure and descending colon. (Courtesy of The Stamford Hospital.)

(con't)	POSITION OF PART	CENTRAL RAY DIRECTED	STRUCTURES INCLUDED/ BEST SEEN
RAO	Patient PA, obl ≈40°, centered to midline, cassette centered to level of iliac crest	⊥ mid-cassette	Right PA obl proj of the colon, demonstrates *ascending colon and hepatic flexure;* see Fig. 7–99

Routine: (1) 14 × 17

LAO	Patient PA obl ≈40°, centered to midline, cassette centered to level of iliac crest	⊥ mid-cassette	Left PA obl proj of the colon, demonstrates *descending colon and splenic flexure*

Note: *RPO* will demonstrate *descending colon and splenic flexure, LPO* will demonstrate *ascending colon and hepatic flexure.*
Routine: (1) 14 × 17

LAT	Patient lat recumbent, midaxillary line centered to grid, cassette centered at level ≈2" above pubic symphysis	⊥ mid-cassette	L or R lat proj, especially for *rectum* and *rectosigmoid* area

Routine: (1) 10 × 12

Figure 7–100. Right lateral decubitus view of the air and barium-filled colon. The heavier barium sulfate moves toward the dependent side, while air rises to fill the remainder of the barium-coated lumen. Thus, the right lateral decubitus demonstrates double contrast of the "left-sided walls" of the ascending and descending colons (ie, lateral side of descending colon and medial side of ascending colon). (Courtesy of The Stamford Hospital.)

POSITION OF PART	CENTRAL RAY DIRECTED	STRUCTURES INCLUDED/ BEST SEEN
LAT Decubitus (R and L) Patient lat recumbent, (AP or PA), MSP ⊥ and centered to upright grid at iliac crest	Horizontal and ⊥ midcassette	Air rises to provide double-contrast delineation of *lateral walls of colon;* both decubitus are routinely performed; see Fig. 7–100

Routine: (2) 14 × 17

7. Terminology and Pathology.

The following is a list of radiographically significant abdominal and digestive conditions and devices with which the student radiographer should be familiar.

Achalasia
Appendicitis
Ascites
Colostomy
Crohn's disease
Diverticulitis
Diverticulosis
Dysphagia
Enteritis
Esophageal atresia
Esophageal reflux
Esophageal varices
Gastric tube
Gastritis
Gastroenteritis

Hiatal hernia (see Fig. 7–101)
Hirschsprung's disease
Ileostomy
Imperforate anus
Intussusception
Irritable-bowel syndrome
Levin tube
Miller–Abbott tube
Peptic ulcer
Peritonitis
Pneumoperitoneum
Polyp
Pyloric stenosis
Ulcerative colitis
Volvulus

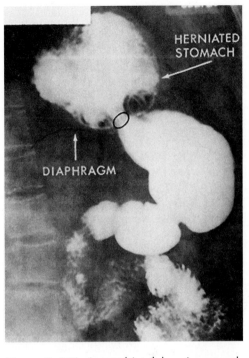

Figure 7–101. Large hiatal hernia extending up through the (circled) diaphragmatic esophageal hiatus. (From Way, LW. *Current Surgical Diagnosis & Treatment,* 10th ed. East Norwalk, CT: Appleton & Lange, 1994.)

A&U Chapter Review Questions

⭐ *Congratulations! You have completed a large portion of this chapter. You may go on to the "Registry-type" multiple-choice questions that follow. For greatest success, be sure also to complete the short answer questions found at the end of this chapter.*

1. During a gastrointestinal examination, the AP recumbent projection of a stomach of average shape will usually demonstrate:
    1. barium-filled fundus
    2. double-contrast body and antral portions
    3. retrogastric portion of the duodenum

    (A) 1 only
    (B) 1 and 2 only
    (C) 1 and 3 only
    (D) 1, 2, and 3

2. The salivary gland located near the angle of the mandible is the:
   (A) parotid
   (B) submaxillary gland
   (C) sublingual gland
   (D) Wharton's gland

3. Which of the following projections of the abdomen should be used to demonstrate air or fluid levels when the erect position cannot be obtained?
   (A) AP Trendelenburg
   (B) AP supine
   (C) lateral decubitus
   (D) lateral recumbent

4. Which of the following best describes the relationship between the esophagus and trachea?
   (A) esophagus is posterior to the trachea
   (B) trachea is posterior to the esophagus
   (C) esophagus is lateral to the trachea
   (D) trachea is lateral to the esophagus

5. To demonstrate esophageal varices, the patient must be examined in the:
   (A) recumbent position
   (B) erect position
   (C) anatomic position
   (D) Fowler's position

6. The usual preparation for an upper GI series is:
   (A) clear fluids 8 hours prior to exam
   (B) npo after midnight
   (C) enemas until clear before exam
   (D) light breakfast day of the exam

7. What instructions might be given after a GI examination?
   1. drink plenty of fluids
   2. take a mild laxative
   3. withhold fluids for 6 hours
   (A) 2 only
   (B) 1 and 2 only
   (C) 2 and 3 only
   (D) 1, 2, and 3

8. In which of the following positions are the pyloric canal and duodenal bulb best demonstrated during a GI series?
   (A) RAO
   (B) left lateral
   (C) recumbent PA
   (D) recumbent AP

9. What position is frequently used to project the GB away from the vertebrae in the asthenic patient?
   (A) RAO
   (B) LAO
   (C) left lateral decubitus
   (D) PA erect

10. Which of the following barium/air-filled anatomic structures is best demonstrated in the RAO position?
    (A) splenic flexure
    (B) hepatic flexure
    (C) sigmoid colon
    (D) iliocecal valve

Answers and Explanations

1. (D) With the body in the AP recumbent position, barium flows easily into the fundus of the stomach, displacing it somewhat superiorly. The fundus, then, is filled solely with barium, while the air that had been in the fundus is displaced into the gastric body, pylorus, and duodenum, thus illustrating them in double-contrast fashion. Air contrast delineation of these structures allows us to see through the stomach, to retrogastric areas and structures.

2. (B) There are three groups of salivary glands. The largest are the parotid glands, which lie below and anterior to the ear and are emptied by Stenson's duct. The submaxillary glands are located near the angle of the mandible and are emptied by Wharton's duct. The sublingual gland, as its name implies, is located under the tongue; a group of ducts (of Rivinus) empty the gland. The largest of these is Bartholin's duct.

3. (C) Air or fluid levels will be clearly demonstrated only if the CR is directed parallel to them. Therefore, to demonstrate air or fluid levels, erect or decubitus positions should be used. A "three-way abdomen" study is often performed to evaluate possible obstruction or free air or fluid within the abdomen and usually consists of AP recumbent, AP erect, and left lateral decubitus projections of the abdomen.

4. (A) The trachea (windpipe) is a tube-like passageway for air that is supported by C-shaped cartilaginous rings. The trachea is part of the respiratory system and is continuous with the main stem bronchi. The esophagus, part of the alimentary canal, is a hollow tube-like structure connecting the mouth and stomach, and lies posterior to the trachea. If one inadvertently aspirates food or drink into the trachea, choking occurs.

5. (A) Esophageal varices are tortuous dilatations of the esophageal veins. They are much less pronounced in the erect position and must always be examined with the patient recumbent. The recumbent position affords more complete filling of the veins, as blood flows against gravity.

6. (B) The upper GI tract must be empty for best x-ray evaluation. Any food or liquid mixed with the barium sulfate suspension can simulate pathology. Preparation therefore is to withhold food and fluids for eight to nine hours before the exam, typically after midnight, as fasting exams are usually performed first thing in the morning.

7. (B) Barium can dry and harden in the large bowel, causing symptoms from mild constipation to bowel obstruction. It is therefore essential that the radiographer provide clear instructions of follow-up care, along with its rationale, especially to out-patients. To avoid the possibility of fecal impaction, the patient should drink plenty of fluids for the next few days and take a mild laxative such as milk of magnesia.

8. (A) The RAO position affords a good view of the pyloric canal and duodenal bulb. It is also a good position for the barium-filled esophagus, projecting it between the vertebrae and heart. The left lateral projection of the stomach demonstrates the left retrogastric space; the recumbent PA is used as a general survey of the gastric surfaces, and the recumbent AP with a slight left oblique affords a double-contrast of the pylorus and duodenum.

9. (B) There are four types of body habitus. Listed from largest to slightest they are: hypersthenic, sthenic, hyposthenic, asthenic. The position, shape, and motility of various organs can differ greatly from one body type to another. The typical asthenic gallbladder is situated low and medial, often very close to the midline. To move the GB away from the midline, the LAO position is used. The GB of hypersthenic individuals occupies a high lateral, and transverse position.

10. (B) In the prone oblique positions (RAO, LAO) the flexure disclosed is the one closer to the film. Therefore, the RAO position will open up the hepatic flexure. The AP oblique positions (RPO, LPO) demonstrate the side away from the film.

D. URINARY SYSTEM

1. Introduction. Two of the functions of the urinary system (Fig. 7–102) are to remove wastes from the blood and eliminate it in the form of urine. The tiny units within the renal substance that perform these functions are called *nephrons*. The major components of the urinary system are the kidneys, ureters, and bladder. The paired *kid-*

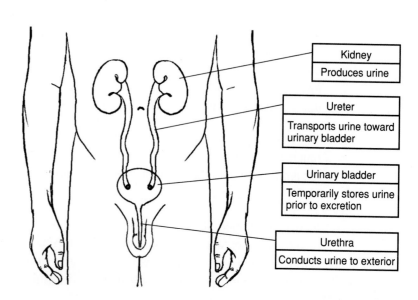

Figure 7–102. Components of the urinary system.

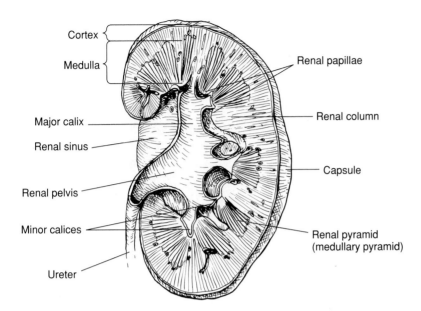

Cortex

Medulla

Renal papillae

Major calix

Renal column

Renal sinus

Capsule

Renal pelvis

Minor calices

Ureter

Renal pyramid
(medullary pyramid)

Figure 7–103. Section through the left renal pelvis.

neys are **retroperitoneal**, and embedded in adipose tissue between ◄ the vertebral levels of T12 and L3. The right kidney is usually 1″ to 2″ lower than the left because of the presence of the liver on the right. The kidneys move inferiorly 1″ to 3″ when the body assumes an erect position; they move inferiorly and superiorly during respiration. The slit-like opening on the medial renal surface is the *hilum,* which opens into a space called the *renal sinus* (Fig. 7–103). The renal artery and vein pass through the hilum. The upper, expanded portion of the ureter is called the *renal pelvis,* or *infundibulum,* and also passes through the hilum; it is continuous with the major and minor calyces within the kidney.

Within each kidney, the renal **parenchyma** is divided into two ◄ parts; the outer *cortex* and inner *medulla.* The cortex is compact and has a grainy appearance as a result of the many *glomeruli* within its tissues. The medulla contains 10 to 14 *renal pyramids* with a characteristic striated appearance that is due to the *collecting tubules* within (Fig. 7–103).

The proximal portion of each *ureter* is at the renal pelvis. As the ureter passes inferiorly, three normal constrictions can be observed: at the ureteropelvic junction, at the pelvic brim, and at the ureterovesicular junction. Urine is carried through the ureters by peristaltic activity. If a ureter is obstructed by a kidney stone, **hydronephrosis** occurs. The ureters enter the *urinary bladder* posteroinferiorly (Fig. 7–104). The base of the bladder rests on the pelvic floor. The triangular-shaped area formed by the *ureteral* and *urethral orifices* is called the *trigone.* Micturition is the process of emptying the urinary bladder of its contents through the *urethra.* The male urethra is about 7 to 8″ long and is divided into prostatic, membranous, and penile portions. The female urethra is about 1-1/2″ in length.

A common complication of regional enteritis or diverticular disease is the formation of a **fistula** between the urinary bladder and small or large intestine. Fistulous tracts may often be evaluated radiographically with contrast media.

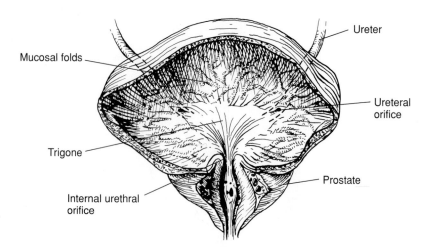

Figure 7–104. Bladder trigone (anterior portion of bladder removed).

Figure 7–105. A preliminary or scout film of the abdomen is taken before the start of an IVU. The radiograph is checked for residual barium from previous contrast studies, patient preparation (including barium from previous studies; note residual barium in patient's appendix), location of kidneys, technical factors, and any calcifications. (Courtesy of The Stamford Hospital.)

Routine radiographic procedures of the urinary system are generally performed via the intravenous route. When performed in the retrograde manner, **cystoscopy** is required.

Routine intravenous procedures are most correctly referred to as *intravenous urography* (IVU), or *excretory urography,* although they are still commonly referred to as intravenous *pyelography (pyel* refers only to renal *pelvis).* Intravenous procedures demonstrate *function* of the urinary system. Retrograde studies demonstrate only the *structure* of the part and are generally performed to evaluate the lower urinary tract (lower ureters, bladder, and urethra).

2. Patient Preparation.
Investigation of the urinary tract requires patient preparation sufficient to rid the intestinal tract of gas and fecal material. Typical preparation usually begins the evening before the examination with a light dinner, a gentle laxative, and nothing to eat or drink (NPO) after midnight. Immediately before beginning the IVU, the patient must be instructed to empty his or her bladder; this prevents dilution of opacified urine in the bladder. If the patient has a urinary catheter, it is generally clamped just before the injection and unclamped before the post-void radiograph. The IVU is preceded by a preliminary scout film of the abdomen to evaluate patient preparation and reveal any calcifications (renal or gallstones), position of kidneys, and accuracy of technical factor selection (Fig. 7–105).

Because the urinary structures have so little subject contrast, artificial contrast material must be employed for better visualization of these structures. Contrast agents used for urographic procedures can have unpleasant, and (rarely) even lethal, side effects. Intravenous injection of contrast frequently produces a warm, flushed feeling, a bitter or metallic taste, or mild nausea. These side effects are of short duration and usually pass as quickly as they come. More serious side effects include **urticaria,** respiratory discomfort and distress and, rarely, **anaphylaxis.** An **antihistamine** is appropriate treatment for simple side effects, but the radiographer must always be prepared to deal quickly and efficiently with patients experiencing more serious reactions. *Nonionic* contrast agents are far less likely to produce side

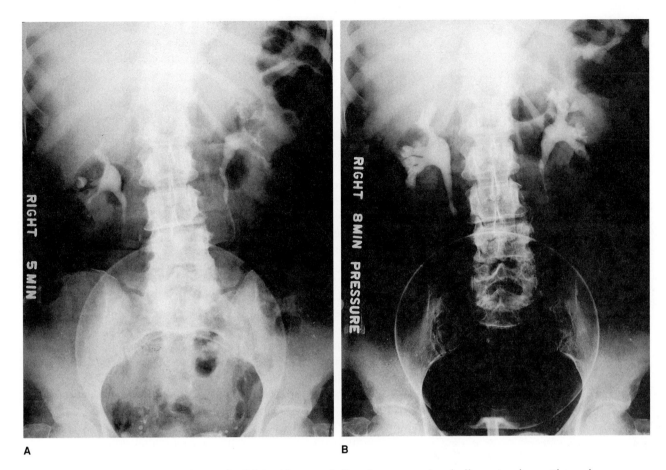

A   **B**

Figure 7–106. **(A)** 5-min IVU with an uninflated compression balloon in place. The collecting system within the kidneys, renal pelves, and ureters are perceptible but not fully distended. **(B)** The 8-min film, taken 3 min following inflation of the balloon, which serves to partially obstruct the ureters and promote more complete distention of the renal collecting system, pelves, and ureters. Tubes associated with body systems such as ureters, calyces, the esophagus, the common bile duct, and blood vessels are most accurately evaluated when filled and slightly distended. Observe the difference in radiographic density seen through the inflated balloon and the uninflated balloon. These may be likened to similar density differences that can occur between inspiration and expiration projections of the chest made with identical exposure factors. (From the American College of Radiology Learning File. Courtesy of the ACR.)

effects. Contrast agents and their side effects are more thoroughly discussed in Chapter 1.

The selected contrast agent is injected intravenously and successive radiographs are made at specified intervals. A time-interval marker must be included on each radiograph to indicate the post-injection time elapsed. Injection and post-injection protocol varies with the institution, radiologist, patient condition, and diagnosis. The contrast may be rapidly injected in a *bolus* to obtain a 30-second *nephrogram.* Radiographs collimated to the kidneys (11 × 14 crosswise) may be required at 1, 3, and 5 minutes to evaluate a diagnosis of **renal hypertension.** Both obliques and tomograms may be required to evaluate a suspected **tumor** or **lesion.** AP and oblique kidney, ureter, and bladder films (KUBs) are usually required at 10 to 15 minutes after injection. Maximum concentration of the contrast material usually occurs at 15 to 20 minutes after injection, but varies with degree of patient hydration. A prone KUB is frequently requested at 20 minutes.

3. Types of Examinations.

Compression over the distal ureters (delaying contrast or urine travel to bladder) may be required to more completely fill the kidneys with contrast medium or to visualize the contrast-filled kidneys for a longer period of time (Fig. 7–106). *Tomograms* are often useful to remove superimposed shadows from kidneys and better evaluate the renal collecting system. Patients having a condition interfering with renal function will often require delayed films to demonstrate the collecting system and/or ureters. Since the lower poles of the kidneys and the ureters are more anterior structures, the prone position is often used to demonstrate filling of these structures. An erect radiograph is occasionally requested to demonstrate renal mobility and ureteral tortuosity. An AP post-void bladder film is usually required to detect any *residual urine* in the evaluation of tumor masses or enlarged prostate glands.

Retrograde urograms require catheterization of the ureter(s). Radiographs that include the kidney(s) and ureter(s) in their entirety are made after retrograde filling of the structures. A cystogram or (voiding) *cystourethrogram* requires urethral catheterization only. Radiographs are made of the contrast-filled bladder and frequently of the contrast-filled urethra during voiding. *Cystoscopy* is required for location and catheterization of the vesicoureteral orifices.

Excretory and retrograde urography involve accurate positioning of the abdomen to include the kidneys, ureters, and bladder. If these structures cannot fit on a single film, a second radiograph is generally taken for the bladder. The following is a review of abdomen KUB positioning and an overview of bladder positioning.

4. KUB (Kidney, Ureter, and Bladder)

POSITION OF PART	CENTRAL RAY DIRECTED	STRUCTURES INCLUDED/ BEST SEEN
Patient supine, MSP ⊥ centered to grid, cassette centered to iliac crest	⊥ to midline at level of crest	AP proj of abdomen shows size and shape of kidneys, liver, spleen, psoas muscles, and, any calcifications or masses; should include from top of kidneys through symphysis pubis (see Fig. 7–107); obliques may be performed at 30°

Note: The 30° oblique KUB places the kidney of the side *away* from the film *parallel* to the film.
Routine: (1) 14 × 17

Figure 7–107. This KUB is a 5-min IVU film. Good collimation is evident and the kidneys, ureters, and bladder are included in their entirety. *Review the contents of the abdominal cavity* by correctly identifying each of the lettered structures. (Courtesy Bob Wong, RT.)

5. Bladder

	POSITION OF PART	CENTRAL RAY DIRECTED	STRUCTURES INCLUDED/ BEST SEEN
AP	Patient supine, MSP ⊥ centered to grid, lower edge of cassette just below pubic symphysis	⊥ to center of cassette	AP proj shows contrast-filled or post-void bladder
Routine: (1) 10 × 12			
AP *(Voiding Studies)*	Patient supine, MSP ⊥ centered to grid, cassette centered to pubic symphysis	⊥ to midline at level of pubic symphysis	AP projection of bladder and proximal urethra; used for voiding cysto-urethrograms (see Fig. 7–108); a 5° caudal angle may be used to project bladder neck and urethra below pubis; obl proj are obtained at 40 to 60°

Figure 7–108. AP projection of voiding cystourethrogram demonstrating complete left vesicoureteral reflux. Because pediatric voiding disorders are frequently associated with vesicoureteral reflux, it is often necessary to include most of the abdomen in the radiograph. (Reproduced with permission from Way, LW, ed. *Current Surgical Diagnosis & Treatment,* 10th ed. East Norwalk, CT: Appleton & Lange, 1994.)

6. Terminology and Pathology. The following is a list of radiographically significant urinary conditions and devices with which the student radiographer should be familiar.

Cystitis	Polycystic kidney
Double collecting system	Prostatic hypertrophy
Double ureter	Pyelonephritis
Fistula	Renal calculi
Foley catheter	Renal hypotension
Horseshoe kidney	Staghorn calculus (see Fig. 7–109)
Hydronephrosis	Supernumerary kidney
Hydroureter	(see Fig. 7–110)
Incontinence	Uremia
Nephroptosis	Ureteral stent
Nephrostomy tube	Ureterocele
Pelvic kidney	Vesicoureteral reflux

E. FEMALE REPRODUCTIVE SYSTEM

1. Introduction. The female reproductive system consists of the ovaries, oviducts, and uterus. The broad, suspensory, round, and ovarian ligaments are all associated with support of the reproductive organs.

The *ovaries* are the female gonads that function to release ova (female reproductive cells) during ovulation and produce various female hormones including estrogen and progesterone. The *oviducts,* or Fallopian tubes, are 3 to 5″ long, arise from the uterine cornu (angles) and extend laterally to arch over each ovary. The oviduct lateral extremities are broader than their medial ends and are bordered by motile *fimbriae* (see Fig. 7–111 on p. 201). The fimbriae sweep over the ovary and function to collect the liberated ovum. *Fertilization* of the ovum usually occurs in the outer portion of the oviducts. Ova are propelled through the oviduct by peristaltic motion. **Salpingitis** is possibly the most common cause of female sterility; if fertilization does occur, the zygote is unable to traverse the oviduct due to its scarred or narrowed condition. Occasionally, a fertilized ovum will become implanted in the oviduct, a condition known as **ectopic,** or **tubal, pregnancy.** This condition is a gynecologic emergency because, if left untreated, the patient can die from internal hemorrhage.

The most superior, arched, portion of the *uterus* is the fundus. The angle on each side is the cornu, and marks the point of entry of the oviducts. The *body* is the large central region and the narrow inferior portion is the *cervix.*

2. Hysterosalpingogram. The most commonly performed radiologic examination of the reproductive system is hysterosalpingography, which is employed for evaluation of the uterus, oviducts, and ovaries of the female reproductive system. The procedure serves to delineate the position, size, and shape of the structures and demonstrate pathology such as **polyps, tumors,** and **fistulas.** However, it is most often used to demonstrate *patency* of the oviducts in cases of **infertility,** and is sometimes therapeutic in terms of opening a blocked oviduct.

Hysterosalpingograms should be scheduled about 10 days after the start of menstruation. This is the time just *before* ovulation,

A

B

Figure 7–109. Although radiograph **(A)** may appear to be part of an IVU examination, no urine-filled ureter or bladder is associated with the opaque right kidney; the opaque area is associated with formation of a staghorn calculus. Radiograph **(B)** is a 1-hr IVU film demonstrating both collecting systems. Staghorn calculi are usually associated with chronic infection and alkaline urine. They may be associated with a single calyx or an entire renal pelvis, and may be unilateral or bilateral. Whenever possible, staghorn (named for their shape, resembling a stag's antlers) calculi are removed because they can cause partial obstruction of the calyces and/or ureteropelvic junction. (From the American College of Radiology Learning File. Courtesy of the ACR.)

when there should be little chance of irradiating a newly fertilized ovum.

After the cervical canal is cannulated, an iodinated organic contrast agent is injected via the cannula into the uterine cavity. If the oviducts are patent, contrast will flow through them and into the peritoneal cavity. Fluoroscopy is performed during injection and spot films are taken. Overhead radiographs may be performed following the fluoroscopic procedure.

	POSITION OF PART	CENTRAL RAY DIRECTED	STRUCTURES INCLUDED/ BEST SEEN
AP	Patient supine, MSP centered to grid, and a point 2″ above the pubic symphysis centered to the cassette	⊥ midcassette	AP proj of uterus and oviducts; 30° obliques may be taken as required; see Fig. 7–112

A

B

C

Figure 7–110. Radiograph **(A)** of this retrograde urogram shows a diminished collecting system with an oversized kidney shadow. A second ureterovesicular orifice was found within the bladder. The upper system was drained of contrast and the second one filled **(B)**. Radiograph **(C)** is a superimposition of film **(A)** on film **(B)**, and shows the two separate excretory systems from calyces to ureteral orifices. Two separate systems within one kidney, or duplication of the renal pelvis, is a congenital anomaly called a *supernumerary kidney*. It is of no clinical significance, is usually asymptomatic, and requires no treatment; any urinalysis or renal function test would be normal. The ureters of supernumerary kidneys may join at some point or may continue to two separate orifices in the bladder, as in this case. (Courtesy of The Stamford Hospital.)

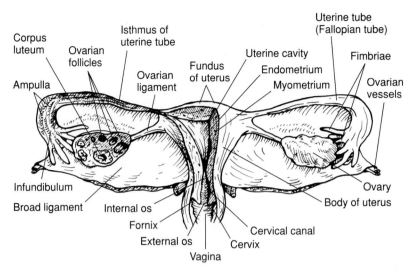

Figure 7–111. Uterus, uterine tubes (oviducts), and ovaries.

Figure 7–112. AP projection of hysterosalpingogram study. Contrast-filled uterus and oviducts are shown. (Courtesy of The Stamford Hospital.)

3. Terminology and Pathology. The following is a list of radiographically significant reproductive conditions with which the student radiographer should be familiar.

Bicornuate uterus	Leiomyoma
Ectopic pregnancy	Pelvic inflammatory disease
Endometriosis	Placenta previa
Infertility	Salpingitis

Chapter Review Questions

⭐ ***Congratulations!*** *You have completed your review of a large portion of this chapter. You may go on to the "Registry-type" multiple-choice questions that follow. For greatest success, be sure also to complete the short answer questions found at the end of this chapter.*

1. In what order should the following radiographs be performed?
    1. barium enema
    2. intravenous pyelogram
    3. upper GI
   (A) 3, 1, 2
   (B) 1, 3, 2
   (C) 2, 1, 3
   (D) 2, 3, 1

2. Which of the following will best demonstrate the size and shape of the liver and kidneys?
   (A) lateral abdomen
   (B) AP abdomen
   (C) dorsal decubitus abdomen
   (D) ventral decubitus abdomen

3. Which of the following examinations require(s) restriction of the patient's diet?
    1. GI series
    2. abdominal survey
    3. pyelogram
   (A) 1 only
   (B) 1 and 2 only
   (C) 1 and 3 only
   (D) 1, 2, and 3

4. During IV urography, the prone position is generally recommended to demonstrate:
   1. filling of obstructed ureters
   2. the renal pelvis
   3. the superior calyces
   (A) 1 only
   (B) 1 and 2 only
   (C) 1 and 3 only
   (D) 1, 2, and 3

5. Which of the following examinations require(s) catheterization of the ureters?
   1. retrograde urogram
   2. cystogram
   3. voiding cystogram
   (A) 1 only
   (B) 1 and 2 only
   (C) 2 and 3 only
   (D) 1, 2, and 3

6. Some common mild side effects of intravenous administration of water-soluble iodinated contrast agents include:
   1. flushed feeling
   2. bitter taste
   3. urticaria
   (A) 1 only
   (B) 1 and 2 only
   (C) 1 and 3 only
   (D) 1, 2, and 3

7. Hysterosalpingograms may be performed for the following reason(s):
   1. demonstration of fistulous tracts
   2. investigation of infertility
   3. demonstration of tubal patency
   (A) 1 only
   (B) 1 and 2 only
   (C) 1 and 3 only
   (D) 1, 2, and 3

8. A post-void radiograph of the urinary bladder is usually requested at the completion
   of an IVP, and may be helpful in demonstrating:
   1. residual urine
   2. prostate enlargement
   3. ureteral tortuosity
   (A) 1 only
   (B) 1 and 2 only
   (C) 1 and 3 only
   (D) 1, 2, and 3

9. During routine intravenous urography, the oblique position demonstrates the:
   - (A) kidney of the side up parallel to the film
   - (B) kidney of the side up perpendicular to the film
   - (C) urinary bladder parallel to the film
   - (D) urinary bladder perpendicular to the film

10. To better demonstrate contrast-filled distal ureters during intravenous urography, it is helpful to:
    1. use a 15° AP Trendelenburg position
    2. apply compression to the proximal ureters
    3. apply compression to the distal ureters
    - (A) 1 only
    - (B) 2 only
    - (C) 1 and 2 only
    - (D) 1 and 3 only

Answers and Explanations

1. (C) When scheduling patient examinations it is important to avoid the possibility of residual contrast medium covering areas of interest on later exams. The IVP should be scheduled first because the contrast medium used is excreted rapidly. The BE should be scheduled next. The GI series is scheduled last. Any barium remaining from the previous BE should not be enough to interfere with the stomach or duodenum, though a preliminary scout film should be taken in each case.

2. (B) The AP projection provides a survey of the abdomen, showing the size and shape of the liver, spleen, and kidneys. When performed erect, it should demonstrate both hemidiaphragms. The lateral projection is sometimes requested and is useful for evaluating the prevertebral space occupied by the aorta. Ventral and dorsal decubitus positions provide a lateral view of the abdomen useful for demonstration of air-fluid levels.

3. (C) A patient having a GI series is required to be npo for at least 8 hours prior to the exam; food or drink in the stomach can simulate disease. A patient scheduled for a pyelogram must have the preceding meal withheld so as to avoid the possibility of aspirating vomitus in case of allergic reaction. An abdominal survey does not require the use of contrast medium and no patient preparation is required.

4. (B) The kidneys lie obliquely in the posterior portion of the trunk, with their superior portions angled posteriorly and their inferior portions and ureters angled anteriorly. Therefore, to facilitate filling of the most anteriorly placed structures, the patient is examined in the prone position. Opacified urine then flows to the most dependent part of the kidney and ureter—the ureteropelvic region, inferior calyces, and ureters.

5. (A) Retrograde urograms require catheterization of the urethra and/or ureter(s). Radiographs that include the kidney(s) and ureter(s) in their entirety are made after retrograde filling of the structures. A cystogram or (voiding) cystourethrogram requires *urethral* catheterization only. Radiographs are made of the contrast-filled bladder and frequently of the contrast-filled urethra during voiding. Cystoscopy is required for location and catheterization of the vesicoureteral orifices.

6. (B) Because the urinary structures have so little subject contrast, artificial contrast material must be employed for better visualization of these structures. Contrast agents used for urographic procedures can have unpleasant, and (rarely) even lethal, side effects. Intravenous injection of contrast frequently produces a warm, flushed feeling, a bitter or metallic taste, or mild nausea. These side effects are of short duration and usually pass as quickly as they come. More serious side effects include urticaria, respiratory discomfort/distress and, rarely, anaphylaxis. An antihistamine is appropriate treatment for simple side effects, but the radiographer must always be prepared to deal quickly and efficiently with patients experiencing more serious reactions. Nonionic contrast agents are far less likely to produce side effects.

7. (D) The most commonly performed radiologic examination of the reproductive system is hysterosalpingography, which is employed for evaluation of the uterus, oviducts, and ovaries of the female reproductive system. The procedure serves to delineate the position, size, and shape of the structures and demonstrate pathology such as polyps, tumors, and fistulas. However, it is most often used to demonstrate *patency* of the oviducts in cases of *infertility,* and is sometimes therapeutic in terms of opening a blocked oviduct.

8. (B) An AP post-void bladder film is usually required to detect any *residual urine* in the evaluation of *tumor masses* or *enlarged prostate glands.* An erect radiograph is occasionally requested to demonstrate renal mobility and ureteral tortuosity.

9. (A) During intravenous urography, both oblique positions are generally obtained. The 30° oblique KUB places the kidney of the side *away* from the film *parallel* to the film. The kidney closer to the film is placed perpendicular to the film. The oblique positions provide an oblique projection of the urinary bladder.

10. (A) A 15 to 20° AP Trendelenburg position during IV urography is often helpful in demonstrating filling of the distal ureters and the area of the vesicoureteral orifices. In this position, the contrast-filled urinary bladder moves superiorly, encouraging filling of the distal ureters and superior bladder, and provides better delineation of these areas. The CR should be directed perpendicular to the cassette. Compression of the *distal* ureters is used to prolong filling of the renal pelvis and calyces. Compression of the *proximal* ureters is not advocated.

F. CENTRAL NERVOUS SYSTEM

1. Introduction. The central nervous system (CNS) is composed of the *brain* and *spinal cord* (Fig. 7–113), enclosed within the bony skull and vertebral column. The brain consists of the cerebrum (largest part), *cerebellum, pons varolii,* and *medulla oblongata.* The *gray matter* of the brain consists of neuron cell bodies; the *white matter* consists of tracts (pathways) of axons. In transverse section, the spinal cord is seen to have an H-shaped configuration of gray matter internally, surrounded by white matter (Fig. 7–114). The brain and spinal cord work together in the perception of sensory stimuli, in integration and correlation of stimuli with memory, and in neural actions resulting in coordinated motor responses to stimuli.

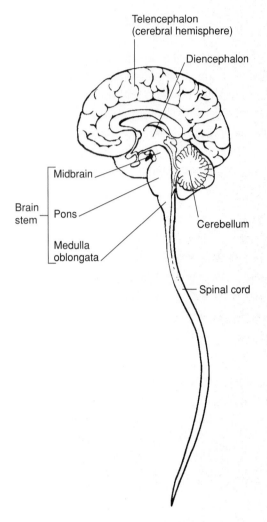

Telencephalon
(cerebral hemisphere)

Diencephalon

Midbrain

Brain
stem

Pons

Medulla
oblongata

Cerebellum

Spinal cord

Figure 7–113. The CNS: brain and spinal cord.

The CNS is enclosed within three tissue membranes, the *meninges.* The *pia mater* is the innermost, vascular membrane, which is closely attached to the brain and spinal cord. The *arachnoid mater* is a thin layer outside the pia mater and attached to it by web-like fibers. The *subarachnoid space* is between the pia and arachnoid mater and is filled with cerebrospinal fluid (CSF). The brain and spinal cord float in CSF, which acts as a shock absorber. **Cerebral artery hemorrhage** will leak blood into the CSF. *Lumbar puncture* is performed (between L3 and L4 or L4 and L5) to remove small quantities of CSF for testing and to introduce contrast medium during myelography. The *dura mater* is a double-layered fibrous membrane outside the arachnoid mater. The *subdural space* is located between the arachnoid and dura mater; it does not contain CSF. The *epidural space* is located between the two layers of dura mater.

The cylindrical spinal cord is a continuation of the medulla oblongata, extending through the foramen magnum and spinal canal to its termination at the *conus medullaris* (about the level of L1). The lumbar and sacral nerves have long roots that extend from the spinal cord as the *cauda equina* (horse's tail).

2. Procedures. Routine radiographic examination of the bony components of the CNS includes studies of the skull and vertebral column and, occasionally, tomography of these structures. Computerized tomography (CT) and magnetic resonance imaging (MRI) procedures have replaced many plain radiographic procedures in the diagnosis and management of traumatic injuries and pathologic processes of the brain and spinal cord.

3. Myelogram. Nevertheless, *myelography* remains a valuable diagnostic tool to demonstrate the site and extent of **spinal cord tumors** and **herniated intervertebral discs.** Rupture of an intervertebral disc can be caused by trauma or degeneration. The *nucleus pulposus* protrudes posteriorly through a tear in the *annulus fibrosus* and impinges on nerve roots (Fig. 7–115). Over 90% of disc ruptures occur at the L4–L5 and L5–S1 interspaces. Narrowing of the affected disc space may often be detected radiographically and the defects caused by the rupture can generally be demonstrated through myelography, CT, or MRI.

Water-soluble nonionic iodinated contrast agents are the most widely used contrast media for myelography. Advantages of water-soluble contrast agents (over non–water-soluble) include better visualization of the nerve roots (see Fig. 7–116 on p. 208) and absorption properties that allow it to be left in the subarachnoid space after the examination (because it is easily absorbed by the body). However, the use of water-soluble contrast agents for myelography does require that radiographs be made accurately and without delay, because it is absorbed fairly quickly.

Foot and shoulder supports must be securely attached to the x-ray table. The patient should receive a complete explanation of the examination and must be instructed about the importance of keeping his or her chin extended when the table is lowered into the Trendelenburg position.

A lumbar puncture is performed (usually at the fourth intervertebral space with the patient in the prone or flexed lateral position), a small quantity of CSF is removed from the subarachnoid space and sent to the laboratory for testing, and an equal amount of contrast agent is injected. The position of the contrast column will change according to gravitational forces, and its movement is observed fluoroscopically as the x-ray table is angled to varying degrees of Trendelenburg and Fowler's positions. Fluoroscopic spot films are taken as needed, followed by overhead radiographs. Routine protocol generally includes an AP or PA and a horizontal beam (cross-table) lateral view of the vertebral area examined.

4. Terminology and Pathology.

The following is a list of radiographically significant CNS conditions with which the student radiographer should be familiar.

Degenerative disc disease	Parkinson disease
Herniated nucleus pulposus	Meningitis
Hydrocephalus	Meningomyelocele
Meningioma	Spondylosis

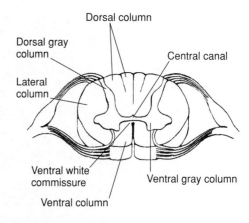

Figure 7–114. Cross-section of the spinal cord.

G. CIRCULATORY SYSTEM

1. Introduction.

The circulatory system consists of the *heart* and vessels (arteries, capillaries, veins) that distribute blood throughout the body (see Fig. 7–117 on p. 209). The heart is the muscular pump, the *arteries* conduct oxygenated blood throughout the body; the *capillaries* are responsible for diffusion of gases and exchange of nutrients and wastes; and the *veins* collect deoxygenated blood and return it to the heart and lungs. Contraction of the heart muscle as it pumps blood is called *systole;* relaxation is called *diastole;* these values are measured with a *sphygmomanometer.* Accompanying the contraction and expansion of the heart is contraction and expansion of arterial walls—called *pulse.*

The heart wall is made up of the external *epicardium,* the middle *myocardium,* and the internal *endocardium.* The *pericardium* is the fibroserous sac enclosing the heart and roots of the great vessels. The heart has four chambers. The two upper chambers are the *atria,* and the two lower chambers are the *ventricles.* The apex of the heart is the tip of the left ventricle.

Venous blood is returned to the right atrium of the heart via the *superior* (from the upper part of the body) and *inferior* (from the lower body) *vena cavae* and the *coronary sinus* (from the heart substance; see Fig. 7–118 on p. 210). Upon atrial systole, the blood passes through the *tricuspid valve* into the right ventricle. During ventricular systole, the blood is pumped through the *pulmonary semilunar valve* into the *pulmonary artery* (the only artery to carry deoxygenated blood) to the lungs for oxygenation. Blood is returned via the *pulmonary veins* (the only veins to carry oxygenated blood) to the left atrium. During atrial systole, blood passes through the *mitral* (bicuspid) *valve* into the left ventricle. During ventricular systole, the oxygenated blood is pumped through the *aortic semilunar valve* into the aorta. When blood pressure is reported, as for example "130 over 85," the top number (130) represents the systolic pressure and the lower number (85) represents the diastolic pressure.

Figure 7–115. Myelograms demonstrating herniated L4–L5 disc. (Reproduced with permission from deGroot, J. *Correlative Neuroanatomy,* 21st ed. East Norwalk, CT: Appleton & Lange, 1991.)

A

B

Figure 7–116. **(A)** Non–water-soluble contrast (Pantopaque) myelography. **(B)** Water-soluble contrast myelography; observe improved visualization of nerve roots seen at the level of each pedicle as linear radiolucencies within the small inferolateral extensions of the contrast agent. (**(A)** courtesy of the Stamford Hospital; **(B)** from the American College of Radiology Learning File. Courtesy of the ACR.)

The *aorta* is the trunk artery of the body; it is divided into the ascending aorta, aortic arch (Fig. 7–119), descending thoracic aorta, and abdominal aorta. Many arteries arise from the aorta to supply destinations throughout the body. The *superior* and *inferior vena cavae* and the *coronary sinus* are the major veins, collecting venous blood from the upper and lower body areas and heart substance respectively. The formation of sclerotic plaques (as in **atherosclerosis**) and other conditions that impair the flow of blood can lead to ▶ *ischemia* and tissue *infarction*. Atherosclerosis of the coronary arteries can cause **angina pectoris** and **myocardial infarction.**

The four divisions of the aorta and their major branches are the following.

Ascending Aorta

- L and R coronary arteries

Aortic Arch (Fig. 7–119)

- Brachiocephalic (innominate) artery gives rise to:
- R common carotid artery

Pulmonary Circulation
- Unoxygenated blood from the right side of the heart is directed to the lungs for oxygenation, then to the left side of the heart.

Systemic Circulation
- Oxygenated blood from the left side of the heart is pumped to the body tissues then back to the right side of the heart.

Figure 7–117. The major arteries of the cardiovascular system.

Figure 7–118. The four chambers of the heart and the major blood vessels. Directions of blood flow are indicated.

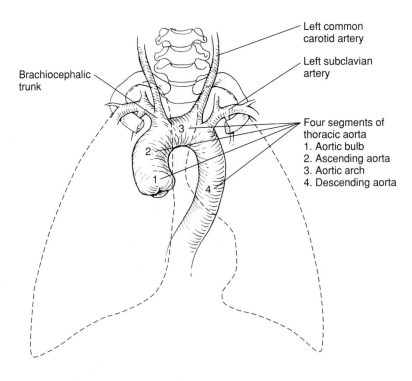

Figure 7–119. Thoracic aorta illustrating major branches of aortic arch.

- R subclavian artery
- L common carotid artery
- L subclavian artery

Thoracic Aorta

- Intercostal arteries
- Superior phrenic arteries
- Bronchial arteries
- Esophageal arteries

Abdominal Aorta

- Inferior phrenic arteries
- Celiac (axis) artery gives rise to:
- Common hepatic artery
- L gastric artery
- Splenic artery
- Superior mesenteric artery
- Suprarenal arteries
- Renal arteries
- Gonadal arteries (testicular or ovarian)
- Inferior mesenteric artery
- Common iliac arteries give rise to lower extremity arteries:
    - Internal iliac arteries
    - External iliac (hypogastric) arteries

Arteries of the Lower Extremity:

- Internal iliac arteries
- External iliac arteries give rise to:
- femoral arteries give rise to:
- popliteal arteries give rise to:
- anterior tibial arteries
  and posterior tibial arteries
  give rise to:
    - dorsalis pedis arteries
    - posterior tibial arteries
- give rise to:
    - peroneal arteries
    - medial and lateral plantar arteries

Figure 7–120. Lower-extremity arteriogram demonstrating popliteal aneurysm. (Reproduced with permission from Way, LW, ed. *Current Surgical Diagnosis & Treatment*, 10th ed. East Norwalk, CT: Appleton & Lange, 1994.)

The majority of peripheral and visceral angiographic procedures are performed in a specially equipped angiographic suite by cardiovascular-interventional technologists (Figs. 7–120 and 7–121). Many cardiovascular suites today have equipment available for digital subtraction angiography (DSA). *Subtraction* is a technique that removes unnecessary structures such as bone from superimposition on contrast-filled blood vessels. DSA is subtraction achieved by means of a computer, which can also permit manipulation of contrast and other image characteristics by the technologist. The student radiographer, while not performing most of these examinations, should be familiar with the names of the most common procedures and the conditions and disorders for which they are performed.

2. Venogram.

The one vascular procedure that is still commonly performed in general radiography is the lower extremity *venogram*

Figure 7–121. The renal arteriogram is one of many types of procedures performed by specially trained teams of health care professionals. (From the American College of Radiology Learning File. Courtesy of the ACR.)

Figure 7–122. AP projection of a lower extremity venogram demonstrating multiple intraluminal filling defects. (Way, LW, ed. *Current Surgical Diagnosis & Treatment,* 10th ed. East Norwalk, CT: Appleton & Lange, 1994.)

(Fig. 7–122). This examination is generally performed to confirm a suspected deep vein thrombosis in an effort to avoid the complications of a pulmonary embolism.

The patient should be examined on a radiographic table that can be tilted to a semierect position of at least 45°. Tourniquets are used to force contrast medium into the deep veins. Sterile technique must be rigorously maintained. An injection of 50 to 100 ml at 1 to 2 ml/sec is usually made through a superficial vein in the foot. Radiographs are made at about 5 to 10-sec intervals of the lower leg, thigh, and pelvis.

3. Terminology and Pathology. The following is a list of radiographically significant circulatory conditions with which the student radiographer should be familiar.

Aneurysm
Angina pectoris
Atherosclerosis
Atrial septal defect
CVA (Cerebrovascular accident)
Coarctation of aorta
Congestive heart failure
Coronary artery disease
Hypertension
Myocardial infarction

Patent ductus arteriosus
Pericardial effusion
Phlebitis
Pulmonary edema
Pulmonary embolism
Rheumatic heart disease
Tetrology of Fallot
Thrombophlebitis
Ventricular septal defect

A&U Chapter Review Questions

☆ *Congratulations! You have completed your review of a large portion of this chapter. You may go on to the "Registry-type" multiple-choice questions that follow. For greatest success, be sure also to complete the short answer questions found at the end of this chapter.*

1. Which of the following statements regarding myelography is (are) correct?
    1. spinal puncture can be performed in the prone or flexed lateral position
    2. contrast medium distribution is regulated through table angulation
    3. the patient's head must be in acute flexion during Trendelenburg positions
   (A) 1 only
   (B) 1 and 2 only
   (C) 1 and 3 only
   (D) 1, 2, and 3

2. The contraction and expansion of arterial walls in accordance with forceful contraction and relaxation of the heart is called:
   (A) hypertension
   (B) elasticity
   (C) pulse
   (D) pressure

3. The method by which contrast-filled vascular images are removed from superimposition upon bone is called:
   (A) positive masking
   (B) reversal
   (C) subtraction
   (D) registration

4. Indicate the correct sequence of oxygenated blood as it returns from the lungs to the heart:
   (A) pulmonary veins, left atrium, left ventricle, aortic valve
   (B) pulmonary artery, left atrium, left ventricle, aortic valve
   (C) pulmonary veins, right atrium, right ventricle, pulmonary semilunar valve
   (D) pulmonary artery, right atrium, right ventricle, pulmonary semilunar valve

5. In myelography, the contrast medium is generally injected into the:
   (A) cisterna magna
   (B) individual intervertebral discs
   (C) subarachnoid space between the first and second lumbar vertebrae
   (D) subarachnoid space between the third and fourth lumbar vertebrae

6. Lower extremity venography requires an injection of iodinated contrast medium into the:
   (A) superficial veins of the foot
   (B) deep veins of the foot
   (C) femoral vein
   (D) popliteal vein

7. Myelography is a diagnostic examination used to demonstrate:
    1. posterior protrusion of herniated intervertebral disc
    2. anterior protrusion of herniated intervertebral disc
    3. internal disc lesions
    (A) 1 only
    (B) 2 only
    (C) 1 and 2 only
    (D) 1 and 3 only

8. The four major arteries supplying the brain include the:
    1. brachiocephalic artery
    2. common carotid arteries
    3. vertebral arteries
    (A) 1 and 2 only
    (B) 1 and 3 only
    (C) 2 and 3 only
    (D) 1, 2, and 3

9. Which of the following statements is (are) true regarding lower extremity venography?
    1. the patient is often examined in the semi-erect position
    2. tourniquets are used to force contrast medium into the deep veins
    3. all radiographs are AP projections
    (A) 1 only
    (B) 1 and 2 only
    (C) 1 and 3 only
    (D) 1, 2, and 3

10. The apex of the heart is formed by the:
    (A) left atrium
    (B) right atrium
    (C) left ventricle
    (D) right ventricle

Answers and Explanations

1. (B) Myelography is the radiologic examination of structures within the spinal canal. Opaque contrast medium is usually used. Following injection, the contrast medium is distributed to the vertebral region of interest by gravity; the x-ray table is angled Trendelenburg for visualization of the cervical region and in the Fowler's position for visualization of the thoracic and lumbar regions. While the table is Trendelenburg, care must be taken that the patient's head be kept in acute *extension* in order to compress the cisterna magna and keep contrast medium from traveling into the ventricles of the brain.

2. (C) As the heart contracts and relaxes while functioning to pump blood from the heart, those arteries that are large and those in closest proximity to the heart will feel the effect of the heart's forceful contractions in their walls. The arterial walls pulsate in unison with the heart's contractions. This movement may be detected with the fingers in various parts of the body, and is referred to as the *pulse.*

3. (C) Superimposition of bony details frequently make angiographic demonstration of blood vessels less than optimal. The method used to remove these superimposed bony details is called *subtraction. Digital* subtraction can accomplish this through the use of a computer, but *photographic* subtraction may also be performed using films from an angiographic series. *Registration* is the process of matching one series image exactly over another. A reversal film, or *positive mask,* is a reverse of the black and white radiographic tones, obtained using special single emulsion film.

4. (A) Deoxygenated blood is returned by way of the inferior and superior vena cava to the right side of the heart. The blood is emptied into the right atrium, passes through the tricuspid valve, and enters the right ventricle. It is forced through the pulmonary semilunar valve into the pulmonary artery (by contraction of the right ventricle) and passes to the lungs for reoxygenation. From the lungs it is collected by the *pulmonary veins,* which carry the oxygenated blood to the *left atrium,* where it travels through the mitral valve into the *left ventricle.* Upon contraction of the left ventricle, blood passes through the *aortic valve* into the aorta and to all parts of the body.

5. (D) Generally, contrast medium is injected into the subarachnoid space between the 3rd and 4th lumbar vertebrae. Since the spinal cord ends at the level of the 1st or 2nd lumbar vertebrae, this is considered to be a relatively safe injection site. The cisterna magna can be used, but the risk of contrast entering and causing side effects increases.

6. (A) Lower extremity venography requires an injection of contrast medium into the superficial veins of the foot. The skin on top of the patient's foot is very sensitive and every precaution should be taken to minimize the pain involved. Explain the procedure fully and soak the foot in warm water to make the veins more accessible for injection.

7. (A) Rupture of an intervertebral disc can be caused by trauma or degeneration. The nucleus pulposus protrudes *posteriorly* through a tear in the annulus fibrosus and impinges on nerve roots and can be demonstrated by placing positive or negative contrast media into the subarachnoid space. Internal disc lesions can only be demonstrated by injecting contrast into the individual discs (this procedure is termed *discography*). Anterior protrusion of a herniated intervertebral disc does not impinge on the spinal cord, and is not demonstrated in myelography.

8. (C) Major branches of the common carotid arteries (internal carotids) function to supply the anterior brain, while the posterior brain is supplied by the vertebral arteries (branches of the subclavian arteries). The brachiocephalic (innominate) artery is unpaired and is one of three branches of the aortic arch, from which the right common carotid artery is derived. The left common carotid artery comes directly off the aortic arch.

9. (B) To increase the concentration of contrast medium in the deep veins of the leg, a Fowler's position is used with the table angle approximately 45°. Tourniquets can also be used to force the contrast into the deep veins of the leg. Filming may be performed with or without fluoroscopy and may include AP, lateral, and 30° obliques of the lower leg in internal rotation.

10. (C) The heart wall is made up of the external epicardium, the middle myocardium, and the internal endocardium. The pericardium is the fibroserous sac enclosing the heart and roots of the great vessels. The heart has four chambers. The two upper chambers are the atria, and the two lower chambers are the ventricles. The *apex* of the heart is the tip of the left ventricle.

Chapter Exercises

 Congratulations! *You have completed the entire chapter. If you are able to answer the following group of very comprehensive questions, you should feel confident that you have really mastered this section. You can refer back to the indicated pages to check your answers and/or review the subject matter.*

1. Identify the bony structures composing the appendicular skeleton *(pp. 89–94, 103–111).*

2. Describe the (a) method of positioning, (b) direction and point of entry of the CR, (c) principle structures visualized, and (d) pertinent traumatic or pathologic conditions and any technical adjustments they may necessitate relative to the appendicular skeleton, to include routine and special views of the:

    A. hand and wrist *(pp. 98, 99, 100)*

    B. forearm and elbow *(pp. 100, 101)*

    C. humerus and shoulder *(pp. 100, 101, 102)*

    D. clavicle and scapula *(pp. 103, 104, 105)*

    E. foot and ankle *(pp. 112, 113, 114)*

    F. lower leg and knee *(pp. 114, 115, 116, 117)*

    G. femur and hip *(pp. 118, 119)*

    H. pelvis and sacroiliac joints *(pp. 95, 119–120)*

    I. long bone measurement *(p. 121)*

    J. arthrography *(pp. 121, 122)*

3. Identify the bony structures comprising the axial skeleton *(pp. 129–131, 138–139, 141–149).*

4. Describe the (a) method of positioning, (b) direction and point of entry of the CR, (c) principle structures visualized, and (d) pertinent traumatic and pathologic conditions and any technical adjustments they may necessitate relative to the axial skeleton, to include routine and special views of the:

    A. cervical spine *(pp. 132–134)*

B. thoracic spine *(p. 134)*

C. lumbar spine *(p. 136)*

D. sacrum, coccyx *(p. 138)*

E. scoliosis series *(p. 139)*

F. sternum and ribs *(pp. 140–141)*

G. cranial and facial bones *(pp. 149–154)*

H. mastoids and petrous portions *(pp. 157–159)*

I. paranasal sinuses *(pp. 155–157)*

5. Identify the principle structures comprising the respiratory system and their function(s) *(pp. 163–164).*

6. Describe the (a) method of positioning, (b) direction and point of entry of the CR, (c) principle structures visualized, and (d) pertinent traumatic and pathologic conditions and any technical adjustments that may be required relative to the routine and special views of the chest (PA, lat, obl, lordotic, decubitus) and airway *(pp. 164–169).*

7. Identify the principle structures comprising the biliary system and their function(s) *(pp. 173–174).*

8. Describe the (a) method of positioning, (b) direction and point of entry of the CR, (c) principle structures visualized, and (d) pertinent traumatic and pathologic conditions and any technical adjustments that may be required relative to the routine and special views of the biliary system, including:

A. OCG *(pp. 174–176)*

B. OR and T-tube cholangiograms *(p. 176)*

C. ERCP *(p. 176)*

9. Identify the principle structures comprising the digestive system and their function(s) *(pp. 177–180).*

10. Describe the (a) method of positioning, (b) direction and point of entry of the CR, (c) principle structures visualized, and (d) pertinent traumatic and pathologic conditions and any technical adjustments that may be required relative to the routine and special views of the digestive system, to include:

A. abdomen *(pp. 181–182)*

B. esophagus *(p. 184)*

C. stomach and small intestine *(pp. 184–186)*

D. large intestine *(pp. 186–188)*

11. Identify the principle structures comprising the urinary system and their function(s) *(pp. 192–194).*

12. Describe the (a) method of positioning, (b) direction and point of entry of the CR, (c) principle structures visualized, and (d) pertinent traumatic and pathologic conditions and any technical adjustments that may be required relative to the routine and special views of the urinary system, to include:

A. KUB *(pp. 196–197)*

B. retrograde examinations *(p. 196)*

C. compression *(p. 195)*

D. bladder *(pp. 197)*

13. Identify the principle structures comprising the female reproductive system and their function(s) *(pp. 198–201).*

14. Describe the (a) method of positioning, (b) direction and point of entry of the CR, (c) principle structures visualized, and (d) pertinent traumatic and pathologic conditions and any technical adjustments that may be required in hysterosalpingography *(pp. 198–201).*

15. Identify the principle structures comprising the CNS and their function(s) *(pp. 205–206).*

16. Describe the (a) method of positioning, (b) direction and point of entry of the CR, (c) principle structures visualized, and (d) pertinent traumatic and pathologic conditions and any technical adjustments that may be required in myelography *(pp. 206–208).*

17. Identify the principle structures comprising the circulatory system and their function(s) *(pp. 207, 209, 210).*

18. List the kinds of specialized examinations that might be performed to demonstrate various traumatic and pathologic conditions of the circulatory system *(pp. 211–212).*

part
III

Radiation Protection

Radiation Protection Considerations

I. IONIZING EFFECTS OF X-RAYS

A. ELECTROMAGNETIC RADIATION

A review of electromagnetic radiation and energy is essential to the study of x-rays and other forms of ionizing radiation. ***Electromagnetic*** ◄

221

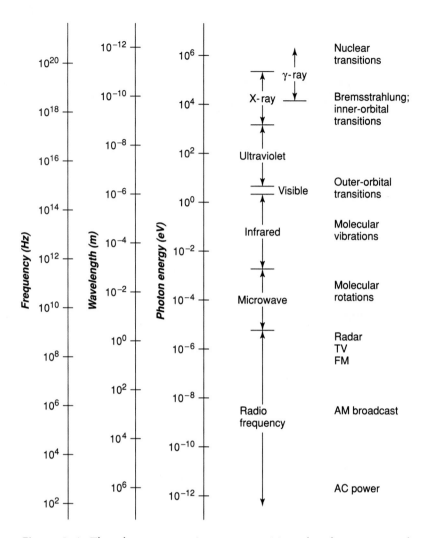

Figure 8–1. The electromagnetic spectrum. Note that frequency and photon energy are directly related and that they are inversely related to wavelength.

▶ **radiation** can be described as wavelike fluctuations of electric and magnetic fields. There are many kinds of electromagnetic radiation; Figure 8–1 illustrates that visible light, microwaves, and radio waves are within the *electromagnetic spectrum*. All the electromagnetic radiations have the same velocity, 186,000 miles per second; however, they differ greatly in wavelength.

▶   **Wavelength** refers to the distance between two consecutive
▶ wave crests (Fig. 8–2). **Frequency** refers to the number of cycles per second (cps); its unit of measure is the *hertz* (Hz), which is equal to 1 cps.

Frequency and wavelength are closely associated with the relative *energy* of electromagnetic radiations. More energetic radiations have shorter wavelengths and higher frequency. The relationship among frequency, wavelength, and energy is illustrated in the electromagnetic spectrum (Fig. 8–1). Some radiations are energetic

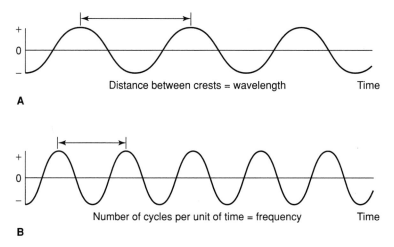

Figure 8–2. Wavelength versus frequency. *Wavelength* is described as the distance between successive crests. The shorter the wavelength, the more crests/cycles per unit of time (eg, per second). Therefore, the shorter the wavelength the greater the *frequency* (number of cycles/second). Wavelength and frequency are inversely related.

enough to rearrange atoms in materials through which they pass, and can therefore be hazardous to living tissue.

Some radiations are called *ionizing* because they have the energetic potential to break apart electrically neutral atoms, resulting in the production of negative and positive **ions.** Humans have always been exposed to ionizing radiation. Some ionizing radiations (such as those emitted by uranium) occur naturally in the earth's crust and in its atmosphere (from the sun and cosmic reactions in space). These radiations are present in the structures in which we live and in the food we consume; radioactive gas is present in the air that we breathe, and there are traces of radioactive materials in our bodies themselves. These radiations are referred to as **natural background** (environmental) **radiation.** The levels of natural background radiation vary greatly from one location to another. The greatest portion of our exposure to background radiation comes from naturally occurring sources such as these.

In addition to background radiation, we are also exposed to sources of radiation created by humans. *Artificial,* or **man-made** **radiation** includes sources such as medical and dental x-rays, nuclear testing fallout, and radiation associated with nuclear power plants. Figure 8–3 illustrates the approximate quantity of radiation received from natural and man-made sources.

X-ray **photons** are infinitesimal bundles of energy that deposit some of their energy within matter as they travel through it. This deposition of energy and subsequent **ionization** has the potential to cause chemical and biologic damage.

B. PRODUCTION OF X-RAYS AT THE TUNGSTEN TARGET

Diagnostic x-rays are produced within the x-ray tube as high speed **electrons** are rapidly decelerated by the tungsten target. The source of electrons is the heated cathode filament; they are driven across to

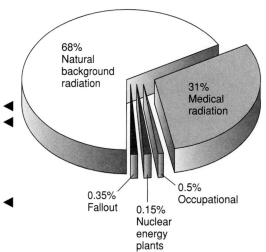

Figure 8–3. The population's exposure to various sources of radiation. Natural background radiation (the earth, the sun, building materials) compose the majority of our exposure. Medical irradiation is the largest portion of our exposure to man-made sources of radiation. Occupational radiation, nuclear energy, and fallout are responsible for only a minute portion of our total exposure.

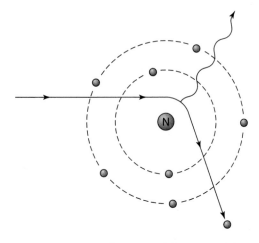

Figure 8–4. Production of bremsstrahlung (brems) radiation. A high-speed electron is deflected from its path and the loss of kinetic energy is emitted in the form of an x-ray photon.

the anode focal spot when high voltage (kVp) is applied. When the high speed electrons are suddenly stopped at the focal spot, their kinetic energy is converted to x-ray photon energy. This happens in two ways.

1. Bremsstrahlung (Brems) or "braking" **radiation.** A high speed electron, passing through a tungsten atom is attracted (braked) by the positively charged nucleus, and therefore is deflected from its course with a resulting loss of energy. This energy loss is given up in the form of an x-ray photon (Fig. 8–4). The electron may not give up all its kinetic energy in one such interaction; it may go on to have several more interactions deeper in the target, each time giving up an x-ray photon having less and less energy. This is one reason the x-ray beam is heterogeneous (ie, has a spectrum of energies). Brems radiation comprises 70 to 90% of the x-ray beam.

2. Characteristic radiation. In this case, a high speed electron encounters the tungsten atom and ejects a K-shell electron (Fig. 8–5A), leaving a vacancy in the K shell (Fig. 8–5B). An electron from the shell above (that is, the L shell) fills the vacancy and in doing so emits a K *characteristic ray* (Fig. 8–5C). The energy of the characteristic ray is equal to the difference in energy between the K and L shell.

C. BASIC INTERACTIONS BETWEEN X-RAY PHOTONS AND MATTER

The gradual decrease in exposure rate as radiation passes through tissues is called *attenuation.* Attenuation is principally attributable to the two major types of interactions that occur between x-ray photons and tissue in the diagnostic range.

1. In the *photoelectric effect,* a relatively *low* energy (low kVp) x-ray photon uses all its energy (true absorption) to eject an *inner shell* electron, leaving an orbital vacancy. An electron from the shell above drops down to fill the vacancy and, in doing so, gives up energy in the form of a *characteristic ray* (Fig. 8–6).

The photoelectric effect is more likely to occur in absorbers of high *atomic number* (eg, bone, positive contrast media) and contributes significantly to patient dose, as all the photon energy is absorbed by the patient (and for the latter reason, is responsible for the production of short-scale contrast).

2. In *Compton scatter,* a fairly *high* energy (high kVp) x-ray photon ejects an *outer shell* electron (Fig. 8–7). Though the x-ray photon is deflected with somewhat reduced energy (modified scatter), it retains most of its original energy and exits the body as an energetic scattered photon.

Since the scattered photon exits the body, it does not pose a radiation hazard to the patient. It can, however, contribute to *film fog* and pose a *radiation hazard to personnel* (as in fluoroscopic procedures).

Summary

- **The radiations of the electromagnetic spectrum all travel at the same velocity, 186,000 mps, but differ in wavelength.**
- **Wavelength is the distance between two consecutive wave crests.**

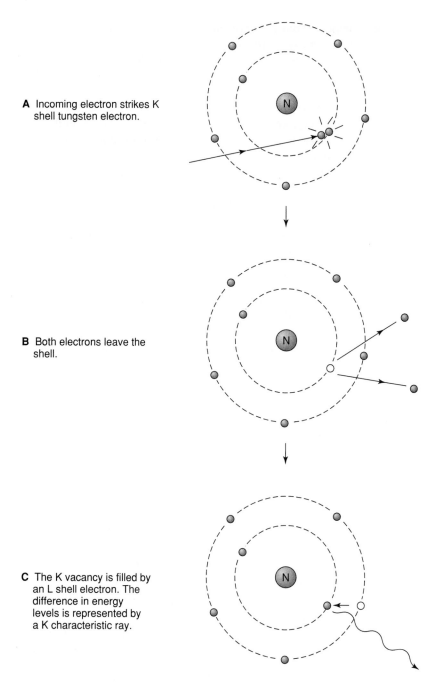

A Incoming electron strikes K shell tungsten electron.

B Both electrons leave the shell.

C The K vacancy is filled by an L shell electron. The difference in energy levels is represented by a K characteristic ray.

Figure 8–5. Production of characteristic radiation. A high speed electron (**A**) ejects a tungsten K-shell electron, leaving a K shell vacancy (**B**). An electron from the L shell fills the vacancy and emits a K characteristic ray (**C**).

- The number of cycles and crests per second is frequency; its unit of measure is the Hz.
- Wavelength and frequency are inversely related.
- Natural background and artificial (man-made) are the two kinds of radiation sources; natural sources account for the largest human exposure to radiation.

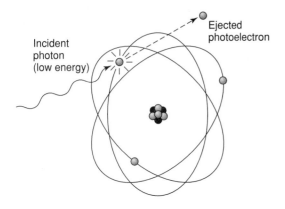

Figure 8–6. In the photoelectric effect, the incoming (low energy) photon releases all its energy as it ejects an inner shell electron from orbit.

- Medical radiation exposure is the largest source of artificial radiation exposure for humans.
- Ionization is caused by high-energy, short-wavelength electromagnetic radiations that break apart electrically neutral atoms.
  - Two types of radiation are produced at the anode through energy conversion processes: brems and characteristic radiation; brems radiation predominates.
- Characteristics of photoelectric effect:
  - Low-energy x-ray photon gives up all its energy ejecting an inner shell electron.
  - Produces a characteristic ray.
  - Major contributor to patient dose.
  - Occurs in absorbers of high atomic number.
  - Produces short-scale contrast.
- Characteristics of Compton scatter:
  - High-energy x-ray photon uses a portion of its energy to eject an outer shell electron.
  - Responsible for scattered-radiation film fog.
  - Radiation hazard to personnel.
- Exposure dose depends on the type of interaction between x-ray photons and tissue and attenuation, therefore, is affected by radiation quality and the subject being irradiated (ie, thickness and nature of part).

II. DOSE–RESPONSE RELATIONSHIP

A. DOSE–RESPONSE CURVES

The association between a dose of ionizing radiation and the magnitude of the resulting response or effect is referred to as a
▶ *dose–response relationship.*

Dose–response, or dose–effect, curves are used to illustrate the relationship between exposure to ionizing radiation and possible biologic effects (Fig. 8–8). The two most frequently utilized dose–response curves in radiation protection are the *linear, nonthreshold* and the *linear, threshold.* The Committee on Biologic Effects of Ionizing Radiation (BEIR) has evaluated the linear and linear quadratic

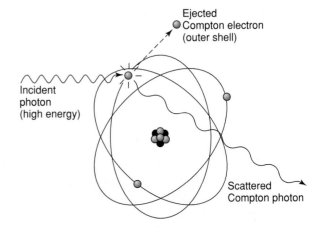

Figure 8–7. In the Compton scatter process the incoming (high energy) photon uses part of its energy to eject an outer shell electron; in doing so, the photon changes direction (scatters) and retains much of its original energy.

nonthreshold curves and has pronounced the linear nonthreshold curve (the more conservative of the two) as the curve of choice for radiation protection standards.

B. LINEAR, NONTHRESHOLD

The linear, nonthreshold curve is used to illustrate responses such as leukemia, cancer, and genetic effects. These are sometimes referred to as **stochastic effects.** Stochastic effects occur randomly and are "all-or-nothing" type effects, that is, they do not occur with degrees of severity. It must be noted that *in a nonthreshold curve there is no safe dose,* that is, no dose below which there will definitely be no biologic response. Theoretically, even one x-ray photon can cause a biologic response. This is the curve of choice to predict effects of low level (eg, medical and occupational) exposure to ionizing radiation.

C. LINEAR, THRESHOLD

A linear, threshold curve illustrates that a certain dose of ionizing radiation must be received before an effect will be manifested, ie, there is a **threshold** dose—a dose below which no biologic effects are likely to occur. This is the case in somatic conditions such as skin erythema. These effects are predictable and sometimes referred to as **nonstochastic effects.**

D. LATE (LONG-TERM) EFFECTS

Occupationally exposed individuals are concerned principally with *late* (ie, *long term,* or *delayed*) effects of radiation, such as **genetic** **effects,** *leukemia,* and *cancers,* which can occur many years following initial exposure to low levels of ionizing radiation. These long-term, or delayed, effects are represented by the linear, nonthreshold dose–response curve. History provides us with many examples of the delayed effects of ionizing radiation: many of the early radiologists and radiation scientists, A-bomb survivors of Hiroshima and Nagasaki, and ankylosing spondylitis patients in Great Britain in the 1940s developed leukemia and other life-span–shortening diseases as a result of exposure to varying quantities of radiation over a period of time. Some children irradiated in the 1940s for enlarged thymus glands developed thyroid cancer as adults 20 years later. Many radium watch-dial painters in the 1920s developed a variety of bone cancers following a latent period of 20 to 30 years. These are all delayed effects of radiation and are represented by the linear, nonthreshold dose–response curve.

Cataractogenesis is another late effect of exposure to ionizing radiation, but is represented by the linear, threshold dose–response curve. An acute dose of about 200 **rad** would be required to cause radiogenic cataracts. A far greater occupational (ie, fractionated) dose of about 1000 rad would be required to induce cataracts.

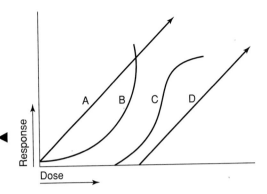

Figure 8–8. Dose–response curves. **(A)** Linear, nonthreshold curve. **(B)** Nonlinear, nonthreshold curve. **(C)** Nonlinear, threshold curve. **(D)** Linear, threshold curve.

Summary

- **Ionization of living tissue can cause chemical and biologic damage to somatic and/or genetic cells.**
- **A nonthreshold dose–response curve indicates that there is no safe dose of radiation below which there will be no effects.**

- The linear, nonthreshold dose–response curve illustrates stochastic responses (cancer, genetic effects) and is the curve of choice for occupational exposure.
- Occupationally exposed workers are concerned with late effects of radiation such as carcinogenesis, cataractogenesis, and life-span shortening.

III. BIOLOGIC EFFECTS OF RADIATION

Before beginning our review of somatic and genetic effects of radiation, a brief review of **radiobiology** is in order. Radiobiology is the study of the effects of ionizing radiation on biologic material at the cellular level.

A. LAW OF BERGONIÉ AND TRIBONDEAU

Two scientists, Bergonié and Tribondeau, proposed in 1906 that certain cellular qualities made tissues more or less radiosensitive. The Law of Bergonié and Tribondeau states that the following cells are particularly radiosensitive:

1. Young, immature cells
2. Stem (undifferentiated, or precursor) cells
3. Highly mitotic cells

Thus, very young cells, stem cells, and cells having the most reproductive activity are highly **radiosensitive.** An example of highly radiosensitive tissue is that of the rapidly developing embryo and fetus.

B. QUALITY FACTOR

Ionization causes the removal of electrons from some atoms and the addition of electrons to other atoms. Thus the stage is set for biologic effects; as a result of the ionization, appropriate chemical bonds cannot be maintained.

Similar absorbed doses of *different kinds* of radiation can cause different biologic effects. A *quality factor* **(QF)** is a number assigned to different types of ionizing radiations so that their effect(s) may be better determined. The QF accounts for differences in biologic effect between different kinds of radiation. For example, to equate the rad with the **rem,** the following formula is used.

$$rad \times QF = rem$$

C. LINEAR ENERGY TRANSFER VERSUS BIOLOGIC DAMAGE

Radiation deposits energy as it passes through tissue. The rate at which this occurs is described as *linear energy transfer* **(LET).** LET is another means of expressing radiation quality and determining QF; it expresses the ability of radiation to do damage. *Diagnostic x-rays are considered low LET radiation.* The more penetrating the radiation, the lower the LET and QF. As the LET of radiation increases, the radiation's ability to produce biological damage also increases. This is described quantitatively by *relative biologic effectiveness* **(RBE).** LET and RBE are directly related.

NCRP Recommended QF Values	
Type of Radiation	**QF**
χ	1
β	1
γ	1
thermal neutrons	5
α	20
protons	20

Energy transferred to tissue can cause molecular damage. The manifestation of that damage will depend on the extent of molecular disruption and the type of tissue affected.

D. Molecular Effects of Radiation

The interactions that serve to form the radiologic image, the photoelectric effect and Compton scatter, are ionization processes producing photoelectrons and ***recoil electrons*** that traverse tissue and subsequently ionize molecules. This action can lead to molecular damage in the form of *impaired function* or *cell death*.

1. Direct Effect. The two major types of effects that occur are the ***direct effect*** and the ***indirect effect.*** The direct effect usually ◄ occurs with high LET radiations and when ionization occurs at the DNA molecule.

2. Indirect Effect. The indirect effect (which occurs most frequently) happens when the ionization takes place remote from the DNA molecule, but the energy from the interaction is transferred to the molecule via a *free radical* (formed by radiolysis of cellular water).

Damage to the DNA molecule can be varied. A single-strand break on the DNA molecule is *repairable*. A double-strand break, widely spaced, may repair with difficulty or may result in *cell death*. A double-strand break on the same "rung" of the DNA ladder results in *irreparable* damage or *cell death*. Damage to the nitrogenous bases results in alteration of base sequence, causing a cell ***mutation.*** ◄ Any subsequent divisions result in daughter cells with incorrect genetic information.

E. Cellular Radiosensitivity

These types of molecular damage can occur to any of the ***somatic*** ◄ cells or to genetic cells. For example, high levels of radiation exposure to the bone marrow (where blood cells are produced) can cause a decrease in the number of circulating blood cells. *Lymphocytes,* a type of white blood cell that play an important role in the immune system, are particularly radiosensitive. If lymphocytes suffer radiation damage, the body loses its ability to fight infection and becomes more susceptible to disease.

Epithelial tissue, which lines the respiratory system and intestines, is also a highly radiosensitive tissue. In contrast, muscle and nervous tissue are comparatively insensitive to radiation. Because nerve cells in the adult do not undergo mitosis, they comprise the most ***radioresistant*** somatic tissue. However, nervous tis- ◄ sue *in the fetus* (particularly the second to eighth week) is highly mitotic and hence, highly *radiosensitive*.

The *genetic cells* of the gonads are considered especially radiosensitive tissues. Exposure to ionizing radiation can cause temporary or permanent sterility or mutations in succeeding generations. In particular, the reproductive cells of the fetus and young children are exceptionally radiosensitive. Other factors that determine tissue response to irradiation include the following.

1. ***Fractionation***/protraction: The longer the period of ◄ time over which a dose of radiation is delivered, the less its effect. (The greatest effect of irradiation will be

observed if a *large quantity* of radiation is delivered in a *short time* to the whole body.)

2. Oxygen: The greater the oxygen content of tissues, the greater their radiosensitivity.

3. Age: Fetal tissue is most radiosensitive. As the individual ages, tissue sensitivity decreases. Radiosensitivity increases again in old age, but only slightly.

It is well established that sufficient quantities of ionizing radiation can cause a number of serious *somatic* and/or *genetic* effects. What is not clear, however, are the long term effects of low-level (diagnostic and occupational) x-radiation.

Health care professionals involved in prescribing and delivering radiologic examinations have an obligation to keep nonproductive radiation exposure to all individuals as low as possible. Possible abusive overuse of radiologic (and other diagnostic) examinations is currently being scrutinized by many health care facilities as part of a continuous quality improvement (CQI) program. Some formerly routine examinations are now considered excessive and unnecessary, eg, routine chest x-ray films on admission to the hospital are no longer performed unless the patient is admitted to the pulmonary medicine or surgical service; pre-employment chest and/or lumbar spine examinations are also considered to have little benefit. In states having no *licensure* requirements for radiographers, physicians and hospitals often assume the responsibility of hiring only credentialed radiographers. Participation in *quality assurance* ensures that imaging equipment is functioning optimally. Radiographers must consider patient dose when selecting exposure factors. One component of a radiographer's professionalism, as stated in the seventh principle of the *ARRT Code of Ethics,* is to consistently employ every means possible to decrease radiation exposure to the population.

▶ Radiographers must follow the ***ALARA*** principle (keeping exposure As Low As Reasonably Achievable) as they carry out their tasks. The radiologic facility must undergo appropriate radiation surveys. Staff must be properly oriented and regular inservice training on radiation safety must take place. Proper radiation monitoring and review of monthly radiation reports is essential.

Summary

- **The Law of Bergonié and Tribondeau states that the most radiosensitive cells are young, stem, and highly mitotic cells.**
- **LET is another means of expressing quality and determining QF.**
- **Identical absorbed doses of different kinds of radiation will cause different biologic effects, hence the need for a QF.**
- **Diagnostic x-radiation is low-energy, low-LET radiation.**
- **Radiation effect on cells is named according to the interaction site, namely: direct effect, indirect effect, radiolysis of water.**
- **The most radiosensitive cell is the lymphocyte.**
- **As radiation professionals, we are obligated to keep radiation exposure to our patients and ourselves ALARA.**

IV. GENETIC EFFECTS

A. PREGNANCY

There are a number of situations that require the radiographer's special attention. Irradiation during *pregnancy,* especially in early pregnancy, must be avoided. The fetus is particularly radiosensitive during the first trimester, during much of which time pregnancy may not even be suspected. Especially high-risk examinations include pelvis, hip, femur, lumbar spine, cystograms and urograms, upper GI series, barium enema examinations, and GB series.

During the first trimester, specifically the second to eighth week of pregnancy (ie, during major organogenesis), if the radiation dose is sufficient, fetal anomalies can be produced. *Skeletal anomalies* usually appear if irradiation occurs in the early part of this time period, and *neurologic anomalies* are formed in the latter part; *mental retardation* and childhood *malignant diseases,* such as cancers or leukemia, can also result from irradiation during the first trimester. Fetal irradiation during the second and third trimester is not likely to produce anomalies, but rather, with sufficient dose, some type of childhood malignant disease. Fetal irradiation during the first two weeks of gestation can result in *spontaneous abortion.*

It must be emphasized, however, that the likelihood of producing fetal anomalies at doses below 20 rad is exceedingly small and that most general diagnostic examinations are likely to deliver fetal doses of less than 1 to 2 rad.

B. FEMALES

1. LMP (Last Menstrual Period).   Therefore, in consideration of the potential risk, female patients of child-bearing age should be questioned regarding their *last menstrual period (**LMP**)* and the possibility of their being pregnant. ◄

2. Ten-day Rule. In addition to supporting the ALARA concept, many institutions also use the ***10-day rule*** as a guide for scheduling ◄ x-ray examinations, ie, they are scheduled during the first 10 days following the onset of the menstrual period because that is the time when the presence of a recently fertilized ovum is least likely.

Facilities offering radiologic services should make inquiries of their female patients regarding LMP and advise them of the risk associated with radiation exposure during pregnancy. In many institutions this information is part of a consent form that the patient signs prior to the radiologic examination. Most facilities will also post signs in waiting rooms, dressing rooms, and radiographic rooms cautioning the pregnant patient to advise the radiographer of her condition so that proper precautions may be taken.

Concern is occasionally expressed regarding dose received during diagnostic *mammography.* Yet the risk associated with the x-ray dose received is minimal compared to the benefits of early detection of breast cancer. The use of dedicated mammography equipment with screen–film technique performed by credentialed radiographers will deliver the lowest skin and glandular dose of any mammographic method available.

C. MALES

Due to location of the gonads and *shielding* restrictions thus imposed in the female patient, the female gonads (ovaries) receive more radiation exposure than the male gonads (testes) undergoing similar examinations. The ovaries lie within the abdominal cavity and frequently cannot be effectively shielded during abdominal, pelvic, and lumbar spine radiography. Therefore, they receive far more organ dose than the testes (which are located outside the abdominal cavity) during diagnostic examinations of the abdominal region (eg, lumbar spine, upper and lower GI, intravenous, or retrograde pyelography).

It is important to note that the ovarian stem cells, the oogonia, reproduce only during fetal life. During child-bearing years there are only 400 to 500 mature ova accessible for fertilization, ie, one ovum per menstrual cycle for each of the fertile years. The male germ cells, spermatogonia, are being produced continuously and longevity of fertility is quite different than in the female.

D. CHILDREN

The female oogonia of fetal life and early childhood, and male spermatogonia, are especially radiosensitive due to their immature stage of development, and therefore particular care should be taken to adequately shield the reproductive organs of pediatric patients. All too often a radiographer will conscientiously shield adult patients of reproductive age, but fail to consider children whose reproductive cells are particularly radiosensitive and whose reproductive lives are ahead of them.

Very sizable doses of radiation to children are also thought to be associated with increased incidence of leukemia and other radiation-induced malignancies. Examples of high-risk examinations might include pelvic and abdominal radiography and examinations requiring periodic follow-ups, such as scoliosis series. It is advisable to shield the hematopoietic bones of children to reduce radiation dose to blood-forming cells.

E. GSD (GENETICALLY SIGNIFICANT DOSE)

Each member of the world's population bears a particular genetic dose of radiation. Its sources include environmental exposure, radiation received for medical and dental purposes, and occupational exposure. The quantity of exposure to each individual depends on that individual's geographic location (environmental radiation and elevation of terrain), overall general health, the accessibility of health care, and the occupational worker's adherence to radiation protection guidelines. Generally speaking, the genetic dose to an *individual* is very small. Some individuals may receive no genetic dose in a given year, some individuals are past their reproductive years, some individuals will not or cannot bear children. Even if some individuals receive larger quantities of radiation exposure, its impact is "diluted" by the total number of population. This concept is referred
▶ to as *genetically significant dose (GSD),* defined as the average annual gonadal dose to the population of child-bearing age, and estimated to be 20 mrem.

It is appropriate to mention *repeat radiographs* at this time. Poor radiographs resulting from technical error (eg, incorrect positioning, improper selection of technical factors) or equipment malfunction must be repeated, thereby subjecting the patient to twice the necessary exposure dose. An exceedingly important feature with significant impact on patient dose is appropriate *collimation*. An important part of radiation protection, then, is care and attention to detail to avoid technical errors requiring repeat radiographs. Another component is a quality assurance program (through an ongoing preventative maintenance program and appropriate inservice education) that assures proper equipment function and compliance with established standards.

V. SOMATIC EFFECTS

Somatic effects of radiation are those that affect the irradiated body itself. Somatic effects are described as being *early* or *late,* depending on the length of time between irradiation and manifestation of effects.

Early somatic effects are manifested within minutes, hours, days, or weeks of irradiation and only occur following a very large dose of ionizing radiation. It must be emphasized that doses received from diagnostic radiologic procedures are not sufficient to produce these early effects. An exceedingly high dose of radiation delivered to the whole body in a short period of time is required to produce early somatic effects. Examples of such situations include the fairly recent nuclear reactor accident in Chernobyl and the atomic bomb explosions in Nagasaki and Hiroshima during World War II.

A. CARCINOGENESIS

Late somatic effects are those that can occur years after initial exposure, and are caused by low, chronic exposures. Occupationally exposed personnel are concerned with the late effects of radiation exposure. Some somatic effects like **carcinogenesis** have been ◄ mentioned earlier: the bone *malignancies* developed by the radium watch-dial painters, the thyroid cancers of the individuals irradiated as children for thymus enlargement, the leukemia eventually developed by patients whose pain from ankylosing spondylitis was relieved by irradiation, and the skin cancers developed by early radiology pioneers working so closely with the "unknown ray." These malignancies are also examples of somatic effects of radiation.

B. EMBRYOLOGIC EFFECTS

Embryologic effects are those experienced by the body of the ◄ developing embryo or fetus. Spontaneous abortion, skeletal or neurologic anomalies (mental retardation and microcephaly), and leukemia are examples of embryologic somatic effects.

C. CATARACTOGENESIS

Another example of somatic effects of radiation is *cataract* formation to the lenses of eyes of those individuals accidentally exposed to sufficient quantities of radiation (eg, early cyclotron experimentors).

D. LIFE-SPAN SHORTENING

The lives of many of the early radiation workers were several years shorter than the lives of the general population. Statistics revealed that radiologists, for example, had a shorter life span than physicians of other specialties. *Life-span shortening,* then, *was* another somatic effect of radiation. Certainly, these effects should *never be experienced today.* So much has been learned about the biologic effects of radiation since its discovery and a part of what we have learned has, sadly, been as a result of the experiences of the radiology pioneers.

Summary

- Delivery of ionizing radiation during early pregnancy is particularly hazardous.
- There are five responses of concern to irradiation in utero: spontaneous abortion, congenital anomalies, mental retardation, microcephaly, and childhood malignancies.
- Female patients of childbearing age should be questioned regarding LMP and possible pregnancy.
- The 10-day rule may be employed to schedule elective radiography for female patients.
- Gonadal shielding is easier in the male patient because the reproductive organs are located externally.
- Genetic effects refer to damage to reproductive cells, affecting the reproductive capacity of the individual, or creating mutations that will be passed on to future generations.
- The genetic dose of radiation borne by each member of the reproductive population is called the genetically significant dose.
- Somatic effects include those manifesting themselves in the exposed individual and can be described as early or late effects.
  - Early somatic effects can occur only after a very large single exposure of radiation to the whole body.
  - Late somatic effects include carcinogenesis, cataractogenesis, embryologic effect, and life-span shortening.
- Occupationally exposed personnel are concerned with the late effects of radiation exposure.

Chapter Exercises

 Congratulations! *You have completed this chapter. If you are able to answer the following group of very comprehensive questions, you should feel confident that you have really mastered this section. You are then ready to go on to "Registry-type" questions that follow. For greatest success, do not go to the multiple choice questions without first completing the short answer questions below.*

1. List various kinds of electromagnetic radiation **(p. 222).**

2. Identify the way in which all electromagnetic radiations are similar and in what respect they differ **(p. 222).**

3. Define the terms *wavelength* and *frequency* **(p. 222).**

4. How are wavelength and energy related; frequency and energy **(p. 222).**

5. Describe what is meant by the term *ionizing* radiation and how it differs from other electromagnetic radiations **(pp. 222–223).**

6. Give examples of natural and artificial (man-made) background radiations and identify the percentage each contributes to the population's annual dose **(pp. 222–223).**

7. What are the two ways in which x-ray photons are produced at the tungsten anode? Describe each. Which occurs more often **(pp. 223, 224)?**

8. Describe the photoelectric effect and Compton scatter. The following should be included in your description **(pp. 223–224).**

    A. energy required for production of each

    B. electron shell involved

    C. any electron shell vacancy or occupancy changes

    D. type of absorber (atomic number) most likely involved

    E. retention or loss of energy of incoming photon

    F. interaction associated with a recoil electron

    G. effect on radiographic contrast

    H. impact on patient dose

9. Describe the difference between threshold and nonthreshold dose–response curves *(pp. 226–227)*.

10. Differentiate between stochastic and nonstochastic effects *(p. 227)*.

11. Name the type of dose–response curve that identifies *no* safe dose *(p. 227)*.

12. Explain why occupationally exposed individuals are mainly concerned with the late, or long-term, effects of radiation exposure *(p. 227)*.

13. List possible long-term effects of radiation exposure *(p. 227)*.

14. List the three types of cells described by Bergonié and Tribondeau in 1906 to be the most radiosensitive *(p. 228)*.

15. What is described as the rate at which radiation deposits energy in tissue *(p. 228)*?

16. Why is a QF assigned to different types of radiation *(p. 228)*?

17. How may the terms *rad* and *rem* be equated *(p. 228)*?

18. How are LET and RBE related *(p. 228)*?

19. With respect to the molecular effects of radiation, describe the difference between the direct and indirect effect; identify the one that occurs more frequently in the diagnostic range *(p. 229)*.

20. What type(s) of DNA damage is/are repairable; which can result in cell death; mutation *(p. 229)*?

21. Identify each of the following as either radiosensitive or radioresistant: muscle, nerve (fetal and adult), and epithelial tissue; lymphocytes; and reproductive cells *(p. 229)*.

22. How does each of the following affect the response of tissue to irradiation: tissue age, oxygen content, fractionation/protraction of radiation delivery *(p. 229–230)*.

23. Identify the meaning of the acronym, ALARA, and how it relates to the radiographer *(p. 230)*.

24. What is the most radiosensitive portion of the human gestational period; list four possible results of excessive radiation exposure during this period *(pp. 231–232)*.

25. What can result from excessive radiation exposure during the second and third trimester of pregnancy *(p. 231)*?

26. How much radiation exposure is necessary to produce fetal anomalies; about how much fetal radiation do most diagnostic examinations deliver *(p. 231)*?

27. Explain the value of determining the LMP and/or using the 10-day rule for female patients of childbearing age *(p. 231)*.

28. Describe the effectiveness of gonadal shielding in the male versus female patient; discuss the importance of shielding children *(pp. 231–232)*.

29. Describe the concept of GSD *(p. 232)*.

30. Why are we concerned with genetic dose; when do genetic effects manifest themselves *(p. 234)?*

31. Distinguish between early and late somatic effects; when does each occur with respect to initial exposure; can you give historic examples of each? *(p. 233)*.

32. What kind of radiation exposure would be required to cause early somatic effects; state examples of early somatic effects *(p. 233)*.

33. What kind of radiation exposure is characteristic of late somatic effects; give examples of late somatic effects *(p. 233)*.

A&U Chapter Review Questions

1. How are wavelength and energy related?
   - (A) directly
   - (B) inversely
   - (C) chemically
   - (D) empirically

2. The beam of x-ray photons leaving the x-ray tube focus can be described as having what sort of nature?
   - (A) homogeneous
   - (B) heterogeneous
   - (C) homologus
   - (D) focused

3. Which of the following accounts for x-ray beam heterogeneity?
   1. incident electrons interacting with several layers of tungsten target atoms
   2. electrons moving to fill different shell vacancies
   3. its nuclear origin
   - (A) 1 only
   - (B) 1 and 2 only
   - (C) 1 and 3 only
   - (D) 1, 2, and 3

4. The type of dose–response curve used to predict genetic effects is the:
   (A) nonlinear nonthreshold
   (B) nonlinear threshold
   (C) linear nonthreshold
   (D) nonlinear nonthreshold

5. Long-term effects of radiation include:
   1. formation of cataracts
   2. cancer
   3. genetic effects
   (A) 1 only
   (B) 1 and 2 only
   (C) 2 and 3 only
   (D) 1, 2, and 3

6. Linear energy transfer (LET) is:
   1. a method of expressing radiation quality
   2. a measure of the rate at which radiation energy is transferred to soft tissue
   3. absorption of polyenergetic radiation
   (A) 1 only
   (B) 1 and 2 only
   (C) 1 and 3 only
   (D) 1, 2, and 3

7. In 1906, Bergonié and Tribondeau established a law which states that cells are more radiosensitive if they:
   1. have a low proliferation rate
   2. are stem cells
   3. are young
   (A) 1 only
   (B) 1 and 2 only
   (C) 2 and 3 only
   (D) 1, 2, and 3

8. What is the effect on relative biologic effectiveness (RBE) as linear energy transfer (LET) increases?
   (A) as LET increases, RBE increases
   (B) as LET increases, RBE decreases
   (C) as LET increases, RBE stabilizes
   (D) LET has no effect on RBE

9. A dose of 25 rad to the fetus during the seventh or eighth week of pregnancy is more likely to cause which of the following:
   (A) spontaneous abortion
   (B) skeletal anomalies
   (C) neurologic anomalies
   (D) organogenesis

10. The effects of radiation to biologic material are dependent on several factors. If a quantity of radiation is delivered to a body over a long period of time:
    (A) the effect will be greater than if it were delivered all at one time
    (B) the effect will be less than if it were delivered all at one time
    (C) the effect has no relation to how it is delivered in time
    (D) the effect is solely dependent on the radiation quality

Answers and Explanations

1. (B) Frequency and wavelength are closely associated with the relative energy of electromagnetic radiations. *More energetic radiations have shorter wavelengths and higher frequency,* thus, they are inversely related. The relationship between frequency, wavelength, and energy is illustrated in the electromagnetic spectrum (Fig. 8–1). Some radiations are energetic enough to rearrange atoms in materials through which they pass, and can therefore be hazardous to living tissue.

2. (B) Electrons may undergo any one of a few types of interactions as they encounter the target. The emitted photons can therefore have a variety of energies and thus are termed heterogeneous or polyenergetic. It is only at extremely high energies that photon energy becomes more homogeneous; only gamma radiation can be accurately termed homogeneous or monoenergetic.

3. (B) The x-ray photons produced at the tungsten target comprise a heterogeneous beam, ie, a spectrum of photon energies. This is accounted for by the fact that the incident electrons have different energies. Also, the incident electrons travel through several layers of tungsten target material, lose energy with each interaction, and therefore produce increasingly weaker x-ray photons. During characteristic x-ray production, vacancies may be filled in the K, L, or M shells, differing with each other in binding energies, and therefore, a variety of energy photons are emitted.

4. (C) The linear-nonthreshold curve is used to illustrate responses such as leukemia, cancer, and genetic effects. These are sometimes referred to as stochastic effects. Stochastic effects occur randomly and are "all-or-nothing" type effects, that is, they do not occur with degrees of severity. Remember that *in a nonthreshold curve there is no safe dose,* that is, no dose below which there will definitely be no biologic response. Theoretically, even one x-ray photon can cause a biologic response. The linear-nonthreshold curve is the curve of choice to predict effects of low level (eg, medical and occupational) exposure to ionizing radiation.

5. (D) Occupationally exposed individuals are concerned principally with *late* (ie, *long-term,* or *delayed*) effects of radiation, such as *genetic effects, leukemia, cancers,* and *cataractogenesis,* which can occur many years following initial exposure to low levels of ionizing radiation. These long-term, or delayed, effects are represented by the linear, nonthreshold dose–response curve, with the exception of cataractogenesis, which is represented by the linear, threshold dose–response curve. An acute dose of about 200 rad would be required to cause radiogenic cataracts. A far greater occupational (ie, fractionated) dose of about 1000 rad would be required to induce cataracts.

6. (B) When biologic material is irradiated, there are a number of modifying factors that determine what kind and how much response will occur in the biologic material. One of these factors is LET, which expresses the rate at which particulate or photon energy is transferred to the absorber. Since different kinds of radiation have different degrees of penetration in different materials, it is also a useful way of expressing the quality of the radiation.

7. (C) The law of Bergonié and Tribondeau states that stem cells (that give rise to a specific type cell, as in hematopoiesis) are particularly radiosensitive as well as young cells and tissues. It also states that cells with a high rate of proliferation (mitosis) are more sensitive to radiation. This law is historically important in that it was the first to recognize that some tissues have greater radiosensitivity than others, for example, the fetus.

8. (A) LET expresses the rate at which photon or particulate energy is transferred to (absorbed by) biologic material (through ionization processes) and is dependent upon the type of radiation and absorber characteristics. RBE describes the degree of response or amount of biologic change we can expect of the irradiated material. As the amount of transferred energy (LET) *increases* (from interactions occurring between radiation and biologic material) the amount of biologic effect or damage will also *increase*. LET and biologic effect are directly related.

9. (C) During the first trimester, specifically the second to eighth week of pregnancy (during major organogenesis), if the radiation dose is at least 20 rad, fetal anomalies can be produced. *Skeletal anomalies* usually appear if irradiation occurs in the early part of this time period, and *neurologic anomalies* are formed in the latter part; mental retardation and childhood malignant diseases, such as cancers or leukemia, can also result from irradiation during the first trimester. Fetal irradiation during the second and third trimester is not likely to produce anomalies, but rather, with sufficient dose, some type of childhood malignant disease. Fetal irradiation during the first two weeks of gestation can result in *spontaneous abortion.*

It must be emphasized that the likelihood of producing fetal anomalies at doses below 20 rad is exceedingly small and that most general diagnostic examinations are likely to deliver fetal doses of less than 1 to 2 rad.

10. (B) The effects of a quantity of radiation delivered to a body is dependent on a few factors: the amount of radiation received, the size of the irradiated area, and how the radiation is delivered in time. If the radiation is delivered in portions over a period of time, it is said to be fractionated and has a less harmful effect than if the radiation was delivered all at once. Cells have an opportunity to repair and some recovery occurs between doses.

Patient Protection

As previously discussed, it is an ethical responsibility to keep radiation exposure to patients (and ourselves) to an absolute minimum. We will review means of achieving this goal.

Statistics indicate that the number of x-ray examinations performed annually is steadily increasing. Although the benefits of these examinations far outweigh the risks, the concern about the risk of possible long-term effects of x-ray exposure obliges us to practice the ALARA principle.

One exceedingly important consideration in reducing patient exposure is *good patient communication*. Explaining the examination and answering the patient's questions will better ensure understanding and cooperation, and reduce the chance for retakes.

Quality control programs are in place to ensure that retakes will not be required as a result of equipment malfunction. Employees receive orientation on new equipment to ensure that it is used to best advantage and to reduce retakes as a result of unfamiliarity with equipment operation. The use of technique charts helps take the guesswork out of selecting exposure factors.

There are several topics discussed in this chapter that can have some kind of impact on patient protection.

I. BEAM RESTRICTION

Beam restriction, or limitation of field size, is probably the single most important factor in keeping patient dose to a minimum. The primary beam must be confined to the area of interest, thus, only tissues of diagnostic interest will be irradiated.

Another benefit of beam restriction is that, because a smaller quantity of tissue is irradiated, less scattered radiation will be produced. Remember, scattered radiation does not carry useful information; it degrades the radiographic image by adding a layer of fog that impairs image visibility.

▶   There are three basic types of **beam restrictors:** aperture diaphragms, cones, and collimators.

A. APERTURE DIAPHRAGMS

▶ The **aperture diaphragm** is the most elementary of the three types, and is frequently used in dedicated-head units and many of today's dedicated-chest units. It is simply a flat piece of lead (Pb) with a central opening with a size and shape that determines the size and shape of the x-ray beam. Whereas head units have a variety of aperture diaphragm sizes available for various types of skull exams and required film sizes, today's dedicated-chest units frequently have a more fixed aperture diaphragm. Regardless of the type, the aperture diaphragm should demonstrate adequate beam restriction by providing an unexposed border around the edge of the radiograph.

B. CONES

▶ **Cones** are circular, lead-lined devices that slide into place in the tube head or onto the collimator housing. They may be the straight *cylinder* type, with proximal and distal diameters that are identical, or the infrequently used *flare* type, with a distal diameter that is greater than its proximal diameter. Cylinder cones are frequently able to extend, like a telescope, by means of a simple thumbscrew adjustment (Fig. 9–1).

A disadvantage of both the aperture and cone is that they have a fixed opening size, that is, a particular diaphragm or cone will provide only one field size at a given distance. To change the size of the field you must change to a different size aperature or cone. Additionally, the cylinder cone can be used only for relatively small field sizes, such as the paranasal sinuses, L5-S1, or other small areas of interest.

C. COLLIMATORS

▶ The **collimator** is, overall, the most efficient beam-restricting device. It is attached to the tube head, and its upper aperture, the first set of shutters, is placed as close as possible to the x-ray tube port window

Figure 9–1. Cylinder cones (especially the extendible type) are generally considered more efficient than aperture diaphragms because they restrict the size and shape of the x-ray beam for a greater distance. The closer the distal end of the beam restrictor is to the area of interest, the greater its efficiency. (Courtesy Burkhart Roentgen, Inc.)

(Fig. 9–2). This is done to control the amount of image-degrading "off-focus" radiation leaving the x-ray tube (ie, radiation produced when electrons strike anode surfaces other than the focal track). The next set of *lead shutters* ("blades" or "leaves") actually consists of two pairs of adjustable shutters—one pair for field length and another pair for field width. It is these shutters that the radiographer adjusts when changing the field size and shape.

D. *Light-localization Apparatus*

Another important part of the collimator assembly is the *light localization apparatus*. It consists of a small light bulb (to illuminate the field) and a mirror. For the light field and x-ray field to correspond accurately, *the x-ray tube focal spot and the light bulb must be exactly the same distance from the center of the mirror* (Fig. 9–2). If the light and x-ray fields do not correspond, film alignment may be off enough to require a repeat examination. Collimator accuracy should be regularly checked as part of the quality assurance program. NCRP guidelines state that collimators must be accurate to within 2% of the source-to-image receptor distance (SID) focal film distance (FFD).

E. *Accuracy*

Cylinder cones are often attached to the tube housing and used in conjunction with collimators. It is important to collimate to the approximate cone opening size; wide-open collimator shutters can lead to excessive scattered radiation production and can degrade the resulting radiographic image.

Figure 9–2. X-ray tube, filters, and collimator. The position of the collimator shutters can be seen. Note the position of the first beam restrictor, located at the x-ray tube port window. The oil coolant surrounding the x-ray tube contributes to inherent filtration. Added filtration includes the aluminum filter, the mirror, and collimator. (From Wolbarst, AB. *Physics of Radiology,* East Norwalk, CT: Appleton & Lange, 1993.)

As a back-up to the illuminated light field, should the light bulb burn out, there is a calibrated scale on the front of the collimator that indicates the x-ray field size at various source-to-image receptor distances (see Fig. 9–5A on p. 249).

An important feature of nearly all collimators today (radiographic and fluoroscopic) is *positive beam limitation (PBL).* Sensors located in the Bucky tray or other cassette holder signal the collimator to open or close, according to the cassette size being used in the Bucky tray. A properly calibrated PBL system will provide a small unexposed border on all sides of the finished radiograph, and is required by NCRP guidelines to be accurate to within 2% of the SID.

Summary

- **Beam restriction is the most important way to reduce patient dose.**
  - **Beam restrictors reduce the production of scattered radiation.**
  - **Types of beam restrictors include aperture diaphragms, cones and cylinders, and collimators (most efficient).**
- **Devices used in most equipment today are PBL.**
  - **A properly calibrated PBL will provide an unexposed border on all sides of the finished radiograph.**
- **For the light and x-ray field to correspond accurately, the focal spot and light bulb must be exactly the same distance from the mirror.**

II. AUTOMATIC EXPOSURE CONTROL

▶ An *automatic exposure control (AEC)* is used to automatically regulate the amount of ionizing radiation delivered to the patient and image recorder, thereby serving to produce consistent and comparable radiographic results time after time. When an AEC is installed in the x-ray circuit, it is calibrated to produce radiographic densities as required by the radiologist. AECs have sensors that signal to terminate the exposure once a predetermined, known-correct exposure has been reached. It is essential to use the correct speed screen/film combination with the AEC—the screen/film combination that it has been programmed for. The AEC cannot compensate for a speed system that it does not "know" about. For example, if the system has been programmed for a 400 system and a 200-speed cassette is used, the image will exhibit half the expected density. There are two types of AECs: *ionization chambers* and *phototimers.*

A. Ionization Chamber

A parallel plate ***ionization chamber*** consists of a radiolucent chamber just beneath the tabletop above the cassette and grid (Fig. 9–3). As x-ray photons emerge from the patient, they enter the chamber and ionize the air within. When a predetermined quantity of ionization has occurred (as determined by the selected exposure factors), the exposure automatically terminates.

B. Phototimer

In the ***phototimer,*** a small fluorescent screen is positioned beneath the cassette (Fig. 9–3). When remnant radiation emerging from the patient exits the cassette, the fluorescent screen emits light. The fluorescent light charges a photomultiplier tube and, once a predetermined charge has been reached, the exposure is terminated.

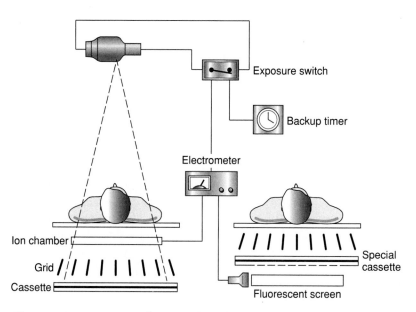

Figure 9–3. Two types of AECs. The ionization chamber is pictured to the left, positioned between the tabletop and cassette. The photomultiplier/phototimer is to the right, located below the cassette. Note that a backup timer, which serves to terminate the exposure in the event of AEC failure, is used in conjunction with both AECs. (From Wolbarst, AB. *Physics of Radiology.* East Norwalk, CT: Appleton & Lange, 1993.)

C. BACKUP TIMER

▶ In either case, the manual timer should be used as **backup timer** so that, in case of AEC malfunction, the exposure would terminate, thus *avoiding patient overexposure and tube overload.*

D. MINIMUM RESPONSE TIME

▶ Another important feature of the AEC to be familiar with is its **mini-**
▶ **mum response** (or, *reaction*) *time,* defined as the length of the shortest exposure possible with a particular AEC. If less than the minimum response time is required for a particular exposure, the radiograph will exhibit excessive density.

Exact positioning and centering is particularly critical when using equipment with AECs. The anatomic part of interest must be positioned (centered) accurately with respect to the AEC's sensors; otherwise, the sensors may react to a different *tissue* density, and result in an undiagnostic *radiographic* density.

Summary

- **When used properly, AECs insure consistency of radiographic density.**
- **There are two types of AECs: ionization chamber type and phototimer (photomultiplier) type.**
- **The ionization chamber type is located between the patient and cassette.**
- **The phototimer/photomultiplier type is located beneath the cassette.**
- **Every AEC has a minimum reaction time.**
- **AECs require accurate positioning and centering to produce predictable results.**
- **The manual timer must be used as backup timer to avoid patient overexposure and tube overload.**

III. EXPOSURE FACTORS

Selection of exposure factors has a significant impact on patient dose. Remember that milliampere-seconds (mAs) is used to regulate the *quantity* of radiation delivered to the patient, and *kVp* determines the *penetrability* of the x-ray beam. As kilovoltage is increased, more high energy photons are produced and the overall average energy of the beam is increased. An increase in mAs will increase the number of photons produced at the target, but is unrelated to photon energy.

Generally speaking then, in an effort to keep radiation dose to a minimum, it makes sense to use the lowest mAs and the highest kVp that will produce the desired radiographic results. An added benefit is that at high kVp and low mAs values, the heat delivered to the x-ray tube is lower and tube life is extended.

IV. FILTRATION

X-ray photons emanating from the target comprise a heterogeneous primary beam. There are many low-energy (or "soft") x-rays that, if not removed, would contribute significantly to patient skin dose.

These low-energy photons are too weak to penetrate the patient and expose the film; they simply penetrate a small thickness of tissue and are absorbed. Filters, usually made of aluminum, are used in radiography to reduce patient dose by removing this low energy radiation, *resulting in an x-ray beam of higher average energy.* Total filtration is composed of **inherent filtration** plus **added filtration.** ◀

A. INHERENT FILTRATION

Inherent filtration, that which is "built-in," and is composed of materials that are a permanent part of the tube housing, ie, the *glass envelope* of the x-ray tube and the *oil coolant* (0.5 or ½ mm aluminum equivalent).

B. ADDED FILTRATION

Added filtration includes the *collimator structures* and *mirror* (1 mm Al equivalent) and *thin sheets of aluminum* that are added to make the necessary total thickness (Fig. 9–2).

C. NCRP GUIDELINES

NCRP guidelines state that equipment operating above 70 kVp must have a minimum total (ie, inherent plus added) filtration of *2.5 mm Al equivalent.* Equipment operating between 50 and 70 kVp must have at least 1.5 mm Al equivalent filtration. X-ray tubes operating below 50 kVp must have at least 0.5 mm Al equivalent filtration. Mammography equipment having a molybdenum target will have 0.025 to 0.03 mm molybdenum (Mo) filtration. For magnification studies, a fractional tungsten (W) target tube, having at least 0.5 mm Al equivalent total filtration, may be used.

   Inherent filtration tends to increase as the x-ray tube ages. With use, *tungsten evaporates* and is deposited on the inner surface of the glass envelope, effectively *acting as additional filtration and decreasing tube output.*

Filtration Summary
< 50 kVp = 0.5 mm Al equiv
50–70 kVp = 1.5 mm Al equiv
> 70 kVp = 2.5 mm Al equiv

Summary

- **Low mAs and high kVp factors keep patient dose to a minimum.**
- **Proper calibration of equipment is essential for predictable results.**
- **Proper selection of technical factors and an effective QA system help reduce radiation exposure.**
- **Filtration removes low-energy x-rays from primary beam, thereby**
   - **Reducing patient dose**
   - **Increasing the average energy of the beam**
- **Filtration is usually expressed in mm of Al equivalent.**
- **Inherent + added filtration = total filtration.**
- **Inherent filtration includes the glass envelope and oil coolant.**
- **Added filtration includes the collimator, mirror, and thin Al sheets.**
- **Equipment operated above 70 kVp must have at least 2.5 mm Al equivalent.**
- **Inherent filtration increases with tube age, thereby decreasing tube output.**

Figure 9–4. Correct placement of shadow shield. (Courtesy of C.B. Radiology Design, Jamestown, NY.)

V. SHIELDING

Protective shielding for especially radiosensitive organs (ie, gonads, blood-forming organs) should be provided whenever possible during radiographic and fluoroscopic examinations (Figs. 9–4 and 9–5).

A. MALE AND FEMALE

Gonadal shielding is far more effective in the male patient because the reproductive organs lie outside the body. Male patients are therefore more easily shielded, and shielding is much less likely to interfere with the diagnostic objectives of the examination. Female reproductive organs are located within the abdominal cavity, where shielding becomes a much less feasible option.

B. GUIDELINES FOR USE

There are three indications for the use of gonadal shields. If the gonads lie in, or within 5 cm, of a well-collimated field, shielding should be used. A patient with reasonable reproductive potential should be shielded; a generally accepted procedure is to include all patients under the age of 55 years. Gonadal shielding should be used if diagnostic objectives permit, ie, as long as the shield does not obscure important diagnostic information.

C. TYPES OF SHIELDS

There are three types of gonadal shields available: *flat, contact shields, shadow shields,* and *contour (shaped) contact shields.*

▶ **1. Flat, Contact.** The simplest type are flat, **contact shields,** such as pieces of lead-impregnated vinyl that are placed over the patient's gonads. Since they are difficult to secure in place, flat contact shields are useful only for AP or PA recumbent positions; they cannot be secured adequately for oblique, lateral decubitus, erect, or fluoroscopic procedures.

▶ **2. Shadow.** *Shadow shields* attach to the x-ray tube head. They consist of a piece of leaded material attached to an arm extending from the tube head (Fig. 9–5). The leaded material casts a shadow within the illuminated field that corresponds to the shielded area. Though shadow shields are initially more expensive, they are likely to be a one-time expense. Shadow shields can be used for more positions than flat contact shields and may also be used without contaminating a sterile field. They cannot be used for fluoroscopic procedures.

▶ **3. Contour (Shaped) Contact Shields.** *Contour* (shaped) **contact shields** are very effective gonadal shields. They are shaped to enclose the male reproductive organs and are held in place by disposable briefs. They are effective for a variety of positions including oblique, erect, and fluoroscopic procedures.

▶ **4. Breast Shields.** *Breast shields* should be used for female patients during scoliosis series; scoliosis series are typically performed at ages when developing breast tissue is particularly radiosensitive. Breast shields are available incorporated in vertebral column compensating filters (Fig. 9–6), and as leaded vinyl vests.

Gonadal Shielding Should Be Used If

- The gonads lie in, or within 5 cm of, a well-collimated field.
- The patient has reasonable reproductive potential.
- Diagnostic objectives permit.

A

B

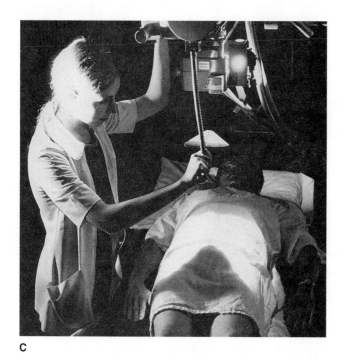

C

Figure 9–5. **(A)** A shadow shield is permanently mounted to the collimator housing. It has a moveable arm that allows a shield of the desired size and shape to be placed in the radiation field over the gonadal area. It is manually operated and swings away when not in use. (Courtesy C.B. Radiology Design, Jamestown, NY.) **(B)** Another type of shadow shield that attaches to the collimator housing. **(C)** Its use. (Courtesy of Nuclear Associates.)

Additional points to remember include the following.

- Lead aprons can be placed under the patient's pillow during GI and BE examinations when the radiographer's assistance is required at the head end of the table during fluoroscopy.
- Half aprons can be used to protect the gonads from ***scattered radiation*** in chest radiography. ◀
- Lead aprons can also be placed over chest/abdomen during radiography of various body parts to protect radiosensitive organs from exposure to scattered radiation.
- Protective shields must be carefully placed; superimposition on diagnostically important anatomic structures can cause retakes and exposure to unnecessary radiation.
- The use of protective shielding during mobile radiography should not be neglected.

Figure 9–6. Spinal column studies are often required for evaluation of adolescent scoliosis, thus presenting a two-fold problem, ie, radiation exposure to youthful gonadal and breast tissues, and significantly differing tissue densities and thicknesses. Both problems can be resolved with the use of a compensating filter (for uniform density) that incorporates lead shielding for the breasts and gonads. **(A)** Film performed without the filter/shield. **(B)** Film performed with the filter/shield. Note the improved visualization of the entire vertebral column and appropriate protection of the breasts and gonads. (Courtesy of Nuclear Associates.)

A   **B**

Summary

- Especially radiosensitive organs include the gonads, lenses, and blood-forming organs.
- Gonadal shielding should be used
  - If the gonads lie in or within 5 cm of collimated beam
  - If the patient has reproductive potential
  - If diagnostic objectives permit
- Three types of gonadal shields are
  - Flat contact
  - Shadow
  - Contour contact
- Male gonads are more easily and effectively shielded.
- Breast shields should be used as needed.

VI. PATIENT POSITION

▶ Since the primary x-ray beam has a ***polyenergetic*** (heterogeneous) nature, the entrance or skin dose is significantly greater than the exit dose. This principle may be employed in radiation protection by placing particularly radiosensitive organs away from the primary beam.

To place the gonads further from the primary beam and reduce gonadal dose, abdominal radiography should be performed in the PA position whenever possible. Dose to the lens is significantly decreased when skull radiographs are performed in the PA position.

The same principle applies when performing scoliosis series on young children in an effort to reduce gonadal dose, and to decrease dose to breast tissue in young girls. Dose to breast tissue during scoliosis survey can also be reduced with the use of breast shields. The PA projection does not generally cause a significant adverse effect on recorded detail and is often advocated to decrease dose to the reproductive organs.

VII. FILM AND SCREEN COMBINATION

The higher the speed of the film and screen system, the smaller the dose of radiation required to produce a diagnostic radiograph. As one component of the effort to reduce population dose, rare-earth phosphors are used almost exclusively today in general radiography. Rare-earth phosphors are at least four times faster than the earlier calcium tungstate phosphors, and the recorded detail they provide is entirely satisfactory. In general, the fastest film and screen combination consistent with diagnostic requirements should be used.

VIII. GRIDS

Grids, both stationary and moving, function to remove a large percentage of scattered (primarily Compton) radiation from the remnant beam before it reaches the image receptor, thereby improving radiographic contrast.

Since scattered radiation often makes a significant contribution to the overall radiographic density, the addition of a grid (or an increase in the grid ratio) must be accompanied by an appropriate increase in exposure factors (usually mAs) to maintain adequate density. The improvement in image quality is usually more significant than the increased exposure to the patient (Fig. 9–7). However, the radiographer should avoid using a high ratio grid with a low kilovoltage; the grid will absorb a portion of the useful beam, requiring an unnecessary and excessive increase in patient dose.

It is interesting to note that, to produce a given density, a moving grid generally requires more exposure than a stationary grid of the same ratio. This is because, as the lead strips continually change position moving back and forth, some of the perpendicular rays will unavoidably be "caught" by the lead strips moving into their path.

IX. AIR-GAP TECHNIQUE

An *air-gap* technique can be used to function similar to, or in place ◄ of, a grid. A distance is introduced between the patient and the film. Scattered photons emerging from the patient will continue to diverge and never reach the film.

A "natural" air gap exists in the lateral projection of the cervical spine, thus, a 72″ SID is used without a grid (Fig. 9–8). Since no air gap is introduced in the AP projection of the cervical spine, it is usually radiographed at 40″ SID with the use of a grid.

The OID required in magnification radiography is an air gap and therefore grids are rarely needed when this special imaging technique is performed.

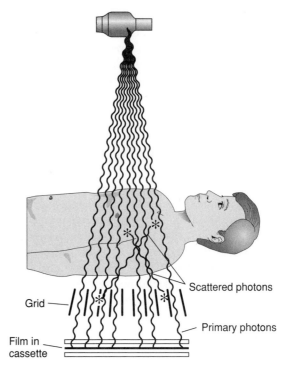

Figure 9–7. Scattered radiation generated within the patient can cause serious degradation of image quality. The improvement in image quality afforded by the use of grids more than makes up for the required increase in patient exposure. (From Wolbarst, AB. *Physics of Radiology.* East Norwalk, CT: Appleton & Lange, 1993.)

Air-gap technique may also be used in place of a grid in chest radiography. However, to maintain optimum recorded detail and avoid excessive magnification, the SID must be increased considerably, followed by a significant increase in mAs. Air-gap technique is limited in use to radiography of fairly thin parts, as dense tissues would require excessive and impractical radiation exposures.

Additionally, equipment must be properly calibrated to produce consistently predictable results; specifically, the equipment must ▶ have **linearity** and **reproducibility.** Linearity refers to consistency in exposure with adjacent mA stations and exposure times adjusted to produce the same mAs. Reproducibility refers to consistency in exposure output during repeated exposures at a particular setting.

A. NCRP Recommendations for Patient Protection

Note: Many of the means of patient protection serve to protect the operator as well. (Further recommendations can be found in section II under "NCRP Guidelines.")

- Equipment operating above 70 kVp must have a minimum total (ie, inherent plus added) filtration of 2.5 mm Al equivalent.
- X-ray intensity at a particular mAs and kVp must be consistent within 20% at all combinations of commonly used mA and exposure times.

- X-ray tube housing must keep leakage radiation to less than 100 mR/hr when measured 1 meter from the tube.
- A device (eg, centering light) must be provided to align the center of the x-ray beam with the center of the image receptor.
- Beam-limiting devices must be provided. The collimated x-ray field must correspond to the visible-light field to within 2% of the SID.
- The x-ray timer must be accurate. Single-phase equipment can be tested with a simple spinning-top test tool. Three-phase equipment is tested with a synchronous spinning top or an oscilloscope.
- Source-to-skin distance (SSD) must not be less than 12″ for all procedures other than dental radiography.
- The SSD must be at least 12″ (preferably 15″) in stationary (fixed) fluoroscopic equipment.
- When more than one x-ray tube can be energized from a single control panel, there must be an obvious indicator on the control panel and on or near each tube housing that indicates which tube is being operated.
- The location of the focal spot must be indicated on the outside of the tube housing.
- The film and screen combination selected should be the fastest possible that is consistent with the diagnostic objectives of the examination.
- Radiographic intensifying screens should be cleaned and checked regularly, at least every 6 months.
- X-ray film must be stored in an adequately protected place.
- Radiographic equipment should undergo regular QA testing.
- The radiographer must be able to see and communicate with the patient at all times.

Summary

- **To reduce exposure to reproductive organs and/or breasts, it is helpful to perform abdominal radiography and scoliosis series in the PA position whenever possible.**
- **The fastest screen and film combination consistent with diagnostic requirements should be used.**
- **Grids improve the radiographic image by reducing the amount of scattered radiation fog, but necessitate an increase in exposure.**
- **An air gap can have the same effect as a low-ratio grid in decreasing the amount of scattered radiation reaching the film; however, SID (FFD), and therefore exposure, must be increased to preserve recorded detail.**
- **There are several important NCRP recommendations governing patient protection with which the radiographer should be familiar.**

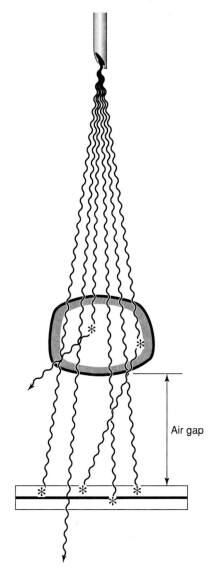

Air gap

Figure 9–8. When an air gap is used, much of the scattered radiation generated within the patient never reaches the image receptor. An air gap may occasionally be used in place of a grid. (From Wolbarst, AB. *Physics of Radiology.* East Norwalk, CT: Appleton & Lange, 1993.)

Chapter Exercises

 Congratulations! *You have completed your review of this chapter. If you are able to answer the following group of very comprehensive questions, you should feel confident that you have really mastered this section. You are then ready to go on to "Registry-type" questions that follow. For greatest success, do not go to the multiple choice questions without first completing the short answer questions below.*

1. What are some methods of achieving the ALARA goal *(pp. 241, 242)?*

2. What is the most important factor in minimizing patient exposure; give an example of how it affects patient dose *(p. 242).*

3. List the three types of beam restrictors; describe the particular use(s) and efficiency of each *(pp. 242–243).*

4. What effect does beam restriction have on the production of scattered radiation *(p. 242)?*

5. What degree of accuracy must a properly calibrated PBL maintain *(p. 243–244)?*

6. How is "off focus" radiation minimized *(p. 242)?*

7. Describe the relationship between the focal spot and collimator light bulb with respect to film alignment *(p. 243).*

8. Explain the importance of a backup timer *(pp. 244–246).*

9. What is meant by the *minimum response time* of an AEC *(pp. 244–246)?*

10. Why is positioning and centering so critical when using AECs *(pp. 244–246)?*

11. What combination of exposure factors can be used, in general, to keep patient dose to a minimum *(pp. 244–246)?*

12. How does filtration affect patient dose *(pp. 244–246)?*

13. Describe the two types of filtration that comprise total filtration *(pp. 244–245).*

14. What are the NCRP filtration requirements *(p. 247)?*

15. How and why does inherent filtration change as the x-ray tube ages; how does it affect tube output *(p. 247)?*

16. List the three criteria for determining when gonadal shielding should be used *(p. 248).*

17. Describe the three types of gonadal shielding and indicate the effectiveness of each *(pp. 248–249).*

18. When might breast or lens shields be used *(p. 248)?*

19. Explain the value of performing scoliosis series, abdominal, and skull radiography in the PA position *(p. 251).*

20. How do screen and film combinations impact patient dose *(p. 251)?*

21. The NCRP makes several recommendations that can impact patient dose. Briefly describe the recommendations for each of the following *(pp. 252–253):*

    A. patient visibility during examination

    B. QA testing

    C. speed and care of intensifying screens

    D. external indication of focal spot

    E. energizing multiple x-ray tubes from one control panel

    F. minimum SSD in fluoroscopy units

    G. x-ray timer testing and accuracy

    H. PBL and accuracy required

    I. beam alignment

    J. leakage radiation

    K. quantity of filtration

    L. linearity and reproducibility

A&U Chapter Review Questions

1. The primary function of filtration is to:
   (A) reduce patient skin dose
   (B) reduce operator dose
   (C) reduce film noise
   (D) reduce scattered radiation

2. Which of the following is (are) feature(s) of x-ray equipment designed especially to eliminate unnecessary radiation to the patient?
   1. filtration
   2. minimum SSD of 10 inches
   3. collimation accuracy
   (A) 1 only
   (B) 1 and 2 only
   (C) 1 and 3 only
   (D) 1, 2, and 3

3. Types of gonadal shielding include which of the following?
   1. flat contact
   2. shaped (contour) contact
   3. shadow
   (A) 1 only
   (B) 1 and 2 only
   (C) 2 and 3 only
   (D) 1, 2, and 3

4. All of the following affect patient dose, EXCEPT:
   (A) inherent filtration
   (B) added filtration
   (C) source-image distance
   (D) focal spot size

5. Which of the following groups of exposure factors will deliver the least amount of exposure to the patient?
   (A) 100 mAs, 100 kVp
   (B) 200 mAs, 90 kVp
   (C) 400 mAs, 80 kVp
   (D) 800 mAs, 70 kVp

6. A backup timer for the automatic exposure control serves to:
   1. protect the patient from overexposure
   2. protect the x-ray tube from excessive heat
   3. increase or decrease inherent filtration
   (A) 1 only
   (B) 1 and 2 only
   (C) 1 and 3 only
   (D) 1, 2, and 3

7. Patient dose can be decreased by using:
   1. high speed film and screen combination
   2. high ratio grids
   3. air-gap technique
   (A) 1 only
   (B) 1 and 2 only
   (C) 1 and 3 only
   (D) 1, 2, and 3

8. The advantages of beam restriction include:
   1. less scattered radiation is produced
   2. less biologic material is irradiated
   3. less total filtration will be required
   (A) 1 only
   (B) 1 and 2 only
   (C) 2 and 3 only
   (D) 1, 2, and 3

9. How does filtration affect the primary beam?
   (A) filtration increases the average energy of the primary beam
   (B) filtration decreases the average energy of the primary beam
   (C) filtration makes the primary beam more penetrating
   (D) filtration increases the intensity of the primary beam

10. The quality assurance term used to describe consistency in exposure with adjacent mA stations and exposure times adjusted to produce the same mAs is:
    (A) automatic exposure control
    (B) positive beam limitation
    (C) linearity
    (D) reproducibility

Answers and Explanations

1. (A) It is our ethical responsibility to minimize radiation dose to our patients. X-rays produced at the target comprise a heterogeneous primary beam. There are many "soft" (low energy) photons that, if not removed, would only contribute to greater patient dose. They are too weak to penetrate the patient and expose the film; they just penetrate a small thickness of tissue and are absorbed. Filters, usually made of aluminum, are used in *radiography to reduce patient dose by removing this low energy radiation,* resulting in an x-ray beam of higher average energy. Total filtration is composed of inherent filtration plus added filtration.

2. (C) According to NCRP regulations, radiographic and fluoroscopic equipment must have a total Al *filtration* of at least 2.5 mm Al equivalent whenever the equipment is operated at 70 kVp or greater, to reduce excessive exposure to low energy radiation. *Collimator*/beam alignment must be accurate to within 2%. The *SSD* must not be less than *12 inches* for all procedures other than dental radiography. Distance is the single best protection from radiation. Excessively short SIDs/SSDs cause a significant increase in patient skin dose.

3. (D) Gonadal shielding should be used whenever appropriate and possible during radiographic and fluoroscopic examinations. *Flat contact* shields (flat sheets of flexible leaded vinyl) are useful for recumbent studies, but when the exam necessitates that oblique, lateral, or erect projections be obtained, they become less efficient. *Shaped contact (contour)* shields are best because they enclose the male reproductive organs, remaining in position in oblique, lateral, and erect positions—but they can be used only for male patients. *Shadow* shields that attach to the tube head are particularly useful for surgical sterile fields.

4. (D) *Inherent* filtration is composed of materials that are a permanent part of the tube housing, ie, the glass envelope of the x-ray tube and the oil coolant. *Added* filtration, usually thin sheets of aluminum, is present in order to make a total of 2.5 mm Al equivalent for equipment operated above 70 kVp. Filtration is used to decrease patient dose by removing the weak x-rays having no value but contributing to skin dose. According to the inverse square law of radiation, exposure dose increases as *distance* from the source decreases, and vice versa. The effect of the *focal spot size* is principally on radiographic detail, having no effect on patient dose.

5. (A) mAs regulates the quantity of radiation delivered to the patient. kVp regulates the quality (penetration) of the radiation delivered to the patient. Therefore, higher energy (more penetrating) radiation—which is more likely to *exit* the patient—accompanied by a lower mAs, is the safest combination for the patient.

6. (B) A parallel plate *ionization chamber* consists of a radiolucent chamber just beneath the tabletop (see Fig. 9–3). As x-ray photons emerge from the patient, they enter the chamber and ionize the air within. When a predetermined quantity of ionization has occurred (as determined by the selected exposure factors), the exposure automatically terminates. In the *phototimer,* a small fluorescent screen is positioned beneath the cassette (see Fig. 9–3). When remnant radiation emerging from the patient exits the cassette, the exposure is terminated. The *manual* timer should be used as *backup timer,* in case the AEC fails to terminate the exposure, *thus protecting the patient from overexposure and the x-ray tube from excessive heat load.*

7. (A) The *higher the speed* of the film and screen system, the *smaller the dose* of radiation required to produce a diagnostic radiograph. As one component of the effort to reduce population dose, rare-earth phosphors are used almost exclusively today in general radiography, as they are at least four times faster than calcium tungstate phosphors.

Grids, both stationary and moving, function to remove a large percentage of scattered (primarly Compton) radiation from the remnant beam before it reaches the image receptor, thereby improving radiographic contrast. Since scattered radiation often makes a significant contribution to the overall radiographic density, the addition of a *grid* (or an increase in the grid ratio) must be accompanied by an appropriate *increase in exposure factors* (usually mAs) in order to maintain adequate density. The improvement in image quality is usually more significant than the increased exposure to the patient (see Fig. 9–7).

Air-gap technique functions similar to, or in place of, a grid. A distance is introduced between the patient and the film. However, to maintain optimum recorded detail and avoid excessive magnification, the SID must be increased considerably, followed by a *significant increase in mAs.*

8. (B) With greater beam restriction (ie, smaller field size), less biologic material is irradiated, thereby reducing the possibility of harmful effects. If less tissue is irradiated, less scattered radiation is produced, resulting in improved film contrast. The total filtration is not a function of beam restriction, but rather, is a radiation protection guideline aimed at reducing patient skin dose.

9. (A) X-rays produced at the target comprise a heterogeneous primary beam. Filtration serves to eliminate the softer, less-penetrating photons leaving an x-ray beam of higher average energy. Filtration is important in patient protection because unfiltered, low-energy photons not energetic enough to reach the film are absorbed by the body and contribute to total patient dose.

10. (C) Equipment must be properly calibrated to produce consistently predictable results; specifically, the equipment must have *linearity* and *reproducibility*. Linearity refers to consistency in exposure with adjacent mA stations (very similar to reciprocity law) and exposure times adjusted to produce the same mAs. *Reproducibility* refers to consistency in exposure output during repeated exposures at a particular setting. Positive beam limitation (PBL) is automatic collimation. The two types of automatic exposure control (AEC) are the photomultiplier and ionization chamber.

Occupational Exposure

KEY TERMS ◀

BUCKY-SLOT COVER

CONTROL BOOTH

DEAD-MAN SWITCH

FETAL MONITOR

FILM BADGE

FLUOROSCOPIC

GESTATIONAL DOSE LIMIT

IMAGE INTENSIFIER

INVERSE SQUARE LAW

LEAD APRON

LEAD GLOVES

LEAKAGE RADIATION

OCCUPATIONAL EXPOSURE

PRIMARY BARRIER

PRIMARY BEAM

PROTECTIVE CURTAIN

SECONDARY BARRIER

SECONDARY RADIATION

TLD

I. GENERAL CONSIDERATIONS

Radiographers must conscientiously avoid unnecessary radiation exposure to themselves as well as strive to keep patient dose to an absolute minimum. The NCRP recommends personal monitoring for individuals who might receive 25% of the occupational dose equivalent limit of 5 rem/yr (50 mSv/yr). The use of radiation-monitoring devices helps us to evaluate the effectiveness of our radiation-protection practices. The periodic reports received from *film badge* or thermolumi- ◀
nescent dosimeter *(TLD)* laboratories are official legal documents that ◀
must be reviewed, and attempts should be made to reduce *any* exposure, no matter how small. Radiographers must follow the ALARA principle as they carry out their tasks. The radiologic facility must undergo appropriate radiation surveys. Staff must be properly oriented and regular inservice education on radiation safety must take place. Proper radiation monitoring (film badges, etc) and review of monthly radiation reports is essential.

II. OCCUPATIONAL RADIATION SOURCES

A. SCATTERED RADIATION

When primary photons intercept an object and undergo a change in direction, scattered radiation results.

The most significant occupational radiation hazard in diagnostic radiology is scattered radiation from the patient, particularly in fluoroscopy, where the use of high kilovoltage results in energetic Compton scatter emerging from the patient poses a real occupational hazard to the radiologist and radiographer. *The intensity of scattered radiation one meter from the patient is about 0.1% of the intensity of the primary beam.* That is why, in terms of radiation protection, the patient is considered the most important source of scatter. Other scattering objects include the x-ray table, the ***Bucky-slot cover**/closer,* and the ***control booth*** wall.

B. LEAKAGE RADIATION

▶ ***Leakage radiation*** is that which is emitted from the x-ray tube housing in directions other than that of the primary beam. Federal regulations (NCRP) state that leakage radiation must not exceed 100 mR/hr at a distance of 1 m from the x-ray tube.

C. NCRP GUIDELINES

NCRP guidelines regulate equipment design, among other things, in an effort to reduce exposure to personnel and patients. Two other guidelines that serve to reduce exposure to personnel are:

- The control panel must somehow indicate when the x-ray tube is energized, (ie, "exposure-on" time) by means of an audible or visible sign.
▶ - The x-ray exposure switch must be a ***"dead-man" switch*** and situated so that it cannot be operated outside the shielded area.

There are some patients who are unable to hold the required position, for example, the elderly, the very ill or incapacitated, infants, and children. Mechanical immobilizing and restraining devices, thoughtfully and intelligently used, will serve admirably in most cases. Additional help, though rarely required, should ideally be a nonpregnant relative or friend (over age 18) or, as last recourse, another hospital employee. Radiology personnel must *never* be used to hold patients.

NCRP recommendations regarding protection of the *patient and/or personnel* during ***fluoroscopic*** procedures include the following.

- During fluoroscopic procedures, the ***image intensifier*** serves as a protective barrier from the primary beam and must be the equivalent of 2.0 mm Pb.
- The exposure switch must be the "dead-man" type.
- With under-table fluoroscopic tubes, a Bucky-slot closer/cover having at least the equivalent of 0.25 mm Pb must be available to attenuate scattered radiation (which is about at gonad level).
- A cumulative timing device must be available to signal the fluoroscopist (audibly, visibly, or both) when a maximum of 5 minutes of fluoroscopy time has elapsed.

Rules for Selecting Someone to Assist the Patient in the Radiographic Room

- A male (over age 18) is preferred; however, a female who is not pregnant may also be employed.
- The individual must be provided with protective apparel.
- The individual must be as far as possible from the useful beam.
- The individual must not stand in the path of the useful beam.

- A leaded screen drape and table-side shield to reduce scatter radiation to the operator must be available having at least 0.25 mm Pb equivalency.
- The tabletop intensity of the fluoroscopic beam must be less than 10 R/min (preferably less than 5 R/min).
- Protective **lead aprons** must be at least 0.5 mm Pb equiva- ◄ lent (according to NCRP Report no. 102) and must be worn by the workers in the fluoroscopy room.
- Protective **lead gloves** must be at least 0.25 mm Pb equiva- ◄ lent. The unshielded hand must not be placed in the unattenuated/useful beam.
- When fluoroscopy is performed with an under-table image intensifier (as in "remote" x-ray units), palpation must be performed mechanically.

Summary

- Time, distance, and shielding are the principle guidelines for reducing radiographic exposure; monitoring evaluates their effectiveness.
- The principle scattering object is the patient; others include the x-ray table, Bucky-slot closer, and control-booth walls.
- It is important to be familiar with pertinent guidelines established by the NCRP regulating equipment design, performance, and use (NCRP Report no. 102); radiation protection for medical and allied health personnel (NCRP Report no. 105); and recommendations on limits for exposure to ionizing radiation (NCRP no. 91).
- Mechanical restraining devices should be used to immobilize patients when necessary during radiographic examinations.
- Persons occupationally exposed to radiation must never assist (hold) patients during radiographic examinations.
- If someone is required to assist a patient during an examination, it is essential that radiation safety guidelines be adhered to.
- There are several NCRP recommendations regarding protection during fluoroscopic procedures with which the radiographer should be familiar.

III. FUNDAMENTAL METHODS OF PROTECTION

A. CARDINAL RULES

The practice of effective radiation control depends chiefly on common sense, that is, to safeguard yourself from something harmful you generally remove yourself from it as soon as possible, stay as far away from it as possible, and keep a barrier between it and yourself. Hence, the cardinal principles of *time, distance* and *shielding.*

B. INVERSE SQUARE LAW

Reducing the length of time exposed to ionizing radiation, as in reducing fluoroscopy time, results in a reduction of **occupational** ◄ **exposure.** Increasing the distance from the source of radiation, as illustrated by the **inverse square law,** results in a reduction of ◄ occupational exposure. Placing a barrier, like a lead wall or lead apron, between you and the source of radiation results in a reduction of occupational exposure.

Examples:

- If 10 mrem is received in 1 hour of fluoroscopic procedures, how much will be received if the fluoroscopic time is reduced to 30 minutes? (If the fluoroscopic exposure time is cut in half, from 60 to 30 minutes, the exposure dose received would be correspondingly one half of the original, or 5 mrem.)
- If 40 mrem is received at a distance of 40 inches from the x-ray source, what dose will be received at a distance of 80 inches from the source? (According to the inverse square law, if the distance from the radiation source is doubled, exposure dose will be one fourth of the original quantity, or 10 mrem.)

To reduce exposure dose to health care professionals, patients, and the general population, we must minimize the time of exposure to the source of radiation, provide effective shielding from the radiation source and, most importantly, maximize the distance from the source of radiation.

IV. PRIMARY AND SECONDARY BARRIERS

A. NCRP GUIDELINES

▶ **Primary barriers** protect against direct exposure from the primary, or useful, x-ray beam and have much greater attenuation capability
▶ than **secondary barriers,** which only protect from leakage and scattered radiation.

Examples of primary barriers are the lead walls and doors of a radiographic room, that is, any surface that could be struck by the useful beam. Primary protective barriers of typical installations generally consist of walls with 1/16″ lead thickness 7 ft high.

▶ **Secondary radiation** is defined as leakage and scatter radiation. The x-ray tube housing protects from leakage radiation as stated previously. The patient is the source of most scattered radiation.

Secondary radiation barriers include that portion of the walls above 7 ft in height; this area requires only 1/32″ lead. The control booth is also a secondary barrier, toward which the primary beam must never be directed (Fig. 10–1). The radiographer must be protected by the control booth shielding during exposures, and the exposure switch or cord must be positioned and attached so that the exposure can only be made *within* the control booth. Leaded glass, usually 1.5 mm Pb equivalent, should be available for patient observation.

B. CARE OF PROTECTIVE APPAREL

During fluoroscopic procedures requiring the radiographer's presence in the radiographic room, the radiographer must wear protective apparel (Fig. 10–2). According to NCRP Report no. 102, lead aprons must provide the equivalent of at least 0.50 mm Pb, and lead gloves at least 0.25 mm Pb equivalent. *Lead aprons and lead gloves are secondary barriers; they will not provide protection from the useful beam!!* Proper care of protective apparel is essential to ensure effectiveness. They should be hung on appropriate racks, not dropped on

Attenuation Specifics of Lead Aprons

Equivalent Pb Thickness	X-ray Attenuation Level (%)		
	100 kVp	75 kVp	50 kVp
0.25 mm Pb	51%	66%	97%
0.50 mm Pb	75%	88%	99.9%
1.0 mm Pb	94%	99%	99.9%

Figure 10–1. The control booth permits the operator to view the patient. The leaded booth and glass protect the operator from exposure to scattered radiation. The control booth is a secondary barrier toward which the primary beam must never be directed. (Courtesy of Nuclear Associates.)

Figure 10–2. Other leaded apparel available for fluoroscopic procedures include thyroid shields and leaded eye wear. (Courtesy of Nuclear Associates.)

Figure 10–3. Movable leaded barriers provide full-body protection for individuals required to remain in the radiographic or fluoroscopic room. Mobile barriers provide protection from secondary radiation and are available in a variety of sizes and lead equivalents. (Courtesy of Nuclear Associates.)

the floor or folded. Careless handling may result in formation of cracks. Lead aprons and gloves should be imaged annually (either fluoroscopically or radiographically) to check for cracks.

C. PROTECTIVE ACCESSORIES

Another device available for individuals required to remain in the fluoroscopy room is a mobile leaded barrier (Fig. 10–3). Mobile barriers provide full body protection from scattered radiation and are available in a variety of lead equivalents.

V. SPECIAL CONSIDERATIONS

A. PREGNANCY

Deserving special consideration in protection from occupational exposure is the *pregnant radiographer.* As soon as the technologist knows she is pregnant, the radiographer should notify her supervisor. At that time, her occupational radiation history will be reviewed and any necessary modifications made in her work assignments.

A radiographer who wears his or her monitor on the collar outside the lead apron usually receives less than 100 mrem/yr. If a *fetal monitor* were worn under the apron at waist level it would receive 10% of that dose or 10 mrem. Since the *gestational dose limit* to the fetus during the gestation period must not exceed *500 mrem,* under typical conditions when sufficient protection measures are taken, modification of work assignments is not necessary. If a fetal, or "baby," monitor is worn, it must be clearly identified and not confused with the radiographer's regular monitor.

However, radiation protection standards should be reviewed at this time and monthly badge reports closely monitored. Many facilities document the counseling received by the pregnant radiographer from the time she advises her supervisor of her pregnancy and make the signed documents part of the employee's records.

The greatest amount of occupational exposure is received in fluoroscopy (including special procedures) and mobile radiography. It is here that the radiographer must place special emphasis on the cardinal rules of radiation protection: time, distance, and shielding. Federal government controls also regulate manufacturing standards for the protection of both personnel and patients.

B. MOBILE UNITS

Each *mobile x-ray unit* should have a *lead apron* assigned to it. The radiographer should wear the apron while making the exposure at the furthest distance possible from the x-ray tube. The mobile unit's exposure cord must permit the radiographer to stand at least *6 ft* from the x-ray tube and patient. In *mobile fluoroscopic* units there must be a source to patient skin distance of at least 12 in (30 cm).

C. FLUOROSCOPIC UNITS AND PROCEDURES

All *fluoroscopic* equipment must provide at least 12 in (30 cm), and preferably 15 in (38 cm), between the x-ray source (focal spot) and the x-ray tabletop (patient), according to NCRP Report no. 102. The *tabletop intensity* of the fluoroscopic beam must not exceed *10 R/min* or 2.1 R/min/mA. Fluoroscopic mA must not exceed 5, although image-intensified fluoroscopy usually operates between 1 and 3 mA. Since the image intensifier functions as a primary barrier, it must have a lead equivalent of at least 2.0 mm.

Beam collimation must be apparent through visualization of unexposed borders on the TV monitor, and *total filtration* must be at least *2.5 mm Al* equivalent. Since occupational exposure to scattered radiation is of considerable importance in fluoroscopy, a ***protective*** ◀ ***curtain*** of at least *0.25 mm Pb* equivalent must be placed between the patient and fluoroscopist.

The effect of kVp and mA adjustment on fluoroscopic images is similar to that on radiographic images. The automatic exposure control automatically varies the exposure required when viewing body tissues of widely differing tissue densities (eg, between the abdomen and chest). *As in radiography, high kVp and low mAs values are preferred in an effort to reduce dose.*

Summary

- **The cardinal principles of radiation protection are time, distance, and shielding.**
- **Primary barriers protect from the useful (primary) beam, eg, the walls and doors of the radiographic room.**
- **Secondary barriers protect from sources of leakage and scattered radiation, eg, x-ray tube housing, the patient.**
- **Secondary barriers (eg, control-panel wall, lead apron) will not afford protection from the primary beam.**
- **There are several NCRP recommendations with which the radiographer should be familiar regarding required thickness and uses of protective shielding (see pages 262, 263).**
- **A pregnant radiographer should advise her supervisor of her condition as soon as possible.**
- **A pregnant radiographer should wear a second monitor at waist level under her lead apron.**
- **Most occupational exposure is received in fluoroscopy, special procedures, and mobile radiography (especially C-arm).**

Chapter Exercises

 Congratulations! *You have completed your review of this chapter. If you were able to answer the following group of very comprehensive questions, you should feel confident that you have really mastered this section. You are then ready to go on to "Registry-type" questions that follow. For greatest success, do not go to the multiple choice questions without first completing the short answer questions below.*

1. What are the three cardinal rules, or principle guidelines, for radiation protection *(p. 263)?*

2. When is personal radiation monitoring required *(p. 261)?*

3. What is the most significant scattering object in fluoroscopy; why? List other scattering objects *(p. 262).*

4. What are the NCRP rulings on leakage radiation; exposure switches; exposure indicators *(p. 262)?*

5. What resources should be employed to assist and immobilize patients during radioscopic examinations *(p. 262)?*

6. What rules apply if an individual is required in the radiographic room for assistance during a procedure *(p. 262)?*

7. Describe the NCRP rules that are in place for patient and personnel protection during fluoroscopic procedures with respect to *(pp. 262–263):*

    A. image intensifier lead equivalent

    B. exposure switch

    C. Bucky-slot cover

    D. cumulative timer

    E. lead drape or curtain

    F. tabletop intensity maximum

    G. apron and glove lead equivalency

    H. palpation with remote fluoroscopy units

8. Distinguish between and give examples of primary and secondary barriers *(p. 264)*.

9. What is the usual recommended thickness of x-ray room walls; the recommended height *(p. 264)?*

10. What protects from leakage radiation *(p. 264)?*

11. Identify each of the following as primary or secondary barriers: x-ray room walls, control panel, lead aprons and gloves *(p. 264)*.

12. How should lead aprons and gloves be cared for *(p. 264)?*

13. Describe how a pregnant radiographer might use a second personal monitor *(p. 266)*.

14. What is the gestational fetal dose limit *(p. 266)?*

15. What kinds of counseling and documentation are recommended for the pregnant radiographer *(p. 266)?*

16. What x-ray areas generally have the highest occupational exposure *(p. 266)?*

17. What NCRP rules govern mobile radiography with respect to availability of lead aprons, the exposure cord, the fluoro SSD *(p. 266)?*

18. What NCRP rules govern fluoroscopy equipment with respect to SSD, tabletop intensity, maximum mA, image intensifier lead equivalent, fluoroscopy exposure switch *(p. 266)?*

19. What NCRP rules govern fluoroscopy equipment with respect to collimation, total filtration, protective curtain, Bucky-slot cover, cumulative timer *(pp. 262, 266)?*

A&U Chapter Review Questions

1. Some patients, such as infants and the elderly, are frequently unable to maintain the necessary radiographic position and require assistance. If mechanical restraining devices cannot be used, who of the following is BEST requested to hold these patients?
   (A) floor nurse
   (B) orderly
   (C) friend or relative
   (D) student radiographer

2. Which of the following is (are) features of fluoroscopy equipment, designed especially to eliminate unnecessary radiation to patient and personnel?
    1. protective curtain
    2. filtration
    3. collimation
   (A) 1 only
   (B) 1 and 2 only
   (C) 1 and 3 only
   (D) 1, 2, and 3

3. The protective booth from which the radiographer makes the x-ray exposure is a:
   (A) primary barrier
   (B) secondary barrier
   (C) useful beam barrier
   (D) remnant radiation barrier

4. Radiation dose to personnel is reduced by the following exposure core guidelines:
    1. exposure cords on fixed equipment must be very short
    2. exposure cords on mobile equipment must be at least 6 feet long
    3. exposure cords on fixed and mobile equipment should be the coiled expandable type
   (A) 1 only
   (B) 1 and 2 only
   (C) 2 and 3 only
   (D) 1, 2, and 3

5. Which of the following groups of exposure factors will deliver the least amount of exposure to the patient?
   (A) 100 mAs, 100 kVp
   (B) 200 mAs, 90 kVp
   (C) 400 mAs, 80 kVp
   (D) 800 mAs, 70 kVp

6. Which of the following is (are) guidelines used to reduce personnel and/or patient dose in fluoroscopy?
    1. maximum tabletop intensity of 10 R/min
    2. maximum SSD of 12 inches
    3. minimum filtration of 2.5 mm Al equivalent
   (A) 1 only
   (B) 1 and 2 only
   (C) 1 and 3 only
   (D) 1, 2, and 3

7. Each time an x-ray beam scatters, its intensity at 1 meter from the scattering object is what fraction of its original intensity?
   (A) 1/10
   (B) 1/100
   (C) 1/500
   (D) 1/1000

8. If an individual received 45 mR while standing at 4 feet from a source of radiation for 2 minutes, which of the options listed below will MOST effectively reduce his or her radiation exposure?
   (A) standing 6 feet from the source for 2 minutes
   (B) standing 5 feet from the source for 1 minute
   (C) standing 4 feet from the source for 1 minute
   (D) standing 3 feet from the source for 2 minutes

9. Primary radiation barriers must be AT LEAST how high?
   (A) 5 feet
   (B) 6 feet
   (C) 7 feet
   (D) 8 feet

10. How much protection is provided from a 75 kVp x-ray beam when using a 0.25 mm lead equivalent apron?
   (A) 51%
   (B) 66%
   (C) 88%
   (D) 99%

Answers and Explanations

1. (C) If mechanical restraint is impossible, a friend or relative accompanying the patient should be requested to hold the patient. If a friend or relative is not available, a nurse or orderly may be asked for help. Protective apparel, such as lead apron and gloves, should be provided to the person(s) holding the patient. *Radiology personnel must NEVER assist in holding patients, and the individual assisting should NEVER be in the path of the primary beam.*

2. (D) The *protective curtain,* usually made of leaded vinyl with at least 0.25 mm Pb equivalent, must be positioned between the patient and fluoroscopist to greatly reduce exposure of the fluoroscopist to energetic scatter from the patient. As with over radiation barrierhead equipment, fluoroscopic total *filtration* must be at least 2.5 mm Al equivalent to reduce excessive exposure to low energy radiation. *Collimator*/beam alignment must be accurate to within 2%.

3. (B) Primary barriers are those that protect us from the primary, or useful, beam and have much greater attenuation capability than secondary barriers, which only protect from leakage and scattered radiation. The radiographic room walls are therefore considered primary barriers because the primary beam could be directed toward them, as in chest radiography. Most control booth barriers, however, are secondary barriers because the primary beam is never directed toward them; they are therefore constructed of four thicknesses of gypsum board and/or 1/2 to 1 inch of plate glass. Remnant radiation penetrates the patient and forms the latent image on the film.

4. (B) Radiographic and fluoroscopic equipment is designed to help decrease the exposure dose to patient and operator. One of the design features is the exposure cord.

Exposure cords on fixed equipment must be short enough to prevent the exposure from being made outside the control booth. Exposure cords on mobile equipment must be long enough to permit the operator to stand at least 6 feet from the x-ray tube.

5. (A) mAs regulates the quantity of radiation delivered to the patient. kVp regulates the quality (penetration) of the radiation delivered to the patient. Therefore, higher energy (more penetrating) radiation—which is more likely to exit the patient—accompanied by lower mAs, is the safest combination for the patient.

6. (C) All *fluoroscopic* equipment must provide at least 12 in (30 cm), and preferably 15 in (38 cm), between the x-ray source (focal spot) and the x-ray tabletop (patient/*SSD*), according to NCRP Report no. 102. The tabletop *intensity* of the fluoroscopic beam must not exceed *10 R/min* or 2.1 R/min/mA. Fluoroscopic mA must not exceed 5, although image-intensified fluoroscopy usually operates between 1 and 3 mA. Since the image intensifier functions as a primary barrier, it must have a lead equivalent of at least 2.0 mm.

Beam collimation must be apparent through visualization of unexposed borders on the TV monitor, and *total filtration* must be at least 2.5 mm Al equivalent. Since occupational exposure to scattered radiation is of considerable importance in fluoroscopy, a protective curtain of at least 0.25 mm Pb equivalent must be placed between the patient and fluoroscopist.

7. (D) One of the radiation protection guidelines for the occupationally exposed is that the x-ray beam should scatter twice before reaching the operator. Each time the x-ray beam scatters, its intensity at one meter from the scattering object is about 0.1% of the intensity of the primary beam, ie, *one-thousandth* of its original intensity. That is why, in terms of radiation protection, the patient is considered the most important source of scatter. Of course, the operator should be behind a shielded booth while making the exposure, but multiple scatterings further reduce danger of exposure from scatter radiation. Other scattering objects include the x-ray table, the Bucky-slot cover/*closer,* and the control booth wall.

8. (B) A quick survey of the distractors reveals that options C and D will increase exposure dose; thus, they are eliminated as possible correct answers. Both A and B will serve to reduce radiation exposure, as distance is increased and exposure time decreased in each case. It remains to be seen then, which is the more effective. Using the inverse square law of radiation, it is found that at 6 feet the individual will receive 20 mR in 2 minutes:

$$\frac{I_1}{I_2} = \frac{D_2^2}{D_1^2}$$

Substituting known values:

$$\frac{12 \text{ R/min}}{x} = \frac{12 \text{ ft}^2}{8 \text{ ft}^2}$$

$$\frac{12}{x} = \frac{144}{64}$$

$$144x = 768$$

$$x = 5.3 \text{ R/min at 12 feet}$$

Note the inverse relationship between distance and dose. As distance from the source of radiation increases, dose rate significantly decreases.

9. (C) Radiation protection guidelines have established that primary radiation barriers must be 7 feet high. Primary radiation barriers are walls that the primary beam might be directed toward. They usually contain 1.5 mm lead, but this can vary depending on use factor, and so on.

10. (B) Lead aprons are worn by occupationally exposed individuals during fluoroscopic procedures. Lead aprons are available with various lead equivalents; 0.25, 0.5, and 1.0 mm are the most common. The *1.0 mm* lead equivalent apron will provide close to 100% protection at most kVp levels, but it is rarely used because it weighs anywhere from 12 to 24 pounds! A *0.25 mm* lead equivalent apron will attenuate about 97% of a 50 kVp x-ray beam, 66% of a 75 kVp beam, and 51% of a 100 kVp beam. A *0.5 mm* apron will attenuate about 99% of a 50 kVp beam, 88% of a 75 kVp beam, and 75% of a 100 kVp beam.

Radiation Monitoring

11

KEY TERMS ◀

DOSE EQUIVALENT (DE)

RADIATION ABSORBED DOSE (RAD)

RADIATION EQUIVALENT MAN (REM)

ROENTGEN

PARTICULATE RADIATION

POCKET DOSIMETER

UNIT OF EXPOSURE

I. UNITS OF MEASURE

W.C. Röntgen's paper, "On A New Kind of Rays," described, among other things, x-rays' ionizing effect on air and their effect on photographic emulsions. We use these principles today to detect and quantify radiation exposure.

The radiation units of measure of greatest importance to the radiographer are the roentgen, rad, and rem. Since the ARRT examination does not use SI units (according to the May, 1993 conventions), they will not be covered here.

A. THE ROENTGEN

The ARRT examination does not capitalize "roentgen" as a unit of measure, and no "s" is used at the end, eg, 10 roentgen, *not:* 10 Roentgens (the same is true for the terms rad and rem, ie, an "s" is not used at the end when referring to more than one). When used to express rate, it is abbreviated R/min or R/hr. The **roentgen** is a ◀ unit of measure of *ionization in air.* It is referred to as the **unit of** ◀ **exposure.** Since x-rays ionize air, all the ions of either sign (positive or negative) formed in a particular quantity of air are counted and equated to a quantity of radiation expressed in the unit *roentgen.* The roentgen is valid only for *x and gamma radiations* at energies up to 3 MeV.

B. THE RAD

▶ *Rad* is an acronym for **radiation absorbed dose.** As radiation passes through matter, a certain amount of energy is deposited. Absorbed dose refers to the amount of energy deposited per unit mass and is strongly related to chemical change and biologic damage. The amount of energy deposited and, thus, the amount of possible biologic damage is dependent upon the following.

- Type of radiation
- Atomic number of the tissue
- Energy of the radiation

▶ *Particulate radiation* (alpha, beta, etc) is highly ionizing; as an internal source of radiation, it increases LET, and a significant biologic effect can result. As an external source of radiation, it is virtually innocuous. As the atomic number of the irradiated tissue increases, more x-ray photons are absorbed by tissues (the photoelectric interaction increases), and LET increases. As the energy of radiation increases, it becomes more penetrating and LET decreases, thereby decreasing the likelihood of biologic effects.

Because the rad does not take into account the biologic effect of various types of radiation, it is not used to express occupational exposure.

C. THE REM

▶ *Rem* is an acronym for **radiation equivalent man.** Rem uses the information collected for the rad, but uses a quality factor (QF) as well to predict biologic effects from different types of radiation. Radiations having a high QF have a higher LET and greater potential to
▶ produce biologic damage. The rem is described as the unit of **dose equivalency** (DE), and is used to express occupational exposure.

II. MONITORING DEVICES

A. NCRP GUIDELINES FOR USE

Radiation monitoring is used to evaluate the effectiveness of the radiation safety policies and practices in place. NCRP Report no. 105 recommends that monitoring should be provided for occupationally exposed individuals in a controlled area who are likely to receive more than *one fourth the dose equivalent limit.*

B. FILM BADGE

The most familiar radiation monitor is probably the *film badge.* It consists of special radiation-dosimetry film packaged like dental film and is enclosed in a special plastic holder. The plastic holder features an open window (through which the user's name appears) and various *filters,* which serve to identify the *type and energy of radiation* (Fig. 11–1).

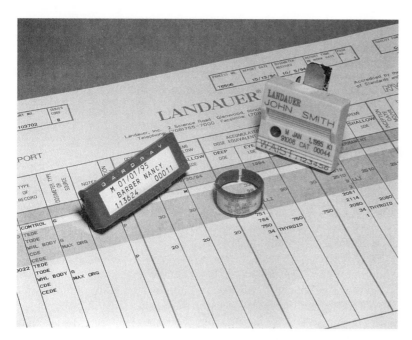

Figure 11–1. The film badge (left) contains filters that function to determine the type and energy of radiation received by the wearer. The TLD (right) contains thermoluminescent crystals that emit quantities of light proportional to their degree of exposure. The ring badge (center) is particularly useful for individuals whose hands are in close proximity to radioactive nuclides or the fluoroscopic x-ray field. A report similar to the one shown is returned monthly, documenting the radiation dose received by each of the personnel monitors. (Courtesy of Landauer, Inc, Glenwood, IL.)

Radiation that exposes film behind an aluminum filter is more energetic than radiation that only passes through the open window, and less energetic than radiation penetrating a copper filter. Film badges are used for *1 month*, collected, and sent to a special laboratory for processing. The degree of exposure is carefully evaluated and equated to a dose, usually expressed in *mrem;* the film badge can measure doses as low as 10 mrem. An official written report is sent to the sponsoring institution (Fig. 11–1).

C. THERMOLUMINESCENT DOSIMETER

A somewhat newer type of personnel radiation monitor is the *thermoluminescent dosimeter (TLD).* The TLD (Fig. 11–1) contains crystalline chips of lithium fluoride (LiF). LiF absorbs and stores the energy associated with exposure to ionizing radiation. When the TLD is returned to the laboratory for processing, the LiF chips are heated. This process causes a release of visible light from the chips in proportion to the amount of ionizing radiation absorbed. The quantity of light emitted is equated to a radiation quantity expressed in mrem on the written report returned to the user. The TLD is more sensitive and precise than the film badge, ie, it can measure doses as low as 5 mrem. The TLD is unaffected by heat and/or humidity and can be worn up to 3 months before processing. However, in the unlikely event that the user had unknowingly received excessive radiation exposure, he or she should be made aware of it as soon as possible, and the event should be recent enough to be able to recall. This is often considered the single disadvantage of the TLD. Both the film badge and TLD measure a variety of energies of x, beta, and gamma radiations.

D. POCKET DOSIMETER

▶ The use of a ***pocket dosimeter*** (Fig. 11–2) is indicated when working with high exposures or large quantities of radiation for a short period of time, so that an immediate reading is available to the user. The pocket dosimeter is sensitive and accurate but has limited application in diagnostic radiography.

The pocket dosimeter, or *pocket isolation chamber,* resembles a pen-light. Within the dosimeter is a thimble ionization chamber. In the presence of ionizing radiation, a particular quantity of air will be ionized and cause the fiber indicator to register radiation quantity in milliroentgen (mR). The self-reading type may be "read" by holding the dosimeter up to the light and, looking through the eyepiece, observing the fiber indicator, which indicates a quantity of 0 to 200 mR. The disadvantage of the pocket dosimeter is that it does not provide a permanent legal record of exposure.

Personnel monitors should be worn consistently in the same place and facing forward (ie, with the open window and user's identification visible). The use of a second monitor is occasionally indicated. The *pregnant radiographer* may wear a second, waist-level, badge under her lead apron to approximate fetal dose. If the first badge is worn at the collar outside the lead apron it will approximate dose to the head and neck and will provide an overestimation of dose to the shielded organs. Some procedures require the hands to be near the useful beam (ie, some fluoroscopic and vascular procedures). A finger, or ring, monitor will provide information on exposure to the hands.

Figure 11–2. The pocket dosimeter contains a small ionization chamber that counts charges in proportion to the exposure received. (Courtesy of Nuclear Associates.)

The radiographer is occupationally exposed to *low energy, low LET* radiation. Monitoring devices are worn only for occupational purposes and never if the individual is exposed for medical or dental reasons.

III. NCRP RECOMMENDATIONS

A part of the professional radiographer's responsibility lies in keeping occupational exposure to a minimum. The use of radiation-monitoring devices helps evaluate the effectiveness of radiation-protection practices. The periodic reports received from film-badge or TLD laboratories are official legal documents that must be reviewed, and an attempt should be made to reduce *any* exposure, no matter how small.

NCRP Report no. 105 recommends that occupationally exposed individuals 18 years of age and older not receive exposures in excess of 5 rem (5000 mrem) annually. A radiography student beginning his or her training before the age of 18 must not receive an annual dose of more than 0.1 rem (100 mrem).

The lifetime cumulative exposure for the occupationally exposed individual is determined using the formula: 1 rem × age in years. Thus, a 26-year-old radiographer's lifetime occupational exposure must not exceed 26 rem. The pregnant radiographer's *gestational* exposure to the fetus must not exceed 0.5 rem (500 mrem), the *monthly* fetal dose must not exceed 0.05 rem (50 mrem).

These are the recommended maximum dose-equivalent limits. The actual mean annual exposure to occupationally exposed medical personnel is 100 to 140 mrem, well below the recommended limit! This seems to indicate that we are performing our tasks in a safe, conscientious, and ethical manner.

Summary

- **The roentgen, or unit of exposure, (R unit) is the unit used to describe quantity of ionization in air.**
- **The rad describes absorbed dose.**
- **The rem is the unit of dose equivalency (DE), used to quantify occupational exposure.**
- **Film badges are convenient, low-cost radiation monitors that are processed monthly.**
- **TLDs utilize LiF crystals to store exposure information. They are more precise and more expensive than film badges and may be processed quarterly.**
- **Film badges and TLDs measure exposure to beta, x, and gamma radiation.**
- **Pocket dosimeters are thimble ionization chambers used to monitor larger quantities of radiation exposure, up to 200 mR.**
- **Radiographers must strive to keep their occupational dose ALARA.**
- **NCRP Report no. 91 recommends limits for exposure to ionizing radiation with which radiographers should be familiar.**

Chapter Exercises

 Congratulations! *You have completed your review of this chapter. If you are able to answer the following group of very comprehensive questions, you should feel confident that you have really mastered this section. You are then ready to go on to "Registry-type" questions that follow. For greatest success, do not go to the multiple choice questions without first completing the short answer questions below.*

1. Discuss the R as a unit of measure; what it measures, the radiation(s) it measures and up to what energy *(p. 275).*

2. What does the acronym *rad* mean? Define rad *(p. 276).*

3. Name the three things influencing the amount of energy deposited (rad) in tissue *(p. 276).*

4. Relate particulate radiation to degree of ionization in tissue, to LET, and to possible biologic effects *(p. 276).*

5. What does the acronym *rem* mean *(p. 276)?*

6. Why can the rem be accurately used to describe occupational DE, whereas the rad cannot *(p. 276)?*

7. Describe the film badge. Include the following in your description *(pp. 276–277):*

   A. construction

   B. purpose of filters

   C. length of time used

   D. type(s) of radiation detected

   E. how it is "read" and in what unit

   F. any advantages or disadvantages

8. Describe the TLD. Include the following in your description *(p. 277):*

   A. construction

   B. type of crystals used; their unique characteristics

C. length of time used

D. type(s) of radiation detected

E. how it is "read" and in what unit

F. any advantages or disadvantages

9. Describe the pocket dosimeter. Include the following in your description *(p. 278):*

A. construction

B. indications for use

C. how it is "read," in what unit, and up to what maximum

D. any advantages or disadvantages

10. What is the NCRP recommended dose limit for occupational exposure in individuals less than 18 years of age; over 18 years of age *(p. 279)?*

11. How is lifetime cumulative occupational exposure determined *(p. 279)?*

12. What is the NCRP recommended dose limit for gestational fetal exposure *(p. 279)?*

A&I Chapter Review Questions

1. During which period of development is the fetus most radiosensitive?
   (A) first trimester
   (B) second trimester
   (C) third trimester
   (D) fourth trimester

2. If a student radiographer who is under 18 years old begins training, what is his or her annual dose limit?
   (A) 0.1 rem (1 mSv)
   (B) 0.5 rem (5 mSv)
   (C) 5 rem (50 mSv)
   (D) 10 rem (100 mSv)

3. The unit of measure used to express occupational exposure is the:
   (A) roentgen (C/Kg)
   (B) rad (Gray)
   (C) rem (Seivert)
   (D) RBE

4. The MPD for occupationally exposed individuals is valid for:
   (A) alpha, beta, and x-radiations
   (B) x and gamma radiations only
   (C) beta, x, and gamma radiations
   (D) all ionizing radiations

5. The purpose of filters in a film badge is:
   (A) to eliminate harmful rays
   (B) to measure radiation quality
   (C) to prevent exposure from alpha particles
   (D) as a support for film contained within

6. Which of the following is a measure of dose to biologic tissue?
   (A) roentgen (C/kg)
   (B) rad (Gy)
   (C) rem (Sv)
   (D) RBE

7. A thermoluminescent dosimetry system would use which of the following crystals?
   (A) silver bromide
   (B) sodium sulfite
   (C) lithium fluoride
   (D) ferrous sulfate

8. What is the established fetal dose–limit guideline for pregnant radiographers during the entire gestation period?
   (A) 0.1 rem
   (B) 0.5 rem
   (C) 5.0 rem
   (D) 10.0 rem

9. The NCRP recommends an annual effective occupational dose equivalent limit of:
   (A) 25 mSv (2.5 rem)
   (B) 50 mSv (5 rem)
   (C) 100 mSv (10 rem)
   (D) 200 mSv (20 rem)

10. The operation of personnel radiation monitoring devices depends on which of the following?
    1. ionization
    2. thermoluminescence
    3. resonance
   (A) 1 only
   (B) 1 and 2 only
   (C) 2 and 3 only
   (D) 1, 2, and 3

Answers and Explanations

1. (A) The first trimester of the developing fetus is the most radiosensitive. Because the fetus is undergoing major organogenesis, very high doses of radiation at this time can cause congenital anomalies. Radiosensitivity gradually decreases through the rest of the pregnancy.

2. (A) Because the established dose limit formula guideline is used for occupationally exposed persons 18 years of age and older, guidelines had to be established in the event a student entered training prior to age 18. The guideline states that the occupational dose limit for students under age 18 is 0.1 rem (100 mrem or 1 mSv) in any given year.

3. (C) *Roentgen* is the unit of exposure; it measures the quantity of ionizations in air. *Rad* is an acronym for **r**adiation **a**bsorbed **d**ose; it measures the energy deposited in any material. *Rem* is an acronym for **r**adiation **e**quivalent **m**an; it includes the relative biologic effectiveness (RBE) specific to the tissue irradiated, thereby being a valid unit of measure of dose to biologic material.

4. (C) The occupational MPD is valid for beta, x, and gamma radiations. Since alpha radiation is so rapidly ionizing, traditional personnel monitors will not record alpha radiation. Because alpha particles are capable of penetrating only a few cm of air, they are practically harmless as an external source.

5. (B) The filters (usually aluminum and copper) serve to help measure radiation quality (energy). Only the most energetic radiation will penetrate the copper; radiation of lower levels will penetrate the aluminum, and the lowest energy radiation will pass readily through the unfiltered area. Thus radiation of different energy levels can be recorded, measured, and reported.

6. (C) Roentgen is the unit of exposure; it measures the quantity of ionization in air. Rad is an acronym for radiation absorbed dose; it measures the energy deposited in any material. Rem is an acronym for radiation equivalent man; it includes the relative biologic effectiveness (RBE) specific to the tissue irradiated, thereby being a valid unit of measure of dose to biologic material.

7. (C) Thermoluminescent dosimeters (TLDs) are personnel radiation monitors that use lithium fluoride crystals. These crystals, once exposed to ionizing radiation and then heated, give off light proportional to the amount of radiation received. TLDs are very accurate personal monitors.

8. (B) The pregnant radiographer poses a special radiation protection consideration, for the safety of the unborn individual must be considered. It must be remembered that the developing fetus is particularly sensitive to radiation exposure. Therefore, established guidelines state that the occupational radiation exposure to the fetus must not exceed 0.5 rem (500 mrem, or 5 mSv) during the entire gestation period.

9. (B) A 1984 review of radiation exposure data revealed that the average annual dose equivalent for monitored radiation workers was approximately 2.3 mSv (0.23 rem). The fact that this is approximately one tenth the recommended limit indicates that the limit is adequate for radiation protection purposes. Therefore the NCRP reiterates its 1971 recommended annual limit of 50 mSv (5 rem). *(NCRP Report No. 105, pp 14–15)*

10. (B) Ionization is the fundamental principle of operation of both the film badge and pocket dosimeter. In the film badge, the film's silver halide emulsion is ionized by x-ray photons. The pocket dosimeter contains an ionization chamber, and the number of ionizations taking place may be equated to exposure dose. Resonance refers to motion, and has no application to personnel radiation monitoring.

part

IV

Image Production and Evaluation

Chapter 13
Automatic Processing and Quality Assurance

I. Film Storage Considerations
  A. Storage Conditions
  1. Temperature and Humidity
  2. Chemicals and Radiation
  3. Expiration Dates
  4. Position of Film Boxes
  5. Film Bin
  B. Safelight Illumination
  1. Types
  2. White Light Leaks

II. Cassettes
  A. Routine Care
  B. Artifacts

III. Identification of Radiographs
  A. Essential Information
  B. Types of Systems

IV. Automatic Film Processing
  A. Chemistry Overview
  1. Developer
  2. Fixer
  3. Wash
  B. Transport System

  C. Replenishment System
  D. Temperature Regulation
  E. Recirculation System
  F. Wash and Dryer Systems
  G. Silver Recovery

Chapter 14
Evaluating Radiographs

I. Evaluation Standards and Image Characteristics
  A. Overview
  B. Recorded Detail and Distortion
  C. Radiographic Density and Contrast
  D. Grid Selection and Use
  E. Film Identification
  F. Collimation and Shielding
  G. Demonstration of Structures

II. Identifying and Correcting Errors
  A. Technical Factor Selection
  B. Equipment Use and Positioning
  C. Patient Variables
  D. Identification of Artifacts
  E. Processing Errors and Malfunction

Radiography students occasionally find the area of technical factors, or technique, to be their first stumbling block. Everything prior to this may have seemed so straightforward and understandable: radiation protection, anatomy, positioning, even physics. Why is it that technique can be so confusing? Perhaps it is because there are so many variables, so many choices to be made, so many factors to consider.

The most obvious variable, and the one in which the least modification is possible, is the patient. Careful and accurate patient evaluation cannot be overemphasized. Body habitus, muscle tone, pathology, trauma, and age all require accurate assessment prior to the intelligent selection of technical factors.

Even in departments using only automatic exposure controls (AECs), the radiographer's accurate evaluation of the patient will result in more efficient use of the AEC. Sometimes, AECs selection will require adjustment or modification; sometimes it will be necessary to use manual technique.

After evaluating the patient, various radiographic accessories must be considered: screen and film combinations, grid ratios, and filters, to name a few. Fortunately, these items are fairly standard from one radiographic room to the next within a given department. When it comes to mobile radiography or being able to move from one department to another, however, a good working knowledge of radiographic accessories and their use is required.

What about circumstances that require deviation from the normal SID, or the introduction of an OID? What if the patient's leg is casted? How does "coning down" (collimating) affect the radiographic image? Why does kVp affect radiographic density as well as regulate radiographic contrast?

This chapter will endeavor to structure, and show the relationship among, these variables to provide a clear understanding and complete review of their impact on the radiographic image.

Technical Factors

12

KEY TERMS ◀

ACTIVE LAYER	FLUORESCENCE	PHOSPHORESCENCE
ACTUAL FOCAL SPOT	FOCAL SPOT	QUANTUM MOTTLE
AFTERGLOW	FORESHORTENING	RARE EARTH PHOSPHORS
ANODE HEEL EFFECT	INTENSIFYING SCREENS	RECORDED DETAIL
BLUR	INVOLUNTARY MOTION	RESOLUTION
CALCIUM TUNGSTATE	LAG	SCREEN SPEED
CONVERSION EFFICIENCY	LINE FOCUS PRINCIPLE	SCREEN–FILM CONTACT
DISTORTION	MAGNIFICATION	SID
EDGE GRADIENT	OID	SPECTRAL MATCHING
EFFECTIVE FOCAL SPOT	OBJECT UNSHARPNESS	UNSHARPNESS
ELONGATION	PHOSPHOR	VOLUNTARY MOTION

I. FACTORS AFFECTING RECORDED DETAIL AND DISTORTION

The term **recorded detail** refers to the *clarity,* or **resolution,** with ◀ which a radiographic image is rendered. If the tiny image details (eg, bony trabeculae, minute calcifications) of a variety of radiographs made under different circumstances were compared, especially with the use of a magnifying glass, it would be noted that the image details

Figure 12–1. Resolution test pattern. Resolution is measured with the use of a *resolution test pattern* and is expressed in line pairs per millimeter (lp/mm). The *star pattern* is generally used for focal spot size evaluation, while the *parallel line* type is used for evaluating intensifying screens. (Courtesy of Nuclear Associates.)

appear with varying degrees of clarity. On some of the radiographs, details would be clearly defined, while on other radiographs, the borders of details would have varying degrees of unsharpness, that is they would not be defined as sharply nor with the same degree of resolution. This is the basic concept of recorded detail.

▶ The term ***distortion*** refers to misrepresentation of the actual
▶ *size (**magnification**)* or *shape (**foreshortening** or **elongation**)* of the structures imaged—which may be partly or wholly due to inherent object unsharpness.

The degree of resolution transferred to the image receptor is a function of the resolving power of each of the system components (and the degree of expertise of the operator) and is expressed in line pairs per millimeter (lp/mm) (Fig. 12–1). Resolution describes how closely fine details may be associated and still be recognized as separate details before seeming to blend into each other and appear "as one" (Fig. 12–2).

A

B

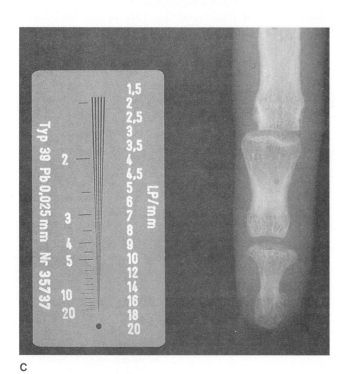

C

Figure 12–2. Magnified views of the first phalanx and resolution test pattern. **(A)** Significant blur or unsharpness of image details; resolution is approximately 6 lp/mm. **(B)** Improved recorded detail; resolution of about 8 lp/mm. **(C)** Best recorded detail (least blur); resolution of about 12 lp/mm. (From the American College of Radiology Learning File. Courtesy of the ACR.)

The term "visibility of detail" refers to *how well the recorded detail can be seen,* eg, excessive density or scattered radiation fog constitutes poor visibility of detail because it obscures the details. Density and fog have no effect on how sharply, or with what degree of clarity, an image detail is rendered. They do, however, determine how easily we are able to recognize those details (ie, *visibility* of detail).

There are a number of technical factors that impact recorded detail. Some of them influence the geometry (size and shape) of the image, and others affect its photographic qualities. Each of the factors having an effect on recorded detail will be discussed further.

Summary

- Recorded detail refers to the sharpness and abruptness of structural detail borders.
- Other terms that refer to *recorded detail* are: resolution, clarity, definition, and sharpness.
- Recorded detail is measured with a *resolution test pattern* and expressed in *lp/mm.*
- Recorded detail is affected by a number of factors; some influence the geometry of the image, while others affect its photographic qualities.
- Anything that affects density or contrast affects *visibility of detail.*
- Distortion relates to the size and shape of the *image* compared to the actual size and shape of the *object.*
- The terms *magnification, elongation,* and *foreshortening* are used when describing distortion.

A. DISTANCES

If you place your hand between a flashlight and the wall of a dimly lighted room, the shadow of your hand will vary in size and clarity as it changes position with respect to the flashlight and wall. As your hand moves farther from the wall, the shadow becomes larger and

Figure 12–3. Effect of distance on magnification and detail. As the finger moves away from the surface (toward the light source), the shadow image becomes magified and blurry.

less distinct. As your hand is brought closer to the wall (and farther from the flashlight) the shadow becomes more like the actual size of your hand and appears with more clarity (Fig. 12–3).

1. OID. This is the effect object-to-image-receptor distance *(OID)* ◄ has on recorded detail. Because (like light) the x-ray beam diverges as it leaves its source, an increase in OID will increase *magnification.* ◄ X-ray photons strike all parts of the object, continue traveling in a divergent fashion, and "deposit" the (now magnified and unsharp) image on the film or other image receptor (Fig. 12–4). *Geometrically recorded detail improves as OID decreases.*

2. SID. A similar example can be used to show the effect of source-to-image-receptor distance *(SID)* on recorded detail. If your ◄ hand is placed a given distance from the wall, any change in the distance between the light source and wall will affect the magnification and clarity of the shadow image. As the flashlight moves closer to your hand, the shadow will become larger and less distinct. As the flashlight is moved farther from the wall, the shadow approaches the actual size of your hand and becomes sharper and more distinct (Fig. 12–5). Similarly, as the distance between the x-ray source and image recorder increases, the x-ray image is less magnified and more distinct (Fig. 12–6). *Geometrically recorded detail improves as SID increases.*

$$M = \frac{IM}{OB} = \frac{SID}{SOD}$$

Figure 12–4. As distance from the object to image receptor (OID) increases, the projected size of the image increases, that is, magnification increases. (Modified from Wolbarst, AB. *Physics of Radiology.* East Norwalk, CT: Appleton & Lange, 1993.)

Figure 12–5. Effect of distance on magnification and detail. As the flashlight moves closer to the finger, the shadow image becomes magnified and blurry.

Figure 12–6. **(A)** PA erect film taken at a distance of 6 ft demonstrates an accurate representation of the heart shadow and various parenchymal and bony structures. **(B)** AP erect at 50 in of the same patient taken within 24 hours and with no change in patient condition. The heart appears markedly larger (15.5 cm on PA and 20 cm on AP) for two reasons: 1. the heart is farther from the film in the AP projection, and 2. the SID is decreased—thus, the heart is magnified. (From the American College of Radiology Learning File. Courtesy of the ACR.)

Summary

- **Recorded detail and magnification are inversely related, that is, recorded detail increases as magnification decreases.**
- **SID and OID regulate magnification and therefore influence the geometric properties, and hence recorded detail, of the radiographic image.**
- **SID is inversely related to magnification (increased SID = decreased magnification) and directly related to recorded detail (increased SID = increased recorded detail).**
- **OID is directly related to magnification (increased OID = increased magnification) and inversely related to recorded detail (increased OID = decreased recorded detail).**

B. INHERENT OBJECT UNSHARPNESS

▶ A certain amount of **object unsharpness** is an inherent part of every radiographic image *due to the position and shape of anatomic structures within the body.*

1. Position Within the Body. Structures within the three-dimensional body lie in different planes. For example, the frontal sinuses

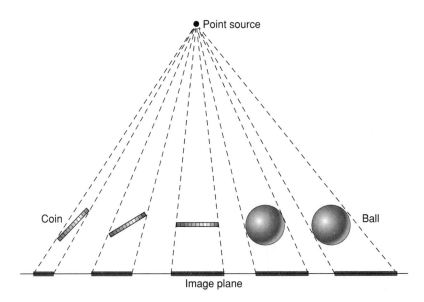

Figure 12–7. The shape of various structures can be radiographically misrepresented (ie, *foreshortened or elongated*) as a result of their position in the body; that misrepresentation can be exaggerated when the part is out of the central axis of the x-ray beam. (From Wolbarst, AB. *Physics of Radiology.* East Norwalk, CT: Appleton & Lange, 1993.)

are more anterior than the sphenoids, the ureters are more anterior than the kidneys, the upper renal poles lie in a plane posterior to the lower renal poles, the fundus of the stomach is more posterior than the body and pylorus, the posterior portions of the sacroiliac joints are more medial than their anterior portions.

2. Structural Shape. Additionally, the three-dimensional shape of solid anatomic structures rarely coincides with the shape of the divergent beam. Consequently, some structures are imaged with more inherent distortion than others and shapes of anatomic structures can be entirely misrepresented. Structures farther from the image receptor will be distorted (ie, *magnified*) more than those closer to the image receptor.

For the shape of anatomic structures to be accurately recorded, the structures must be parallel to the x-ray tube and the image receptor and aligned with the central ray (CR). The shape of anatomic structures lying at an angle within the body or placed away from the CR will be misrepresented on the image receptor (Fig. 12–7).

Unless the edges of a three-dimensional *object* conform to the shape of the x-ray beam, blur or unsharpness will occur at the partially attenuating edge of the object. As Figure 12–8 illustrates, this will be accompanied by changes in optical density, according to the thickness of areas traversed by the x-ray beam.

Summary

■ **Some geometric unsharpness is intrinsic due to the shape and position of the structure of interest within the body.**

Figure 12–8. Blur or unsharpness results when the shape of a three-dimensional object does not coincide with that of the x-ray beam. Blur is accompanied by changes in optical density as a result of differing thicknesses traversed by the x-ray beam. (From Wolbarst, AB. *Physics of Radiology.* East Norwalk, CT: Appleton & Lange, 1993.)

- Structures that do not parallel the x-ray tube and film and/or that lie outside the central axis of the x-ray beam will be foreshortened or elongated.
- Structures within the body lie at varying distances from the x-ray film, producing varying degrees of magnification.

C. Focal Spot Size

▶ Another factor influencing the geometry of the image is *focal spot* size. If x-ray photons were emitted from a single point source, structures would be recorded and resolved with great clarity. However, because x-ray photons emerge from a measurable focus, image details are represented with unsharp edges. As shown in Figures 12–9 and 12–10, photons emerging from various points on a measurable focal spot are responsible for producing blurred, unsharp edges of anatomic details. The extent or size of the unsharp area is directly related to the focal spot size and OID, and inversely related to the SID, ie, unsharpness increases as focal spot size and OID increase and as the SID decreases.

This border of unsharpness around image details is often ▶ referred to as *blur* or *unsharpness,* or *edge gradient.* The smaller the focal spot size, the better the geometrically recorded detail.

▶ A distinction is made between the *actual focal spot* and the ▶ *effective* (projected or apparent) *focal spot.* The actual focal spot is the finite area on the tungsten target that is actually bombarded by electrons from the filament. The effective focal spot is the foreshortened size of the focus as it is projected down toward the image receptor, ie, as it would be seen looking up into the emerging x-ray ▶ beam. This is called *line focusing* or the *line focus principle* (Fig. 12–11). We generally speak in terms of the effective, or projected, focal spot; manufacturers state effective focal spot size.

The angle of the anode can have a significant effect on recorded detail. Differences in anode angle, all other factors remaining constant, will affect the size of the effective focal spot, as illustrated in Figure 12–11C, D, and E. The *actual* focal spots in Figure 12–11C

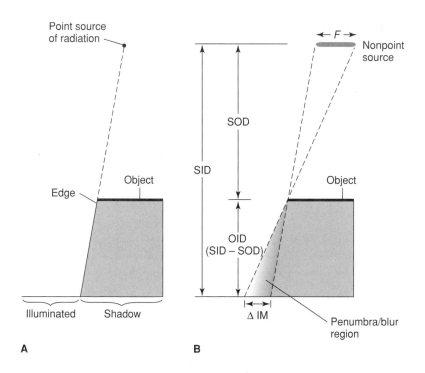

Point source
of radiation

Nonpoint
source

Edge

Object

Object

SID

SOD

OID
(SID − SOD)

Illuminated   Shadow

Δ IM

Penumbra/blur
region

A

B

Figure 12–9. X-ray photons emitted from a point source (**A**) will provide an image having sharply defined borders. X-ray photons emitted from a measurable focal spot (**B**) will produce a zone of blur or unsharpness around each image detail. The degree of blur is directly related to the size of the focal spot. (Modified from Wolbarst, AB. *Physics of Radiology.* East Norwalk, CT: Appleton & Lange, 1993.)

A

FOCAL SPOT SIZE = 1.2 MM (NOM)
MAGNIFICATION = 1.16

B

Figure 12–10. Effect of focal spot on recorded detail. Both images were produced using direct exposure technique to better show the effect of focal spot size on detail, independent of the influence of intensifying screens. (**A**) Magnified image of the first metacarpal, made with a 0.6 mm focal spot. Note the blur or unsharpness associated with bony trabeculae, especially noticeable on the magnified image. (**B**) Film made under identical conditions but using a 1.2 mm focal spot; more severe degradation of recorded detail is demonstrated as a result of blur from the use of a larger focal spot. *Note:* Magnification views must always be made with a 0.3 mm (fractional) focal spot, or smaller, to preserve recorded detail. (From the American College of Radiology Learning File. Courtesy of the ACR.)

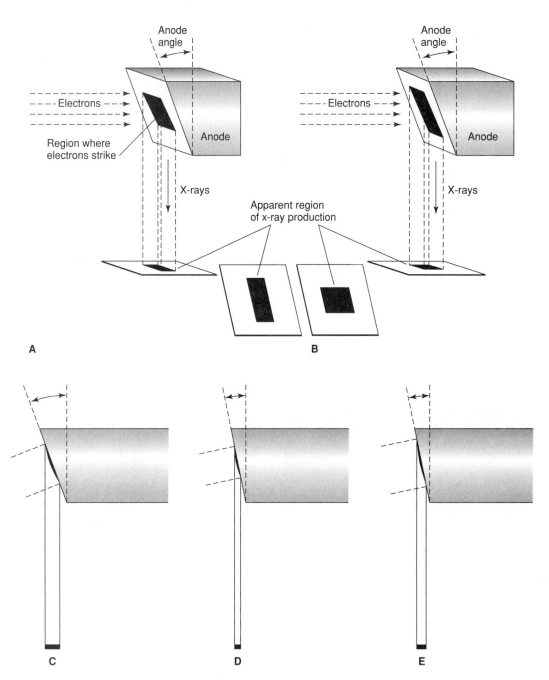

Figure 12–11. **(A)** and **(B)** How the apparent focal spot will differ from the actual focal spot as a result of the line focus principle. **(C)** and **(D)** How the angle/bevel of the actual focal spot will affect the projected focal spot. **(E)** How a small anode angle combined with a large actual focal spot can result in a small effective focal spot. The size of the effective focal spot, with its associated blur, actually varies along the length of the image receptor, being largest at the cathode end of the image receptor and smallest at the anode end (see Figs. 12–12 and 12–13). (**(A)** and **(B)** from Wolbarst, AB. *Physics of Radiology.* East Norwalk, CT: Appleton & Lange, 1993.)

and D are the same size, but the anode *angle* in D is half of that in C. Note how much smaller the *effective* or *projected* focal spot is in Figure 12–11D.

Hence, when using a very small anode angle, a larger actual anode area can be bombarded (Fig. 12–11E) while maintaining a small effective focal spot. Thus, a "fractional" (0.3 mm or smaller) effective focal spot can be maintained, recorded detail is improved, and anode heat-load tolerance is not compromised. This type of x-ray tube is useful in magnification of small blood vessels.

The size of the effective focal spot, with its associated blur or unsharpness, actually varies along the length of the image receptor, being largest at the cathode end of the image receptor and smallest at the anode end (Figs. 12–12 and 12–13).

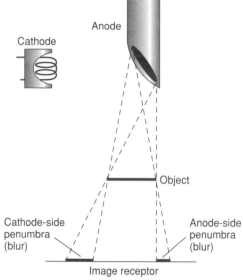

Figure 12–12. Due to the angle of the anode, unsharpness or blur is greatest at the cathode end of the image receptor. (From Wolbarst, AB. *Physics of Radiology.* East Norwalk, CT: Appleton & Lange, 1993.)

Figure 12–13. Variation of effective focal spot size along the longitudinal tube axis. Three images of the third phalanx are shown: one taken at the anode end of the x-ray beam, one at the central portion of the beam, and one at the cathode end. The images clearly illustrate gradual loss of recorded detail toward the cathode end of the x-ray beam. (From the American College of Radiology Learning File. Courtesy of the ACR.)

If the use of a smaller focal spot size provides us with better recorded detail, why isn't the smallest focal spot available always used? Simply because focal spot size is also associated with the buildup of heat within the x-ray tube. Large quantities of heat delivered to the x-ray tube, especially in a short period of time, can be very damaging to the x-ray tube and can shorten its life span.

If the focal spot is small, heat is confined to a tiny area; localized melting of the target material and anode pitting and/or cracking can occur more easily. The larger the focal spot, the greater the surface area available for heat dispersion.

The perfect combination would, of course, be a large actual focus that could withstand heat and still provide a small effective focus for optimum recorded detail. This can be achieved by using an x-ray tube with a small target *angle* of about 7 to 10°. As previously mentioned, the smaller angle enables a larger "face" to be presented to the electron stream, that is, a larger surface area over which to disperse heat (Fig. 12–11). The slight target angle causes significant foreshortening of the actual focal spot, creating a very small *effective* focal spot.

▶ A difficulty associated with the use of a small target angle, however, is maintaining a large (14 × 17) field size. The small target angle produces a pronounced ***anode heel effect*** (Fig. 12–14.) Using a small target angle, a typical radiographic distance of 40″ SID, and a 14″ × 17″ image receptor, there will be approximately 2″ of unexposed film at the anode end of the radiograph. This may be remedied with an increase in SID but, consequently, must be accompanied by an appropriate increase in exposure factors.

Figure 12–14. The anode heel effect. As x-ray photons are produced within the anode, a portion of the divergent beam at its anode end **(A)** is absorbed by the anode's "heel." This represents a decrease in x-ray beam intensity at the anode end of the x-ray beam. The smaller/steeper the target angle/bevel, the more pronounced the heel effect. (From Wolbarst, AB. *Physics of Radiology.* East Norwalk, CT: Appleton & Lange, 1993.)

Summary

- Focal spot size affects detail by influencing the degree of blur or unsharpness: increased focal spot size = increased blur = decreased detail.
- Unsharpness or blur is directly related to focal spot size and OID, and inversely related to SID.
- The use of a small focal spot improves recorded detail but generates more heat at the anode.
- The effective or projected focal spot size is always smaller than the actual focal spot according to the line focus principle.
- Effective focal spot size varies along the longitudinal axis of the image receptor, being largest at the cathode end and smallest at the anode end of the x-ray beam.
- Smaller target angles can permit larger actual focal spot sizes while maintaining small effective focal spot sizes—at the expense of accentuating the anode heel effect.
- Use of a small target angle can limit image receptor coverage at traditional and short SIDs.

D. MOTION

Image blur or unsharpness, as a result of motion, can cause severe degradation of recorded detail (Fig. 12–15). The best method of minimizing **voluntary motion** is through good *communication* and suspended respiration. A patient who understands what to expect and what is expected of him or her is better prepared and more likely to cooperate than a patient whose concerns have been inadequately addressed.

Involuntary motion, such as peristaltic activity, muscle spasms, and heart action, cannot be controlled by the patient. The best way to minimize involuntary motion is by using the shortest possible *exposure time*. Motion is often a problem in mobile radiography with machines of limited output (thereby prohibiting the use of short exposure times).

Special positioning devices (such as pediatric immobilizers), positioning sponges, and carefully placed sandbags are frequently used to assist the patient in maintaining the required position.

Equipment motion can cause an effect similar to that caused by patient motion. Bucky motion can cause motion of the part during tabletop examinations; x-ray equipment often has a switch to turn off the Bucky when doing tabletop work. Bumping an improperly balanced tube head just before making the exposure can result in motion blur or unsharpness if the exposure is made while the tube head is still vibrating. Motion blur is probably the greatest enemy of recorded detail and is most obvious when the motion is close to the film (ie, part motion is more damaging to recorded detail than tube motion; Fig. 12–16).

Deliberate motion is occasionally used to blur out unwanted structures so that the area of interest can be seen to better advantage (Fig. 12–17). The "breathing techniques" of lateral thoracic spine and transthoracic shoulder are typical examples. Another is the more specialized procedure of tomography, in which a preselected structure plane will be clearly delineated while structures above and below that plane are blurred.

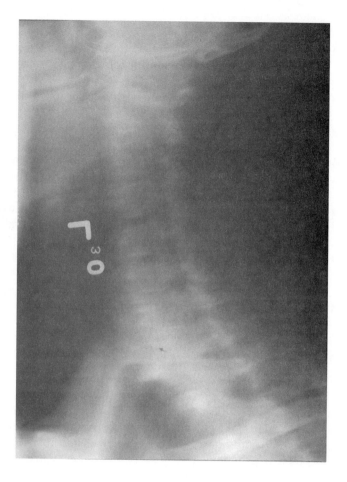

Figure 12–15. Loss of recorded detail as a result of motion of the part. (From the American College of Radiology Learning File. Courtesy of the ACR.)

Summary

- **Motion is the greatest adversary of recorded detail.**
- **Voluntary patient motion can be minimized through good communication.**
- **Involuntary patient motion is best minimized by using the shortest possible exposure time.**
- **Various radiographic accessories are available to help minimize both voluntary and involuntary patient motion.**
- **Equipment motion can also result in loss of recorded detail in the form of image blur.**
- **Special techniques that introduce motion are sometimes employed to see some structures particularly well.**

E. INTENSIFYING SCREENS

Radiographic images produced directly on film emulsion solely by x-rays require many times more x-ray exposure than images produced with the use of intensifying screens. In the very early days of radiography, before **intensifying screens** were available, images were produced by exposure of photographic emulsion to x-rays alone. Tremendously lengthy exposures were required for even the small-

A

B

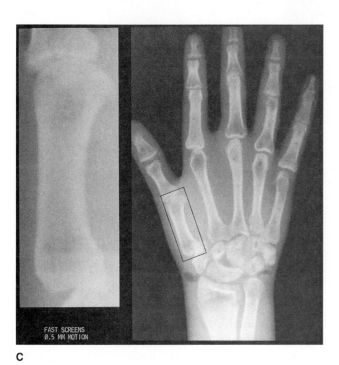

C

Figure 12–16. **(A)** Film made using detail (100 speed) screens; 0.5 mm of motion was introduced. Motion blur is noticeable, particularly in the magnified view of the first metacarpal. Compare the recorded detail of film **A** with that of film **B**. **(B)** Also made using detail/100 speed screens, but having no motion. **(C)** Made with fast/400 speed screens and 0.5 mm motion. Notice how much more obvious detail loss becomes with a faster imaging system, often used in radiology departments today. (From the American College of Radiology Learning File. Courtesy of the ACR.)

A

B

Figure 12–17. **(A)** Plain IVU (also termed IVP or EXU) radiograph with no visible abnormalities. **(B)** An 8-cm tomographic section of the same patient clearly depicting a 7-cm renal cyst overlying the R mid-renal cortex. (From the American College of Radiology Learning File. Courtesy of the ACR.)

est parts. These exposures took their toll on the fragile, scarcely understood equipment and, of course, on the unsuspecting victims of excessive radiation exposure. Direct exposure technique was frequently used through the 1960s and 1970s for examinations of extremities and other small parts not requiring a grid. Due to the excessive patient dose, direct exposure technique is rarely used today.

In 1896, Thomas Edison developed the ***calcium tungstate*** intensifying screen that served to reduce the required exposure to a fraction of that needed without screens. Calcium tungstate screens gained wide acceptance during World War I and were used almost exclusively until the advent of ***rare earth phosphors*** in the early 1970s. ◄

The active ingredient in intensifying screens is the fluorescent ***phosphor,*** which functions to change x-ray photon energy to fluorescent light energy. More than 98% of the exposure received by the film emulsion is from fluorescent light emitted by intensifying screen phosphors. Only a very small fraction of the film density is a result of exposure to x-rays. For every x-ray photon absorbed by the phosphor, many light photons are emitted. They truly *intensify* the action of x-rays, and thus permit the use of much smaller exposures than those required with direct exposure methods.

In the production of intensifying screens, phosphors are ground to a fine powder and mixed with a transparent binding substance. A somewhat-reflective plastic base material is used as a support. The phosphor mixture is spread in a smooth layer onto the plastic base; this is called the ***active/phosphor layer*** (Fig. 12–18). ◄

All phosphors are not created equal. Different types of phosphors have different x-ray-absorbing and fluorescent light-emitting

Rare Earth Phosphors
Gadolinium Lanthanum Yttrium

Figure 12–18. A cross-section of screens and film. The illustration shows how duplitized x-ray film is sandwiched between two intensifying screens. Phosphors of the adjacent intensifying screens absorb x-ray energy and convert it to fluorescent light, which then exposes the neighboring film emulsion as shown in Figure 12–19. Notice that the rear intensifying screen is thicker. As x-ray photons travel through the cassette front and front screen, they are somewhat attenuated and, as a result, their interaction with the rear screen is somewhat diminished. If the rear screen is made thicker, its speed is increased to compensate for the attenuated x-ray beam. (From Wolbarst AB. *Physics of Radiology.* East Norwalk, CT: Appleton & Lange, 1993.)

Intensifying Screen Speed Increases, and Therefore Recorded Detail Decreases, As
• Phosphor size increases • Thickness of the active/phosphor layer increases • Sensitivity of the phosphor increases (ie, calcium tungstate versus rare earth phosphors) • The degree of screen reflectance increases

Recorded Detail Increases As

- Focal spot size increases
- SID increases
- OID decreases
- Motion decreases
- (Shape) distortion decreases
- Screen speed decreases

properties. Some types of phosphors are more efficient than others. Some are able to absorb a greater percentage of the x-ray energy. A particular phosphor's ability to absorb x-ray energy and convert it to ▶ fluorescent light energy is referred to as its ***conversion efficiency.*** Phosphors having greater sensitivity (ie, speed) have greater conversion efficiency.

Factors that contribute to the speed of intensifying screens include type of phosphor, phosphor size, active/phosphor layer thickness, and reflective backing.

1. Phosphors. Phosphors with a *high atomic number* have a greater likelihood of interacting with an x-ray photon, and therefore possess greater speed. How well a particular phosphor detects the presence of x-ray photons is referred to as quantum detection efficiency. The phosphor should have a high *conversion efficiency,* that is, it should emit a liberal measure of fluorescent light for each x-ray photon it absorbs. The greater the conversion efficiency, the greater the speed.

▶ *Fluorescence* should terminate at the same time as the x-ray source; continued fluorescence after termination of exposure is termed ▶ *lag* and contributes to an overexposed radiograph. The wavelength, or color, of light emitted must match the particular sensitivity of the ▶ film emulsion used. This is known as ***spectral matching.*** Calcium tungstate emits a blue-violet fluorescence and *rare-earth phosphors* may fluoresce either green or blue; each must be used with a corresponding green or blue-sensitive film emulsion.

▶ *Phosphorescence* refers to the luminescence from fluoroscopic screen phosphors. Their unique characteristic is the lingering ▶ luminescence *after* the termination of x-ray *(afterglow).* This permits the fluoroscopist to continue viewing the part for a short time as the image slowly fades from the monitor. Thus, the fluoroscopist can use intermittent fluoroscopy to reduce patient dose.

Rare earth phosphors possess a much higher conversion efficiency than calcium tungstate, making them the phosphors of choice today. The rare earth phosphors used in radiography are oxysulfides and oxybromides of *lanthanum, gadolinium,* and *yttrium.* The phosphors used in fluoroscopy are *cesium iodide* and *zinc cadmium sulfide.*

2. Phosphor Size. Screen speed and phosphor size are directly related, ie, as phosphor size increases, more surface area is available for x-ray photon capture, resulting in an increase in ***screen speed.***

3. Active/Phosphor Layer Thickness. Screen speed and active/phosphor layer thickness are directly related, ie, as active layer thickness increases, more x-ray photons are converted to light and, therefore, screen speed increases.

4. Reflective Backing. Screen speed and the degree of reflectance given the base material are directly related, ie, the greater the reflectance, the greater the number of light photons directed toward the film emulsion and, consequently, the greater the screen speed.

Some manufacturers incorporate a *dye* in the phosphor layer that functions to reduce light diffusion, thus improving resolution. It should be noted however, that the addition of dye does sacrifice a little speed.

Loss of recorded detail may be a result of intensifying screen blur or unsharpness. Fluorescent light emerging from the phosphors diffuses and spreads over a larger area (Fig. 12–19A). It is this diffusion of fluorescent light that causes indistinct, blurry anatomic details. *The degree of diffusion, and hence, the degree of blurriness, is primarily dependent on the factors that regulate intensifying screen speed* (Fig. 12–19B).

Screen speed and screen blurriness are directly related, ie, as intensifying-screen speed increases, screen blurriness increases and image resolution/detail decreases.

Radiography departments frequently have more than one speed-intensifying screen available; slower (detail) screens are commonly used for extremity examinations, and faster screens for general radiography.

The use of rare earth phosphors enables the radiographer to greatly reduce patient dose in comparison to exposures required for calcium tungstate screens. The use of rare earth phosphors involves only minimal loss of recorded detail and permits a significant reduction in patient dose; they are, therefore, generally considered the screens of choice.

Another way in which intensifying screens can have a significant impact on recorded detail is through ***screen–film contact.*** Areas of ◄ imperfect screen-film contact result in blurriness that severely degrades recorded detail (Fig. 12–20A). Causes of poor screen–film contact include warped screens, damaged cassette frames, and foreign bodies in the cassette. Elevation of the screen in areas of poor contact allows light to diffuse over a larger area, thus exaggerating screen blur. Larger cassettes are more susceptible to poor screen contact. Proper care of intensifying screens includes periodic evaluation of screen contact using a specially designed wire mesh (Fig. 12–20B).

A related problem associated with screens and resolution is ***quantum mottle.*** As screen speed and kVp are increased, mAs may ◄ be reduced to such a small amount that image *graininess,* or quantum mottle, becomes a problem (Figs. 12–21, 12–22, and 12–23). This graininess becomes apparent and increases as the system speed increases. So few x-ray photons are used (mAs) to produce the image that one can almost count them as the representative black "grains" on the radiographic image!

Summary

- **Intensifying screens serve to decrease patient dose and increase tube life.**
- **As screen speed increases, patient dose decreases and tube life increases.**
- **Intensifying screen phosphors absorb x-ray photons and emit a large quantity of fluorescent light.**
- **Fluorescent light is responsible for more than 98% of the image density.**
- **The color light emitted by the phosphors must be correctly matched with the film emulsion sensitivity (spectral matching).**

- Rare earth phosphors have a greater conversion efficiency than do calcium tungstate phosphors.
- The greater the conversion efficiency and speed of screens, the poorer the recorded detail, as a result of greater fluorescent light diffusion at higher screen speeds.
- Screen speed is influenced by the type and size of phosphor used, the thickness of the active/phosphor layer, and the degree of reflectance given the screen base.
- Quantum mottle is more likely to occur when using fast screens with low mAs and high kVp factors.
- Phosphors that continue to fluoresce after the x-ray source has terminated are said to possess "lag" or "afterglow."
- Phosphorescence is associated with fluoroscopic screens.
- Perfect screen–film contact is required to maintain recorded detail.
- Screens may be tested for screen–film contact with the use of a specially designed wire mesh.

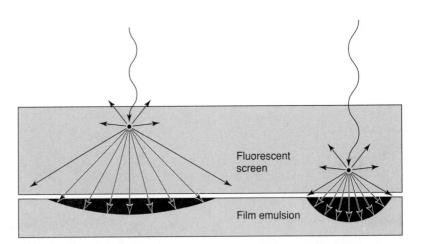

A

Figure 12–19. **(A)** Screen thickness and diffusion of fluorescent light versus recorded detail. As intensifying screen thickness increases, the film is exposed by diffused light from distant phosphors. The phosphors of thinner intensifying screens fluoresce closer to the film; therefore, light is diffused to a lesser degree and recorded detail is maintained. (Modified from Wolbarst, AB. *Physics of Radiology,* East Norwalk, CT: Appleton & Lange, 1993.)

(Continued)

B1

B2

B3

Figure 12–19. *(continued)*. **(B)** Imaging system speed versus required exposure and resolution. Image **1** was made without intensifying screens but required 128 mAs exposure. Image **2** was made using detail (about 100 speed) screens and 10 mAs. Image **3** was made with fast (about 400) screens and 1.33 mAs. Note the progressive loss of recorded detail accompanying the increase in system speed. (From the American College of Radiology Learning File. Courtesy of the ACR.)

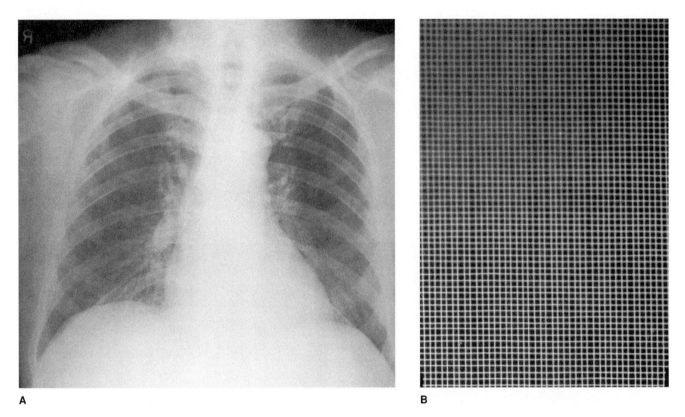

A   B

Figure 12–20. Demonstration of poor screen to film contact. **(A)** Blur due to poor film to screen contact in the apical region of the chest. **(B)** Wire-mesh test of a different cassette illustrates blur due to poor film to screen contact in the central region of the cassette. (From the American College of Radiology Learning File. Courtesy of the ACR.)

A   B

Figure 12–21. **(A)** and **(B)** The contrast-detail quality assurance device imaged illustrates the effect of x-ray exposure and resulting quantum mottle. Image **(B)** was made using a much lower mAs value (fewer x-ray photons) than image **(A);** note the striking graininess in **(B).** (From the American College of Radiology Learning File. Courtesy of the ACR.)

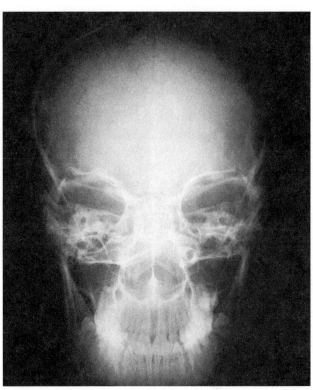

A

B

Figure 12–22. **(A)** and **(B)** The "grainy" appearance of film **(A)** is quantum mottle resulting from a faster screen film combination than film **(B).** (From the American College of Radiology Learning File. Courtesy of the ACR.)

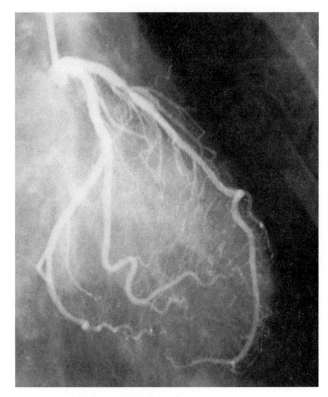

Figure 12–23. Quantum mottle can make visibility of small vessels difficult. (From the American College of Radiology Learning File. Courtesy of the ACR.)

Chapter Review Questions

☆ *Congratulations! You have completed a portion of this chapter. You may go on to the "Registry-type" multiple-choice questions that follow. For greatest success, be sure also to complete the short answer questions found at the end of this chapter.*

1. Which of the following has (have) an effect on recorded detail?
   1. focal spot size
   2. type of rectification
   3. source image distance
   (A) 1 only
   (B) 1 and 2 only
   (C) 1 and 3 only
   (D) 1, 2, and 3

2. If the radiographer is unable to achieve a short object image distance due to structure of the body part or patient condition, which of the following adjustments can be made to minimize magnification distortion?
   (A) smaller focal spot size should be used
   (B) longer source image distance should be used
   (C) faster intensifying screens should be used
   (D) slow intensifying screens should be used

3. When an intensifying screen continues to glow after the x-ray exposure has ended, the screen is said to possess
   (A) fluorescence
   (B) incandescence
   (C) luminescence
   (D) lag

4. Which of the following is (are) considered geometric factor(s) controlling recorded detail?
   1. focal spot size
   2. screen speed
   3. object-film distance
   (A) 1 only
   (B) 2 only
   (C) 1 and 3 only
   (D) 1, 2, and 3

5. Which of the following has an effect on distortion?
   1. source image distance
   2. angulation of the x-ray tube
   3. angulation of the part
   (A) 1 only
   (B) 1 and 2 only
   (C) 2 and 3 only
   (D) 1, 2, and 3

6. Which of the following will result in the BEST recorded detail?
   (A) 1.5 mm focal spot
   (B) 1.0 mm focal spot
   (C) 0.6 mm focal spot
   (D) 0.3 mm focal spot

7. All of the following are related to recorded detail, EXCEPT:
   (A) motion
   (B) screen speed
   (C) object-image distance
   (D) grid ratio

8. Foreshortening may be caused by:
   1. the radiographic object being placed at an angle to the film
   2. excessive distance between the object and the film
   3. insufficient distance between the focus and the film
   (A) 1 only
   (B) 2 only
   (C) 1 and 2 only
   (D) 1, 2, and 3

9. Misalignment of the tube-part-film relationship results in:
   (A) shape distortion
   (B) size distortion
   (C) magnification
   (D) blur

10. Although the stated focal spot size is measured directly under the actual focal spot, focal spot size really varies along the length of the x-ray beam. At which portion of the x-ray beam is the effective focal spot the smallest?
    (A) at its outer edge
    (B) along the path of the central ray
    (C) at the cathode end
    (D) at the anode end

Answers and Explanations

1. (C) Focal spot size affects recorded detail by its effect on blur: the larger the focal spot size the greater the blur produced. Recorded detail is significantly affected by distance changes because of their effect on magnification. As SID increases, magnification decreases and recorded detail increases. The method of rectification has no impact on recorded detail. Single-phase, rectified units produce "pulsed" radiation, whereas three-phase units produce almost constant potential.

2. (B) An increase in SID will help decrease the effect of excessive OID. For example, in the lateral projection of the cervical spine there is normally a significant OID. This effect is decreased by the use of 72 inches SID. However, especially with larger body parts, increased SID usually requires a significant increase in exposure factors. Focal spot size and screen speed are unrelated to magnification.

3. (D) When intensifying screen phosphors absorb x-ray photons, the x-ray photon energy is converted to visible light energy. The light emitted by the phosphors is termed luminescence. There are two types of luminescence: fluorescence and phosphorescence. Fluorescence is luminescent light that ceases to be emitted *as soon as* the x-ray photon stimulation ceases. Phosphorescence, on the other hand, is when the phosphors continue to glow *after* x-ray photon stimulation ceases; another term for this is lag.

4. (C) The relationship among the focal spot, the anatomic part, and the film determines geometric sharpness. That is, effective focal spot size determines the degree of penumbra, and OID and SID determine the degree of magnification. The OID should be as short as possible and the SID should be as long as practical. The anatomic part should be accurately positioned as closely parallel to the film as possible. Screens also lend a degree of unsharpness to the radiograph, but do not affect the *geometry* of the image (ie, size or shape).

5. (D) Distortion can be described as being either size or shape. Size distortion is magnification, caused by either insufficient SID or excessive OID. Shape distortion results from misalignment of the x-ray tube, part, and film. Tube angulation can cause elongation of the part. Angulation of the part with respect to the film will foreshorten the image. Focal spot size is unrelated to distortion, but strongly related to production of penumbral unsharpness.

6. (D) One of the factors influencing geometric sharpness is penumbra, or blur. The production of blur is inversely proportional to recorded detail. As focal spot size increases, blur increases, and recorded detail decreases.

7. (D) Motion is said to be the greatest enemy of recorded detail because it completely obliterates image sharpness. Screen speed can reduce recorded detail according to the degree of light diffusion from the phosphors. Object-image distance causes magnification and blurriness of recorded detail. Grid ratio is related to scatter radiation clean-up; it is unrelated to detail.

8. (A) Size distortion (magnification) is inversely proportional to SID and directly proportional to OID. Decreasing the SID and increasing the OID serve to increase size distortion. Aligning the tube, anatomic part, and film so as to be parallel reduces shape distortion. Angulation of the long axis of the part with respect to the film results in foreshortening of the object. Tube angulation causes elongation of the part.

9. (A) Shape distortion (foreshortening, elongation) is caused by improper alignment of the tube, part, and film. Size distortion, or magnification, is caused by too great an object-image distance or too short a source image distance. Blur is caused principally by use of a large focal spot.

10. (D) X-ray tube targets are constructed according to the *line focus principle,* ie, the focal spot is angled (usually 12 to 17°) to the vertical. As the actual focal spot is projected downward it is foreshortened; thus, the effective focal spot is always smaller than the actual focal spot. As it is projected toward the cathode end of the x-ray beam it becomes larger and approaches its actual size. As it is projected toward the anode end, it gets smaller because of the anode "heel" effect.

II. FACTORS AFFECTING RADIOGRAPHIC DENSITY

KEY TERMS ◀

ADDED FILTRATION	FOCAL RANGE	MOVING GRID
BEAM RESTRICTOR	FOCUSED GRID	OPTICAL DENSITY
BODY HABITUS	FOCUSING DISTANCE	RADIOGRAPHIC DENSITY
BUCKY/GRID FACTOR	GRID	RADIOLUCENT
COLLIMATION	GRID CUTOFF	RECIPROCITY LAW
COMPENSATING FILTERS	GRID LINES	SCATTER RADIATION
CONTRAST IMPROVEMENT FACTOR	GRID RATIO	SELECTIVITY
CONVERGENCE LINE	IMAGE RECEPTOR	SENSITOMETRY
CROSSED GRID	INHERENT FILTRATION	SINGLE-PHASE
DECENTERING	INVERSE-SQUARE LAW	STATIONARY GRID
EXPOSURE RATE	kVp	THREE-PHASE
15% RULE	mAs	

Radiographic density is defined as the overall amount of black- ◀
ening on a radiographic image or a particular portion of the image.
It provides a degree of background blackening for the anatomic
image. Excessive radiographic density can obscure image details;
insufficient radiographic density can mask pathology. Radiographic
density is a *quantitative* factor, ie, it describes an *amount* of image
blackening. Thus, radiographic density is regulated by the ***exposure*** ◀
rate or *number* of photons reaching the film emulsion.

   Optical density is generally thought of as being optimal, ex- ◀
cessive, or insufficient, when in fact it can be precisely measured
and quanitified. Optical density can be described as the relationship between the amount of light incident upon the radiograph (ie,
from the illuminator) compared to the amount of light transmitted
through the radiograph. This relationship is expressed in the following equation.

$$OD = \log_{10} \frac{I_o}{I_t}$$

   OD is optical density expressed as a logarithm, demonstrating the
relationship between the amount of light transmitted through the film
(I_t) compared to the amount of light incident upon (I_o) the film. The
diagnostically useful range of optical density is 0.25 to 2.5 (Fig. 12–24).

A

B

Figure 12–24. **(A)**, **(B)**, and **(C)** The diagnostically useful range of optical densities is about 0.25 to 2.5. Note the range of densities visualized on each of these radiographs as identified by the accompanying characteristic curve on each film. (From the American College of Radiology Learning File. Courtesy of the ACR.) *(Continued.)*

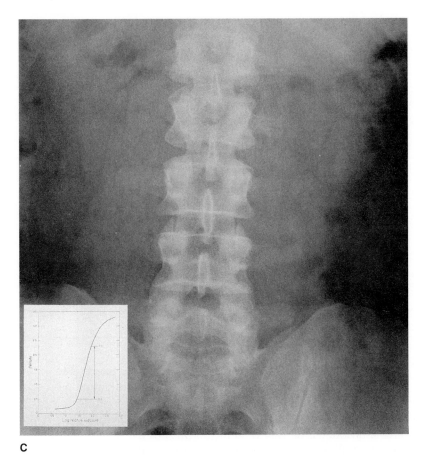

C

Figure 12–24. **(C)** The range of densities visualized lie between 0.5 and 2.5, as indicated by the accompanying characteristic curve. Notice the number and visibility of details imaged here as compared with those imaged in **(A)** (density range about 0.25–0.70) and **(B)** (density range about 0.25–1.5). (From the American College of Radiology Learning File. Courtesy of the ACR.)

A characteristic curve like the one shown (Fig. 12–25) can be used to illustrate the relationship between the x-ray exposure given the film and the resulting radiographic density.

The study of film-emulsion response to exposure is called ***sensitometry.*** The characteristic curve will be discussed further in Section IV: Film, Screen, and Grid Options. ◀

A. MAs

Milliampere-seconds *(mAs)* is the *product* of milliamperes (mA) and ◀ exposure time (seconds). Technical factors are usually expressed in terms of mAs rather than mA and time. This is because there are any number of possible combinations of mA and time that will produce the desired mAs. For example,

> It is known that 10 mAs is required to produce a given radiographic density. Therefore, each of the following combinations should produce the required (and identical) results: 100 mA and 0.1 second, 200 mA and 0.05 second, 300 mA and 0.03 second, 400 mA and 0.025 second, etc.

Any combinations of mA and time that will produce a given mAs (ie, a particular quantity of x-ray photons) will produce identical radiographic density. This is known as the ***reciprocity law.*** ◀

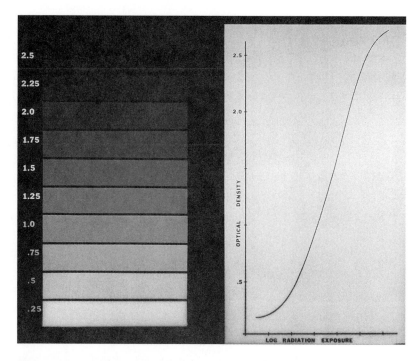

Figure 12–25. Characteristic curve. Notice that the intervals of *exposure* appear in increments of 0.3. This is because doubling the exposure (ie, mAs) results in an increase in log relative exposure of 0.3. For example, 100% of the incident light is transmitted through a film having an optical density of zero (0), 50% of the light is transmitted through a film having an optical density of 0.3, 25% of the light through a film with density of 0.6, etc. (From the American College of Radiology Learning File. Courtesy of the ACR.)

Radiographic density is a quantitative factor because it describes the amount of image blackening. Milliampere-seconds is also a quantitative factor because it regulates x-ray beam *intensity, exposure rate, quantity,* or *number* of x-ray photons produced (mAs is the single most important technical factor associated with radiographic density and is the factor of choice for regulating radiographic density).

mAs is directly proportional to the intensity (exposure rate, number, quantity) of x-ray photons produced, and the resulting radiographic density. If the mAs is doubled, twice the exposure rate and twice the density occurs. If the mAs is cut in half, the exposure rate and radiographic density are cut in half (Fig. 12–26).

It is not surprising then, that, in order to produce just a perceptible change in radiographic density, an mAs change of at least 30% is required. For example,

A particular radiograph was produced using 12 mAs and 78 kVp. The finished radiograph exhibited slightly insufficient background density. What factors would be required to produce a radiograph having satisfactory radiographic density?

Since the radiographic density requires improvement, the mAs is the technical factor requiring manipulation. Since the above information implies that background density is only somewhat lacking, a 30% increase in mAs would most likely remedy the situation. Since

A

B

C

Figure 12–26. Radiographic density is proportional to mAs. **(A)** Radiograph made using 40 mAs. **(B)** Radiograph made of the same subject using 80 mAs, all other factors remaining constant; note that doubling the mAs has produced twice the radiographic density. **(C)** Radiograph made using twice the mAs of film **B** (160 mAs), resulting in another doubling of radiographic density. (From the American College of Radiology Learning File. Courtesy of the ACR.)

30% of 12 mAs is 3.6, a new mAs of 16 should provide adequate radiographic density. If the radiograph were significantly lacking in density, it would have been appropriate to double the mAs.

Summary

- mAs is the product of mA and exposure time.
- Any combination of mA and time that will produce a given mAs will produce identical radiographic density according to the reciprocity law.
- Radiographic density and mAs are quantitative factors and are directly related.
- Doubling the mAs will double the radiographic density; halving the mAs will cut the density in half.
- At least a 30% change must be made in mAs for there to be a perceptible change in radiographic density.

B. SID

As a child you may have been told to "read your book next to the lamp, where you'll have more light." Perhaps your youthful eyes could see just fine where you were, but in fact your advisor was correct in saying that more light was available closer to the lamp.

As distance from a light source increases, the light diverges and covers a larger area; the quantity of light available per unit area becomes less and less as distance increases. The intensity (quantity) ▶ of light decreases according to the **inverse square law,** that is, the intensity of light at a particular distance from its source is inversely proportional to the square of the distance (Fig. 12–27). For example, if you decreased the distance between your book and the lamp from 6 ft to 3 ft, you would have four times as much light available.

Similarly, source-to-image receptor distance (SID) has a significant impact on x-ray beam intensity and, hence, radiographic density. As the distance between the x-ray tube and image receptor increases, exposure rate (and therefore radiographic density) decreases according to the inverse square law.

Notice that, according to the inverse square law the exposure rate is *inversely* proportional to the square of the distance whereas, using the density maintenance formula to determine what the new mAs should be because of the diminished exposure rate, the mAs is *directly* proportional to the distance squared.

▶ In the equations, I represents intensity (a quantitative term refer-
▶ ring to exposure rate or mAs) and D represents distance (SID). The
▶ original intensity (exposure rate or mAs) is represented by I_1, the
▶ original distance squared is represented by D_1^2, and the new distance
▶ squared by D_2^2. I_2 represents the new intensity (ie, the new exposure rate or the new mAs).

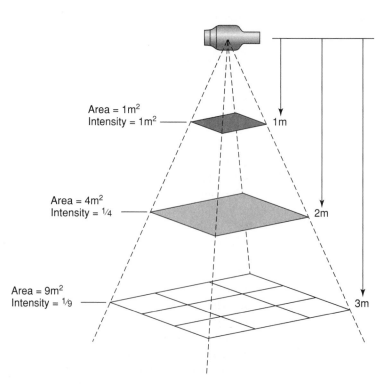

Figure 12–27. The inverse square law. Since x-ray beam coverage (area) increases with the square of the distance, the number of x-ray photons per unit area decreases by the same amount. (From Wolbarst, AB. *Physics of Radiology.* East Norwalk, CT: Appleton & Lange, 1993.)

A radiograph made using a particular group of technical factors at 52-in SID resulted in an exposure rate of 85 mR/min. Another radiograph of the same part will be made at 44-in SID. What is the exposure rate at the new distance?

$$\frac{85}{x} = \frac{1936\,(44^2)}{2704\,(52^2)}$$

$$1936x = 229{,}840$$

$$x = 118.7 \text{ mR/min at 44-in SID}$$

This illustrates the relationship between distance and x-ray intensity. As the distance is decreased, the intensity of the x-ray beam increases (according to the inverse-square law). The resulting increase in radiographic density, will require an adjustment of technical factors, specifically mAs (according to the density maintenance formula), to reproduce the original density.

A particular radiograph was performed at 40-in SID using 12 mAs and 82 kVp. To improve recorded detail, it is necessary to repeat the radiograph using 72-in SID. What new mAs will be required at the new distance in order to maintain the original radiographic density?

Using the distance maintenance formula and substituting known factors:

$$\frac{I_1}{I_2} = \frac{D_1^2}{D_2^2}$$

$$\frac{12}{x} = \frac{1600\,(40^2)}{5184\,(72^2)}$$

$$1600x = 62{,}208$$

$$x = 38.9 \text{ mAs as } (I_2)$$

So, at 72-in SID, 38.9 mAs will be required to produce the same density that was produced at 40-in SID using 12 mAs.

Summary

- **Relatively small changes in SID can have a profound effect on radiographic density.**
- **As the SID increases, exposure rate and radiographic density decrease.**
- **With changes in SID, the *inverse square law* is used to calculate the new exposure rate.**
- **With changes in SID, the *density maintenance formula* is used to calculate the new mAs.**

C. κVP

As kilovoltage is increased, *more* electrons are driven to the anode with greater speed and energy. More high-energy electrons will result in production of *more high energy x-rays*. Thus, **kVp** affects both ◄ quantity and quality (energy) of the x-ray beam. However, although kVp and radiographic density are directly *related,* they are not directly proportional, ie, twice the radiographic density does not

---

Use the Inverse Square Law to Determine

What the new exposure rate is at the new distance, by using the (inverse relationship) equation:

$$\frac{I_1}{I_2} = \frac{D_2^2}{D_1^2}$$

Relationship Between Screen Speed and Tube Wear (Heat Units)

Screen Speed	mAs	Heat Units (HU)
100	60	5400
200	30	2700
400	15	1350

Use the Density Maintenance Formula to Determine

What change in mAs is required to maintain the original radiographic density, by using the (direct relationship) equation:

$$\frac{I_1}{I_2} = \frac{D_1^2}{D_2^2}$$

This is an important concept, since distance changes are frequently an important factor in radiography.

result from doubling the kVp. The effect of kVp on quantity is not proportional because an increase in kVp produces an increase in photons of *all energies.*

With respect to the effect of kVp on radiographic density, there ▶ is one convenient rule (the ***15% rule)*** that can be followed. If it is desired to double the radiographic density, yet impossible to adjust the mAs, a similar effect can be achieved by *increasing the kVp by 15%.* Conversely, the density may be cut in half by decreasing the kVp by 15% (Fig. 12–28).

A radiograph was made using the following technical factors: 400 mA, 0.025 second, and 84 kVp. It is necessary to produce another radiograph with twice the density. The maximum mA available is 400 and the exposure time cannot be increased due to involuntary motion. What alternate kVp can be employed to produce a radiograph with the desired radiographic density?

If twice the original density is needed, the kVp may be increased 15% to produce the desired effect. Fifteen percent of 84 is

A

B

C

Figure 12–28. Illustration of the 15% rule. Film **(B)** was made using 15% more kVp than film **(A)** and demonstrates twice the radiographic density of film **(A).** Similarly, film **(C)** was made using 15% more kVp than film **(B)** and demonstrates twice the radiographic density of film **(B).** (From the American College of Radiology Learning File. Courtesy of the ACR.)

12.6. Therefore, using the same mAs and increasing the kVp to 97 should produce a radiograph with twice the original density. *Note:* changing the kVp will change the scale of contrast (discussed later).

Summary

- **Increased kVp produces more high-energy x-ray photons.**
- **An increase in kVp will result in an increase in radiographic density; a decrease in kVp will result in a decrease in radiographic density.**
- **When mAs manipulation is not possible, radiographic density can be doubled or halved by using the 15% rule.**

D. INTENSIFYING SCREENS

Intensifying screens amplify the effect of x-rays on film emulsion by means of fluorescence. For every one x-ray photon interacting with screen phosphors, many light photons are emitted. This effect becomes more pronounced as screen speed increases.

Therefore, with any given group of exposure factors, as screen speed increases, radiographic density increases.

Screen speed and radiographic density are directly proportional (factors affecting screen speed have been discussed earlier in this chapter). An increase in intensifying screen speed from 200 to 400 doubles the radiographic density and enables the radiographer to cut the mAs in half, thus reducing patient dose (Fig. 12–29) and tube wear (heat units) considerably.

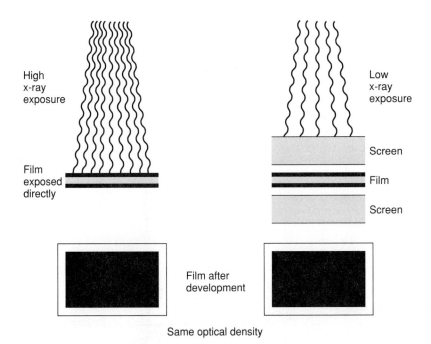

Figure 12–29. Exposure and resulting film density; direct exposure versus intensifying screens. Using intensifying screens, a much smaller patient dose is required to produce the same optical density. (From Wolbarst, AB. *Physics of Radiology.* East Norwalk, CT: Appleton & Lange, 1993.)

Summary

- Intensifying screens amplify the action of x-rays through their property of fluorescence.
- All other factors remaining constant, an increase in screen speed will result in an increase in radiographic density.
- Screen speed and radiographic density are directly proportional.
- Screen speed and patient dose are inversely proportional.
- Screen speed and x-ray tube heat production are inversely related.

E. GRIDS

As x-ray photons travel through a part, they either pass all the way through to expose the film, or they undergo interaction(s) that may result in their being absorbed by the part or deviated in direction. It is those that change direction (scattered radiation) that undermine the image.

Part III discussed the origin of scatter radiation: Compton scatter interactions. Compton scatter can be a personnel radiation hazard, especially in fluoroscopic procedures. With respect to the radiographic image, it is responsible for the scatter radiation that reaches
▶ the film. *Scattered radiation* adds unwanted, degrading densities to the radiographic image.

The single most important way to reduce the production of scat-
▶ tered radiation is to collimate. Although *collimation,* optimum *kVp,* and compression can be used, a large amount of scatter radiation is still generated within the part being radiographed and, because it adds unwanted non–information-carrying densities, it can have a severely degrading effect on image quality, as illustrated in the pelvis radiographs shown in Figure 12–31.

▶ A *grid* is a device interposed between the patient and image receptor that functions to absorb a large percentage of scatter radiation before it reaches the image receptor (Fig. 12–32). It is con-
▶ structed of alternating strips of lead foil and *radiolucent* filler material. X-ray photons traveling in the same direction as the primary beam pass between the lead strips. X-ray photons, having undergone interactions within the body and deviated in various directions, are

---

Origin of Scattered Radiation and Methods for Controlling Its Production (see Fig. 12–30)

- The larger the x-ray field size, the more scatter radiation produced. *Solution:* collimate!
- The higher the kilovoltage, the greater the production of scatter radiation (due to the higher incidence of Compton scatter interactions). *Solution:* use optimum kVp.
- The thicker and more dense the body tissues, the greater the amount of scatter radiation produced. *Solution:* compression of the part or use of the prone position to decrease the effect of fatty tissue.

Amount of scattered radiation depends upon . . . .

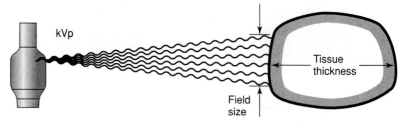

Figure 12–30. Factors affecting the production of SR: kVp level, beam restriction, and thickness and density of tissues. (From Wolbarst, AB. *Physics of Radiology.* East Norwalk, CT: Appleton & Lange, 1993.)

A

B

Figure 12–31. **(A)** Radiograph made at 40 mAs without a grid. Due to the thickness and nature of the part radiographed, a significant amount of scatter radiation was generated and went on to expose the (undiagnostic) film. **(B)** Radiograph made using a 12:1 grid. Although an exposure increase to 400 mAs was required, scatter radiation was removed before it reached the film and a diagnostic radiograph was obtained. (From the American College of Radiology Learning File. Courtesy of the ACR.)

Figure 12–32. Scattered radiation generated in the object is removed (cleaned-up) with the use of a grid. (Modified from Wolbarst, AB. *Physics of Radiology.* East Norwalk, CT: Appleton & Lange, 1993.)

absorbed by the lead strips; this is referred to as "clean-up" of scattered radiation.

The use of grids is recommended for body parts measuring 11 cm and greater. The major exception to this rule is the chest, which may frequently be examined without a grid because its contents (mostly air) do not generate significant quantities of scatter radiation. Even so, many institutions perform most chest examinations using a grid and high kilovoltage factors.

Without the use of a grid, scatter radiation contributes to more than 50% of the total film exposure. If a grid is introduced, there will be significantly *fewer* photons reaching the image receptor, hence a very significant decrease in radiographic *density*. To maintain adequate density then, the addition of a grid must be accompanied by an appropriately substantial increase in *mAs*.

Before beginning a discussion of the impact of grids on technical factors, a more complete study of them is in order. A grid may be *stationary* or *moving*. Stationary grids are the simplest type and usually consist of alternating *vertical* lead strips (ie, a *parallel* grid) and radiolucent interspace filler material. A grid cassette is an example of a stationary grid. Another example is the "slip-on," or "wafer,"
▶ grid that may be placed over a regular cassette. **Stationary grids** are useful in mobile radiography and horizontal beam (cross-table lateral) radiography; they are usually low-ratio. A disadvantage of stationary grids is visibility of grid lines.
▶ If the grid is in motion during the exposure, as it is in the ***moving grid,*** the grid lines are effectively blurred out of the radiographic image. The lead strips and interspace material of a moving grid are slightly *angled* so that, at a given distance from the focal spot, the angle of the lead strips will conform with the divergence of the x-ray
▶ beam. A grid with lead strips that are angled thus is called a ***focused grid;*** if an imaginary line is extended up from each lead strip, the point
▶ of intersection is called the **convergence line,** and the distance from
▶ the convergence line to the surface of the grid is the ***focusing distance*** (Fig. 12–33). That focusing distance is the ideal SID, although
▶ grids usually specify a ***focal range*** in which they can be safely used.

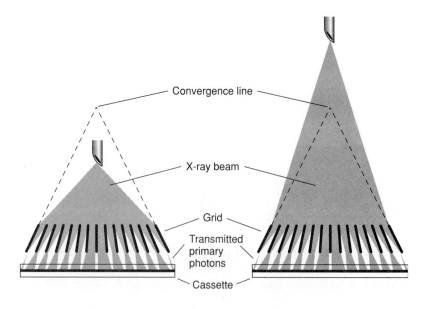

Figure 12–33. Grid cut-off will be apparent if the SID is above or below the specified focal range limits and will be characterized by density loss at the periphery of the image. This is described as an *off-focus error* or *focus-grid distance decentering.* (From Wolbarst, AB. *Physics of Radiology.* East Norwalk, CT: Appleton & Lange, 1993.)

Another type of grid is the ***crossed grid,*** it has a second series ◀
of lead strips aligned perpendicular to the first. Crossed grids may be
parallel or focused, and are extremely efficient in absorbing scattered
radiation; however, their use prohibits any x-ray tube angulation and
requires that the x-ray tube be exactly centered to the center of the
grid. Any misalignment or tube angulation can result in severe ***grid*** ◀
cutoff. Crossed grids are not used in general radiography; they may
have some application in special procedures.

Care must be taken to avoid errors common to the use of
focused grids, including angulation errors, off-level errors, off-focus
errors, off-center errors, and upside-down grid placement.

- *Angulation errors:* The x-ray tube may be safely angled in the
  direction of the lead strips; angulation "against" the lead strips
  causes *grid cut-off,* ie, absorption of the primary beam and
  loss of density similar to that exhibited in off-level errors, ie
  loss of density across image.
- *Off-level errors:* If the planes of the x-ray tube and grid surface are not parallel (ie, cassette centered and perpendicular
  to CR), grid cut-off will occur. This can happen when the x-
  ray tube is tilted (as described). It can also occur when a grid
  cassette is placed inaccurately under a patient during mobile
  radiography; the radiographer must ensure that the grid is
  perpendicular to the central ray.
- *Off-focus errors:* Grid cut-off will occur if the SID is below the
  lower limits, or above the upper limits, of the specified focal
  range. This type of error is also referred to as *focus-grid distance **decentering.*** Off-focus errors are usually characterized ◀
  by loss of density at the periphery of the image.
- *Off-center errors:* If the x-ray beam is not centered to the
  grid, ie, if it is shifted laterally, grid cut-off will occur. This
  type of error is referred to as *lateral decentering,* and is characterized by a uniform density loss across the radiographic
  image (Fig. 12–34).

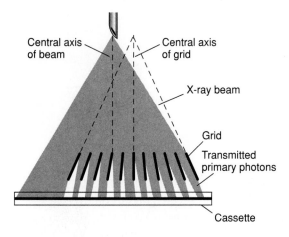

Figure 12–34. A uniform density loss across the radiographic image
will occur if the x-ray beam is off-center laterally. (From Wolbarst, AB.
Physics of Radiology. East Norwalk, CT: Appleton & Lange, 1993.)

If the x-ray beam is both off-center and *off-focus below the focusing distance*, the portion of the image below the focus will show *increased* density; if the x-ray beam is off-center and *off-focus above the focusing distance*, the image below the focus will show *decreased* density.

- *Upside down grid:* A focused grid placed upside down has its lead strips angled exactly opposite the angle of the x-ray beam. So, except for the central area where the lead strips and x-ray beam are vertical, grid cut-off will be severe (Fig. 12–35).

Two of a grid's physical characteristics that determine its degree of efficiency in the removal of scattered radiation are:

▶ - *Grid ratio:* **Grid ratio** is defined as the height of the lead strips compared to the distance between them (Fig. 12–36).

$$\text{Grid ratio} = \frac{\text{height of Pb strip}}{\text{width of interspace material}}$$

For example, a grid having lead strips 1.5 mm tall separated by interspace material 0.15 mm wide has a grid ratio of 10:1.

A

B

Figure 12–35. **(A)** and **(B)** An upside-down focused grid presents its lead strips in the opposite direction to that of the x-ray beam. This results in severe grid cut-off everywhere except in the central portion of the radiographic image. ((**A**) from Wolbarst, AB. *Physics of Radiology.* East Norwalk, CT: Appleton & Lange, 1993; **(B)** from Saia, D. *Appleton & Lange's Review For The Radiography Examination.* East Norwalk, CT: Appleton & Lange, 1997.)

As the lead strips are made taller, scattered radiation is more likely to be trapped before reaching the image receptor. A 12 to 1 ratio grid will absorb more scattered radiation than an 8 to 1 ratio grid.

- *Number of lead strips per inch:* The number of lead strips per inch may also be referred to as grid frequency. The advantage of many lead strips per inch is that there is less *visibility* of the lead strips. As the number of lead foil strips per inch increases, the foil often gets thinner, and therefore less visible. There is, of course, a disadvantage here. If the lead strips get thinner, more energetic scattered radiation can pass through them and reach the ***image receptor.*** So to maintain the efficiency of a grid having many lead strips per inch, its grid ratio is often increased as well, ie, the lead strips are made taller to increase the likelihood of their trapping scattered radiation before it reaches the image receptor.

The radiolucent interspace material is most frequently made of plastic or fiber; some grids use aluminum as the interspace material. Aluminum is more sturdy, gives the radiograph a smoother appearance free of objectionable ***grid lines,*** and can perhaps have an additional filtering effect on scattered radiation. However, because of this filtering effect, a greater increase in patient dose is required with aluminum interspaced grids. Fiber interspace material, on the other hand, can be affected by moisture and result in warping of the grid.

Other ways of expressing and measuring grid efficiency include:

- ***Bucky (grid) factor:*** The *bucky/grid factor* (B) of a particular grid is the ratio of the total amount of radiation (primary and scattered) incident upon the surface of the grid compared to the amount of radiation transmitted through the grid:

$$B = \frac{\text{incident total}}{\text{transmitted total}}$$

The bucky factor is the grid conversion factor, ie, that amount by which the mAs must be increased to compensate for the radiation absorbed by the grid (Fig. 12–37). This will be discussed in further detail later in this section.

- ***Contrast improvement factor:*** The ratio of radiographic contrast obtained with a grid compared to the contrast obtained without a grid is referred to as the contrast improvement factor (CIF).

$$CIF = \frac{\text{contrast with grid}}{\text{contrast without grid}}$$

- ***Selectivity:*** The ratio between the quantity of primary photons transmitted through the grid to the quantity of scattered photons transmitted is referred to as the selectivity (S) of the grid.

$$S = \frac{\text{primary photon transmission}}{\text{scattered photon transmission}}$$

An undesirable but unavoidable characteristic of grids is that they do absorb some primary photons as well as scattered photons

Grid ratio: *T/W*

Figure 12–36. Cross-section of a grid. Grid ratio is defined as the height (T) of the lead strips (S) to width of the interspace material (W). Grid ratio = T/W (Modified from Wolbarst, AB. *Physics of Radiology.* East Norwalk, CT: Appleton & Lange, 1993.)

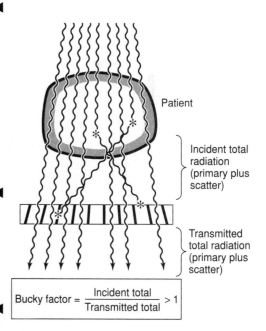

Figure 12–37. The bucky factor (B) is the *grid conversion factor* and describes the total amount of radiation striking the grid surface compared to the amount of radiation transmitted through the grid. (Modified from Wolbarst, AB. *Physics of Radiology.* East Norwalk, CT: Appleton & Lange, 1993.)

and, unfortunately, those more efficient at removing scattered radiation generally also remove more primary photons. The higher the primary to scattered-photon transmission ratio, the more desirable the grid.

- *Lead content:* This is perhaps the form least familiar to the radiographer because it applies little to the practical use of the grid. The definitions of grid ratio and grid frequency do not take into account the thickness of the lead strip; lead content does consider it. Lead content is measured in g/cm², and expresses the amount of lead contained within a particular grid.

How must exposure factors be adjusted to maintain appropriate density when changing from non-grid to grid? How can exposure factors be changed to preserve the density level when changing from one ratio grid to another?

In actual practice, the grid conversion factor varies slightly according to kVp range used. The ARRT recognizes that different textbooks cite slightly different grid conversion factors, and has stated that the distractors in calculation problems will not be so close as to cause conflict with the keyed correct answer. The conversion factors listed in the chart to the left can be used to calculate grid conversions in exposure factor problems.

A particular examination was performed tabletop at 40-in SID using 7 mAs and 90 kVp. In order to reduce the amount of image-degrading scattered radiation, another radiograph will be made using a 12:1 ratio grid. What new mAs factor will be required in order to maintain the original density level?

The grid conversion formula is:

$$\frac{mAs_1}{mAs_2} = \frac{grid\ factor_1}{grid\ factor_2}$$

Substituting known quantities:

$$\frac{7}{x} = \frac{1}{5}$$

$$x = 35\ mAs\ required\ with\ 12:1\ grid$$

A lumbar spine was radiographed laterally at 40-in SID using 40 mAs and 95 kVp and an 8 to 1 ratio grid. To improve scattered radiation clean-up, another radiograph will be made using a 12:1 grid. What new mAs factor will be required in order to maintain the original density level?

Using the grid conversion formula shown, and substituting known quantities:

$$\frac{40}{x} = \frac{4}{5}$$

$$4x = 200$$

$$x = 50\ mAs\ required\ with\ 12:1\ grid$$

An 8:1 grid is satisfactory for radiography up to 90 kVp. A 16 to 1 grid ratio is frequently advocated for radiography over 100 kVp. Routine radiographic equipment generally employs a 10 or 12:1 grid.

Grid Conversion Factors for Various Ratio Grids

Grid Ratio	Conversion Factor
No grid	1
5:1	2
6:1	3
8:1	4
10/12:1	5
16:1	6

The use of high-ratio grids at low kVp levels is discouraged because of the unnecessary patient exposure required.

Remember, to avoid variations in radiographic density, mAs adjustments are essential when changing grid ratios.

A word of caution regarding the use of an *inverted cassette* in place of a grid: the results are unpredictable and this practice is discouraged. Appropriate selection and careful use of a grid provides a far more predictable outcome and a diagnostically superior radiographic image.

An air gap introduced between the object and image recorder can have an effect similar to that of a grid. As energetic scattered radiation emerges from the body, it continues to travel in its divergent fashion and, much of the time, will bypass the image recorder (Fig. 12–38). It is often necessary to increase the SID to reduce magnification caused by increased OID.

Summary

- **Scattered radiation is a result of x-ray photon interaction with tissue via Compton scatter processes.**
- **Scattered radiation adds image-degrading densities to the radiographic image.**
- **The production of scattered radiation increases with an increase in field size, kVp, and thickness and volume of tissue.**
- **The single most important way to decrease the production of scattered radiation is to collimate.**
- **The amount of scattered radiation reaching the film is decreased through the combined use of collimators and grids.**
- **Grids are made of alternating strips of lead and radiolucent material and are placed between the patient and image receptor to stop scattered radiation.**
- **Grids may be stationary or moving, parallel or focused.**
- **Crossed grids are very efficient but require exact centering and prohibit tube angulation.**
- **Focused grids require that**
  - **The correct surface be facing the x-ray tube (ie, not upside down)**
  - **Tube angulation parallels the lead strips**
  - **The long axis of the x-ray tube and grid surface are parallel**
  - **The x-ray tube be within the focusing distance/range**
  - **The x-ray beam not be off-center (laterally) with the center of the grid**
- **If focused grid requirements are not met, the resulting image will demonstrate a loss of density due to grid cutoff (ie, absorption of the primary beam).**
- **The most common way of expressing grid efficency is by grid ratio and number of lead strips per inch.**
- **Since grids remove many x-ray photons that would have contributed to image density, the addition of a grid requires a significant increase in mAs.**
- **When implementing a grid or changing grid ratio, a grid-conversion factor must be used to determine appropriate mAs changes to avoid variations in radiographic density.**

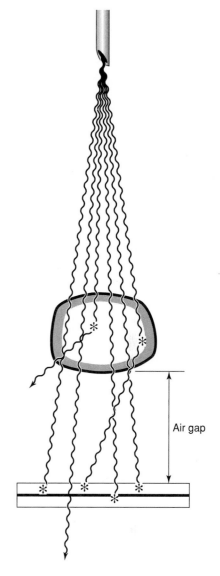

Figure 12–38. Air-gap technique. As scattered radiation emerges from the part, it continues to travel in its divergent fashion, bypassing the image receptor. (From Wolbarst, AB. *Physics of Radiology.* East Norwalk, CT: Appleton & Lange, 1993.)

F. FILTRATION

As discussed in the previous chapter, the primary beam generally has a total filtration of 2.5 mm Al equivalent for patient protection purposes. In general purpose radiographic tubes, the glass envelope usually accounts for about 0.5 mm Al equivalent and the collimator
▶ provides about 1.0 mm Al equivalent. These are considered ***inher-***
▶ ***ent filtration.*** The manufacturer adds another 1.0 mm Al ***(added filtration)*** to meet the minimum requirements of 2.5 mm Al equivalent total filtration for radiographic tubes operated above 70 kVp.

This type of filter serves to remove the diagnostically useless x-ray photons that only contribute to patient dose. Since this radiation is "soft" (low energy) and would not reach the image receptor anyway, the x-ray tube total filtration *has no real effect on radiographic density*. Filtration serves to increase the overall average energy of the beam; it "hardens" the x-ray beam.

▶ ***Compensating filters*** can be used to provide more uniform radiographic density when radiographing structures with widely different x-ray-absorbing properties due to thickness or tissue composition. Usually made of aluminum or clear leaded plastic, they slide into tracks in the tube head similar to a cylinder cone, or attach magnetically to the undersurface of the tube housing.

If a foot radiograph demonstrates well-exposed tarsals, the toes will frequently be overexposed (Fig. 12–39A). Conversely, if the exposure is adjusted to improve the image of the toes, the tarsals will be underexposed. Because the foot varies so greatly in thickness and tissue density along its long axis, it is difficult to achieve uniform radiographic density. A simple *wedge*-shaped compensating filter can remedy the situation (Fig. 12–39E). The filter is attached to the tube head so that the thin portion is over the tarsals and the thick portion over the toes. Exposure factors appropriate for tarsals are used, and the thick portion of the filter removes enough of the primary beam to prevent overexposure of the toes. Thus, a foot radiograph having uniform density throughout is achieved (Fig. 12–39A and B). A wedge filter is also useful for femur examinations and decubitus abdomen films (Fig. 12–39C and D).

Another type of compensating filter is the *trough* filter (Fig. 12–40), so named because its central portion is thin and the portions extending laterally are thicker—thus forming a central trough. A trough filter can be used in chest radiography to permit visualization of the denser mediastinal structures without overexposing the more radiolucent lungs and pulmonary vascular markings.

Another simple, yet effective, application of compensating filtration is the use of a saline bag. The saline bag is placed over the thinner body part and serves to filter out excessive exposure. This technique is effectively employed in the AP projection of the thoracic spine, however its use should be noted on the requisition as its use can cause an artifact.

Summary

- **Ordinary x-ray tube filtration of 2.5 mm Al has no effect on radiographic density.**
- **When anatomic parts vary greatly in thickness or tissue composition, compensating filters may be used to "even out" radiographic densities.**

Figure 12–39. **(A)** Typical foot radiograph performed without the use of a compensating filter; though the tarsals and metatarsals are well demonstrated, the phalanges are significantly overexposed. **(B)** Film made using a compensating filter whose thicker portion was placed over the phalanges to balance radiographic densities. **(C)** Lateral decubitus film of an air and barium-filled colon. Abdominal tissues often shift to the dependent side in the decubitus position, making the "down" side thicker than the "up" side. Excessive density of the air-filled structures can obliterate pathology. **(D)** Use of a wedge-shaped compensating filter can equalize tissue density differences, thus providing more uniform radiographic density and improved visualization of any pathology (a polypoid lesion is demonstrated). **(E)** Compensating (wedge) filter magnetically attached to the x-ray tube housing. (Courtesy of Nuclear Associates.)

A   B

Figure 12–40. **(A)** Film made using conventional filtration. **(B)** Film made using a trough filter; note the improved visualization of mediastinal structures. (From the American College of Radiology Learning File. Courtesy of the ACR.)

- Compensating filters slide into place by means of tracks on the tube housing.
- Compensating filters are available in various shapes: their thicker portions absorb more of the x-ray beam and are therefore placed over thinner body parts, while their thinner portions (absorbing fewer x-rays) are placed over thicker body parts.

G. Structural (Normal Versus Pathologic) Considerations

Normal tissue variants and pathologic processes can alter tissue thickness and composition and thereby have a significant effect on radiographic density. The radiographer must be aware of these variants and processes to make an intelligent and accurate selection of technical factors.

In 1916, R. Walter Mills presented a paper at the American Roentgen Ray Society meeting in Chicago (published in *American Journal of Roentgenology*, April 1917) describing "The Relation of Bodily Habitus to Visceral Form, Position, Tonus and Motility." Here he coined the terms *hypersthenic, sthenic, hyposthenic,* and *asthenic* (defined in Chapter 6) to describe the various body types. He noted that most physicians came into the field prejudiced by their early anatomic teachings and had fixed conceptions, "which the revelations of the roentgen ray ruthlessly outraged."

Radiographers still use these terms today to describe **body** ◀ **habitus** and its normal variants. Knowledge of each of the body types and its associated tissue characteristics, position and tonus of associated organs, and so on helps us to position more accurately and to select appropriate technical factors. The same body part, such as the stomach, in two different individuals will require very different central ray points of entry if one individual is hypersthenic and the other asthenic. The same body part, such as the shoulder, may measure the same on two different individuals, yet it may not be appropriate to select identical exposure factors for each if one is a sthenic athletic build and the other a hyposthenic type with little muscle tone.

Other factors that influence radiographic density, and consequently the selection of technical factors, are age, gender, and pathology. Various abnormal pathologic conditions, disease processes, and trauma can affect tissue density and, hence, radiographic density. Normal variants of muscle development result from different lifestyles, occupations, and age, and will affect radiographic density.

Some pathologic conditions are referred to as *destructive,* such as osteoporosis, pneumoperitoneum, and conditions involving necrosis or atrophy. These conditions can cause an undesirable increase in radiographic density unless they are recognized and appropriate changes made in exposure factors. Other conditions such as ascites, rheumatoid arthritis, and Paget's disease are *additive,* and an increase in exposure factors is required to maintain adequate radiographic density.

> ### Examples of Additive Pathologic Conditions
>
> - Ascites
> - Rheumatoid arthritis
> - Paget's disease
> - Pneumonia
> - Atelectasis
> - Congestive heart failure
> - Edematous tissue

> ### Examples of Destructive Pathologic Conditions
>
> - Osteoporosis
> - Osteomalacia
> - Pneumoperitoneum
> - Emphysema
> - Degenerative arthritis
> - Atrophic and necrotic conditions

Summary

- **Variations in tissue density will be noted as radiographic density variations in the x-ray image.**
- **Normal tissue density differences exist as a result of body habitus, age, gender, and level of activity.**
- **Abnormal density differences exist as a result of trauma or pathologic conditions.**
- **The radiographer must be knowledgeable about the conditions affecting normal and abnormal changes in tissue density to make accurate selection of technical factors.**

H. GENERATOR TYPE

Three-phase x-ray generation is much more efficient than **single-** ◀ **phase** because the voltage never drops to zero. Three-phase equipment has a small voltage ripple, and thus produces more high-energy x-ray photons (Fig. 12–41). Therefore, if two radiographs were made of the same part and using the same factors, one with a single-phase machine and one with three-phase, the three-phase radiograph would show considerably more radiographic density. Consequently, in order to reproduce similar radiographic densities when using different generators, exposure factor adjustment is necessary.

If 92 kVp and 60 mAs were used for a particular abdominal exposure using single-phase equipment, what mAs would be required to produce a similar radiographic image using three-phase, six-pulse equipment?

Figure 12–41. Single-phase (1ɸ) and three-phase (3ɸ) waveforms. Compared to the one useful impulse available per 1/60th sec with alternating current, single-phase rectified current has two useful impulses, 3ɸ 6p rectified has six useful impulses, and 3ɸ 12p has 12.

Correction Factor

Single-Phase	Three-Phase
x mAs	2/3 × (6p)
x mAs	1/2 × (12p)
x kVp	x − 12%

The correction table in the box in this section indicates that only two thirds of the original single-phase mAs would be required to produce similar radiographic density with three-phase equipment. Thus:

$$2/3 \times 60 = 40 \text{ mAs with 3ɸ 6p equipment}$$

(note that kVp is irrelevant)

It should be noted that approximately the same quantity of radiation is delivered to *the film* from each x-ray machine (1ɸ and 3ɸ) to produce similar radiographic images. The entrance skin exposures (ESE), however, differ significantly (Fig. 12–42). This is because the single-phase machine produces many more low-energy photons, contributing only to patient skin dose.

When technical factors are modified for single-phase/three-phase changes, it is usually the mAs that is adjusted, however kVp adjustment is also workable. Changing from single-phase to three-phase requires a 12% decrease in kVp; conversely, from three-phase to single-phase requires a 12% increase in kVp.

Conventional 60 Hz full-wave rectified power is converted to a higher frequency of 500 to 25,000 Hz in the most recent generator design—the high-frequency generator. The high-frequency generator is small in size, in addition to producing an almost constant potential waveform.

Summary

- Three-phase (3ɸ) equipment produces nearly peak potential voltage whereas single-phase (1ɸ) voltage drops periodically to zero between voltage peaks.
- mAs is usually adjusted to compensate for differences between 1ɸ and 3ɸ waveform equipment.
- When changing from 1ɸ to 3ɸ 6p, two-thirds less mAs is required; from 1ɸ to 3ɸ 12p, one-half the original mAs is required (the reverse is true when changing from 3ɸ to 1ɸ).

Single phase
70 kVp
100 mAs
800 mR ESE

A

Single phase
80 kVp
50 mAs
548 mR ESE

B

Three phase
70 kVp
50 mAs
586 mR ESE

C

Figure 12–42. **(A)**, **(B)**, and **(C).** Films **(A)** and **(C)** are good examples of 1φ to 3φ conversion and the difference in entrance skin exposure (ESE). Films **(A)** and **(B)** demonstrate the radiation-protection factor in increasing from 70 kVp at 100 mAs to 80 kVp at 50 mAs; note the big difference in ESE. (From the American College of Radiology Learning File. Courtesy of the ACR.)

I. BEAM RESTRICTION

A change in radiographic density will occur with changes in the size
▶ of the irradiated field, all other factors remaining constant. **Beam restriction** (ie, reducing the volume of tissue irradiated) reduces the production of scattered radiation and, consequently, decreases radiographic density. The reverse is also true: as field size increases, radiographic density increases as a result of increased production of scattered radiation fog. Therefore, as changes are made in the size of the irradiated field, an accompanying change in mAs is required to maintain the same density.

J. ANODE HEEL EFFECT

The anode heel effect was discussed earlier with respect to focal spot size and recorded detail. Figures 12–43 and 12–44 illustrate how a portion of the divergent x-ray beam is absorbed by the anode resulting in diminished radiographic density at the anode end of the radiograph.

When using general radiographic tubes at standard distances, the heel effect is only noticeable when radiographing parts of uneven thickness, such as the femur and thoracic spine. In these cases, the heel effect may be used to advantage by placing the thicker body portion under the cathode end of the x-ray beam, thus having the effect of "evening out" tissue densities.

The Anode Heel Effect is Emphasized Under the Following Conditions

- At short SIDs
- With large cassettes
- With small target-angle x-ray tubes

K. PROCESSING

Radiographic film emulsion is very sensitive to even small changes in chemical processing. A decrease in developer temperature of 2° to 3°F will produce a dramatic decrease in radiographic density (Fig. 12–45) and, conversely, a rise in developer temperature results in a density increase (Fig. 12–46). The impact of developer temperature on the characteristic curve is illustrated in Figure 12–47.

Radiographic density is also directly related to length of development and replenishment rate, ie, density increases as development time increases or as replenishment rate increases.

Summary

- **Changing the size of the irradiated field affects radiographic density as a result of increased or decreased scattered radiation production.**
- **The anode heel effect is characterized by greater x-ray intensity at the cathode end of the beam.**
- **The anode heel effect is most pronounced at short SIDs, with large image receptors, and with x-ray tubes having small target angles.**
- **The anode heel effect can be used to even out densities when radiographing parts of uneven thickness.**
- **Radiographic density increases as developer temperature increases.**
- **Radiographic density increases as the replenishment rate and/or length of development increase.**

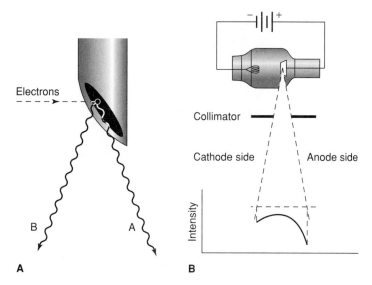

Figure 12–43. The anode heel effect. As x-ray photons are produced within the anode, a portion of the divergent beam is absorbed by the anode's "heel." This represents a decrease in x-ray beam intensity at the anode end of the x-ray beam. (Modified from Wolbarst, AB. *Physics of Radiology.* East Norwalk, CT: Appleton & Lange, 1993.)

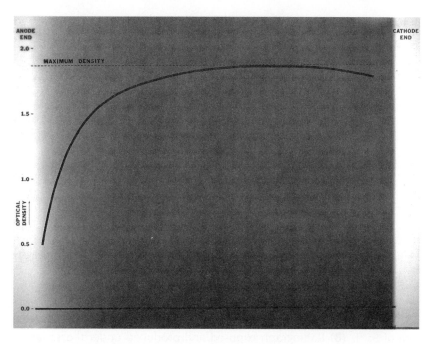

Figure 12–44. Radiographic illustration of the anode heel effect. Note the gradual increase in radiographic density toward the cathode end of the beam. (From the American College of Radiology Learning File. Courtesy of the ACR.)

A

B

C

Figure 12–45. Developer temperature versus image density and patient exposure. **(A)** Radiograph of a chest phantom made using 22 mR and processed at the recommended temperature of 95°F. **(B)** Radiograph exposed and produced under the same conditions except that the developer temperature was 5° lower, at 90°F; note the significant change in radiographic density. **(C)** Radiograph using the same 90°F developer, but with exposure compensated to provide the required density; note the increase in exposure dose to 35 mR. (From the American College of Radiology Learning File. Courtesy of the ACR.)

Figure 12–46. This radiograph was exposed under the same conditions as Figure 12–45A, but was processed at a developer temperature 5° above normal (at 100°F), producing a dark radiograph. Although a diagnostic radiograph might be produced by reducing the film exposure, higher than recommended processing temperatures are not advised because they can produce inconsistent results. (From the American College of Radiology Learning File. Courtesy of the ACR.)

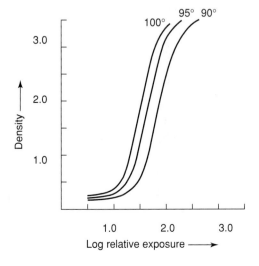

Figure 12–47. The characteristic curve illustrates the effect of developer temperature changes seen in Figures 12–45 and 12–46. The relative position of the lower temperature (90°F) curve is to the right of the optimal temperature (95°F) curve; to achieve the same density, the exposure must be increased to compensate for decreased development. The 100°F curve illustrates a shift to the left of the optimal curve, illustrating that less exposure is required to compensate for decreased development. (Modified from the American College of Radiology Learning File. Courtesy of the ACR.)

A&I Chapter Review Questions

⭐ *Congratulations! You have completed a portion of this chapter. You may go on to the "Registry-type" multiple-choice questions that follow. For greatest success, be sure also to complete the short answer questions found at the end of this chapter.*

1. The quantity of x-ray photons delivered to the patient in a given exposure is PRIMARILY regulated by:
   (A) mAs
   (B) kVp
   (C) SID
   (D) focal spot size

2. Of the following groups of exposure factors, which will produce the greatest radiographic density?
   (A) 200 mA, 0.05 sec, 36 inches SID
   (B) 400 mA, 0.05 sec, 72 inches SID
   (C) 400 mA, 0.10 sec, 72 inches SID
   (D) 200 mA, 0.10 sec, 36 inches SID

3. An exposure was made at 40 inches SID using 300 mA, 0.12 second exposure and 70 kVp with a 200 film/screen combination and an 8:1 grid. It is desired to repeat the radiograph and, in order to produce improved detail, use 48 inches SID and 100 film/screen combination. Using 0.25 second exposure, and with all other factors remaining constant, what mA will be required to maintain the original radiographic density?
   (A) 100 mA
   (B) 200 mA
   (C) 300 mA
   (D) 400 mA

4. If the radiographer is unable to adjust the mAs, yet needs to double the radiographic density on a particular film, which of the following would BEST accomplish this?
   (A) increase the kVp by 50%
   (B) increase the kVp by 15%
   (C) decrease the SID by 25%
   (D) increase the grid ratio

5. Exposure factors of 85 kVp and 10 mAs are used for a particular non-grid exposure. What should be the new mAs if a 12:1 grid is added?
   (A) 20 mAs
   (B) 30 mAs
   (C) 40 mAs
   (D) 50 mAs

6. An image lacking sufficient radiographic density may be attributable to insufficient
   1. SID
   2. developer temperature
   3. kilovoltage
   (A) 2 only
   (B) 1 and 2 only
   (C) 2 and 3 only
   (D) 1, 2, and 3

7. Grid ratio is defined as the relationship between the height of the lead strip and the:
   (A) width of the lead strip
   (B) distance between the lead strips
   (C) number of lead strips per inch
   (D) angle of the lead strip

8. An exposure was made using 200 mA, 0.05 second exposure, and 75 kVp. Each of the following changes will function to double radiographic density, EXCEPT:
   (A) change to 0.1 second exposure
   (B) change to 86 kVp
   (C) change to 20 mAs
   (D) change to 100 mA

9. How is source-image distance related to exposure rate and radiographic density?
   (A) as SID increases, exposure rate increases and radiographic density increases
   (B) as SID increases, exposure rate increases and radiographic density decreases
   (C) as SID increases, exposure rate decreases and radiographic density increases
   (D) as SID increases, exposure rate decreases and radiographic density decreases

10. Focusing distance is associated with which of the following:
    (A) stereoradiography
    (B) chest radiography
    (C) magnification radiography
    (D) grids

Answers and Explanations

1. (A) While mAs is primarily used to regulate x-ray *quantity,* the number of x-ray photons produced in a given exposure, kVp is generally used to regulate x-ray *quality,* the energy or wavelength of x-ray photons produced at the target during a given exposure. Although source-image distance significantly *affects* radiographic density, it is not used to *regulate* the quantity of photons produced. Focal spot size is unrelated to radiation quantity or quality.

2. (D) Using the formula mA × sec = mAs, determine each mAs. The greatest radiographic density will be produced by the combination of greatest mAs and shortest SID. Groups A and C should produce identical radiographic density, according to the inverse square law, since group C is twice the distance and four times the mAs of group A. Group B has twice the distance of group A, but only twice the mAs; it has, therefore, less density than groups A and C. Group D has the same distance as group A, and twice the mAs—making it the group of technical factors which will produce the greatest radiographic density.

3. (D) A review of the problem reveals that three changes are being made: an increase in SID, a change from 200 speed system to 100 speed system, and an increase in exposure time (to be considered last). Since the original mAs was 36, cutting the speed of the system in half (from 200 to 100) will require a doubling of the mAs, to 72, in order to maintain density. Now we must deal with the distance change. Using the inverse square law (and remembering that 72 is now the OLD mAs!) we find that the required new mAs at 48 inches is 103. Since the problem states that we are now using 0.25 second exposure, it is left to determine what mA, used with 0.25 second, will provide 103 mAs.

$$0.25\ x = 103$$

$$x = 412\ \text{mA}$$

4. (B) Radiographic density is proportional to mAs. However, other methods may be used to adjust radiographic density. When adjusting mAs is not possible, an increase in kVp by 15% will effectively double the radiographic density. Decreasing the source-image distance (SID) will increase density, but increased patient dose and size distortion make this an impractical approach. Increasing the grid ratio will decrease radiographic density.

5. (D) To change non-grid to grid exposure, or to adjust exposure when changing from one grid ratio to another, recall the factor for each grid ratio:

$$\text{no grid} = 1 \times \text{original mAs}$$

$$5:1\ \text{grid} = 2 \times \text{original mAs}$$

$$6:1\ \text{grid} = 3 \times \text{original mAs}$$

$$8:1\ \text{grid} = 4 \times \text{original mAs}$$

$$12:1\ \text{grid} = 5 \times \text{original mAs}$$

$$16:1\ \text{grid} = 6 \times \text{original mAs}$$

Therefore, to change from non-grid to 12:1 grid, multiply the original mAs by a factor of five. A new mAs of 50 is required.

6. (C) Insufficient kV can result in underpenetration of an anatomic part and inadequate radiographic density. If developer temperature is too low the developing agents (especially hydroquinone) may become inactive, resulting in an underdeveloped image with insufficient density. Insufficient SID (ie, SID too low) will result in an image with excessive radiographic density.

7. (B) A grid consists of alternate strips of lead and interspace material. The lead strips are used to trap scatter radiation before it reaches the film, thus decreasing the effect of scatter radiation fog on the radiograph. Grid ratio is defined as the height of the lead strip to the distance between the strips (or width of the interspace material).

8. (D) Radiographic density is directly proportional to mAs. If exposure time is *doubled* from 0.05 (1/20) sec to 1/10 sec, radiographic density will double. If the mAs is doubled from 10 to 20 mAs, radiographic density will double. If the kVp is increased by 15%, from 75 to 86 kVp, radiographic density will double according to the 15% rule. Changing to 100 mA will halve the mAs, effectively halving the radiographic density.

9. (D) According to the inverse square law of radiation, the intensity or exposure rate of radiation from its source is inversely proportional to the square of the distance. Thus, as distance from the source of radiation increases, exposure rate decreases. Since exposure rate and radiographic density are directly proportional, if the exposure rate of a beam directed to a film is decreased, the resultant radiographic density would be decreased proportionally.

10. (D) Focusing distance is the term used to specify the optimum source-image distance used with a particular focused grid. It is usually expressed as *focal range,* indicating the minimum and maximum SID workable with that grid. Distances lesser or greater can result in grid cut-off. Although proper distance is important in stereoradiography, chest, and magnification radiography, focusing distance is unrelated to them.

III. FACTORS AFFECTING RADIOGRAPHIC CONTRAST

KEY TERMS ◄

AEC	FILM EMULSION	PATHOLOGY
BACKUP TIMER	FILM LATITUDE	PENETRABILITY
BASE-PLUS-FOG	FIXED kVp TECHNIQUE	SHORT-SCALE CONTRAST
CHARACTERISTIC CURVE	HIGH SUBJECT CONTRAST	SHOULDER
DUPLITIZED	IONIZATION CHAMBER	STRAIGHT LINE PORTION
EXPOSURE LATITUDE	LONG-SCALE CONTRAST	SUBJECT CONTRAST
FILM BASE	LOW SUBJECT CONTRAST	TOE
FILM CONTRAST	MINIMUM REACTION TIME	VARIABLE kVp TECHNIQUE

A. TERMINOLOGY

Radiographic contrast exists whenever two or more different densities are present in a radiographic image. When there is a big difference between shades of densities, radiographic **contrast** is said to ◄ be **high.** When there is little difference between densities, radiographic **contrast** is **low.** ◄

Radiographic contrast is the sum of subject contrast and film contrast.

Subject contrast is a result of differential absorption by tissues ◄ of varying densities and thicknesses. X-ray photons are attenuated to differing degrees by various body tissues, with less exit radiation emerging from thicker, denser structures and more exit radiation from thinner or less dense structures. Hence, subject contrast produces the various density *differences* visible on the radiographic image, and is exhibited as a *scale of grays* having varying tones representative of differential tissue absorption.

Selection of exposure factors and various other techniques are used to *modify* the differential absorption properties of tissue, thereby enabling the radiographer to produce the desired scale of contrast.

A

B

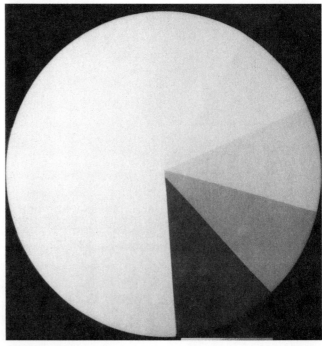

C

Figure 12–48. Contrast serves to make details visible. Radiographs were made of a circular phantom having a variety of wedge-shaped thicknesses; a circular "lesion" of greater density is embedded in each wedge. Note that the level of contrast between adjacent areas is strongly related to the degree of visibility of the "lesions." (A) Illustrates the highest contrast; only two wedges (thicknesses) are visualized and only one "lesion" is barely visible. (B) The contrast scale is a little longer; a third wedge begins to be seen and two "lesions" are visualized. (C) Five wedges are visualized (hopefully the printing process shows them!) and at least three "lesions" can be seen clearly. Methods that can be used to adjust the level of contrast between adjacent areas include: 1. increasing kVp; 2. using compensating filtration; and 3. using lower-contrast (higher-latitude) film. (From the American College of Radiology Learning File. Courtesy of the ACR.)

Subject contrast is regulated by the quality (energy, wavelength, penetrability) of x-ray photons.

Film contrast describes the response of the film emulsion to ◄ the variety of x-ray intensities emerging from the irradiated part. Film contrast is affected by the manufacturing process (film type, base fog), processing conditions, and fluorescent properties of the intensifying screens. Film contrast characteristics are illustrated by the characteristic (D log E) curve.

A radiograph exhibiting a variety of different shades of gray possesses **long-scale** (low) **contrast,** ie, there is *little difference* among ◄ the various shades. One that exhibits only a few shades possesses ◄ **short-scale** (high) **contrast.**

The function of contrast is to make image details visible. Most anatomic structures have an infinite number of details that compose the image and these structural details may represent a variety of tissue densities having different absorption properties. If the anatomic part is represented radiographically by only a few shades of gray, many details are not being visualized at all. If, however, the radiograph displays a wide range of gray tones more anatomic details will be represented and visualized (Fig. 12–48). Hence, long-scale contrast *usually* provides more information (but short scale, ie, high, contrast may be required for certain examinations or body parts; see Fig. 12–49).

A number of factors affect the production of radiographic contrast and each of these will be discussed individually.

Contrast Terminology	
HIGHER CONTRAST shorter scale contrast ↓ IS A PRODUCT OF lower kVp fewer, widely different tissue densities	LOWER CONTRAST longer scale contrast ↓ IS A PRODUCT OF higher kVp many similar tissue densities

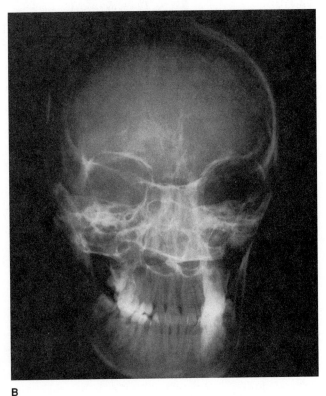

A   **B**

Figure 12–49. **(A)** Example of high, or short-scale, contrast. **(B)** Example of low, or long-scale, contrast. The skull is also rotated in film **(B).** (From the American College of Radiology Learning File. Courtesy of the ACR.)

Summary

- Radiographic contrast refers to the degree of difference between image densities.
- Radiographic contrast is the sum of subject contrast and film contrast.
- Subject contrast is the result of differential absorption of x-rays by body tissues of various thicknesses and densities.
- Film contrast is the result of manufacturing, processing, and intensifying screens.
- Subject contrast is regulated by selection of x-ray beam quality.
- Radiographic images with several different density differences are said to possess long-scale (or low) contrast.
- Radiographic images possessing few density differences, strikingly different from each other, are said to possess short-scale (or high) contrast.

B. kVp

▶ Kilovolts peak (kVp), which governs x-ray **penetrability,** is the primary exposure factor affecting radiographic contrast. In general, as kVp increases so does the scale of contrast (Fig. 12–50).

Figure 12–50. Aluminum step-wedge test. As kVp increases, a greater number of steps (and the subtle differences between them) are discernible. (From the American College of Radiology Learning File. Courtesy of the ACR.)

In general, parts having ***low subject contrast*** will produce ◄ long-scale radiographic contrast and, if high kVp is used to image these parts, unacceptably low radiographic contrast will result.

Scattered radiation fog reduces the visibility of low-contrast objects. When imaging structures that have low subject contrast, the use of lower kVp frequently helps to emphasize what little contrast exists in the subject tissues.

Because kVp determines the penetrating ability of the x-ray photons, low kVp can be used to emphasize the differences between tissue densities, eg, in mammography, foreign-body localization, and iodine-containing renal collecting systems (Fig. 12–51).

Anatomic parts having ***high subject contrast*** will produce ◄ short-scale radiographic contrast and, if low kVp is used to image these parts, unacceptably high radiographic contrast will result (Fig. 12–52). Visibility of structures within the very light and very dark areas is greatly diminished. When imaging structures having high subject contrast, the use of higher kVp will promote more uniform penetration of the part, thus it "evens out" big differences in tissue densities and bringing about visualization of small image details (as in high-kVp chest radiography).

A   **B**

Figure 12–51. In anatomic regions having low subject contrast such as the abdominal viscera, artificial contrast agents are often introduced to demonstrate organs such as the kidneys. **(A)** IVU made using 70 kVp. **(B)** IVU using 110 kVp. The use of too high kVp with iodinated media and the production of more scatter radiation has almost obliterated the contrast-filled collecting systems in film **(B).** (From the American College of Radiology Learning File. Courtesy of the ACR.)

A   **B**

Figure 12–52. PA chest radiographs made using 80 kVp **(A)** and 120 kVp **(B)**. Film **(A)** PA chest radiograph made using 80 kVp demonstrates shorter-scale contrast, and pulmonary vascular markings are not well visualized. **(B)** Chest radiograph made using 120 kVp demonstrates longer-scale contrast, and visualization of pulmonary vascular markings *through* the bony rib details, and requires a smaller patient dose. (From the American College of Radiology Learning File. Courtesy of the ACR.)

C. SCATTERED RADIATION

High kVp may be desirable in terms of patient dose, tube life, and making more details visible, but use of excessively high kVp will result in production of excessive amounts of scatter radiation and fog, resulting in *diminished* visibility of details (Fig. 12–53).

Much of the scatter radiation produced is highly energetic and exits the patient along with useful image-forming radiation. Scattered radiation carries no useful information, but adds noise in the form of fog, thereby impairing visibility of detail.

Since scatter radiation can have such a devastating effect on image contrast, it is essential that radiographers are knowledgeable about methods of reducing its production. The three factors that have a significant effect on the *production of scattered radiation* are:

- Beam restriction
- Kilovoltage
- Thickness/volume and density of tissues

Perhaps the most important way to limit the production of scatter radiation is by limiting the size of the irradiated field, ie, through beam restriction (Fig. 12–54). As the size of the field is reduced, there is less area and tissue volume for scatter radiation to be generated.

A   B

Figure 12–53. Kilovoltage is directly related to the production of scatter radiation. **(A)** Film made using 80 kVp and 75 mAs. **(B)** Film made using 100 kVp and 18 mAs, all other factors remaining the same. As kVp is increased, the percentage of scattered radiation relative to primary radiation increases. Use of optimum kilovoltage for each anatomic part is helpful in keeping scatter to a minimum. (From the American College of Radiology Learning File. Courtesy of the ACR.)

As the volume and/or density of the irradiated tissues increase(s) so does scatter radiation (Fig. 12–55). Thicker and denser anatomic structures will generate more scatter radiation production. Compression of certain parts can occasionally be used to minimize the effect of scatter, but close collimation can always be used effectively.

Introduction of an OID (air gap) can have a noticable effect on radiographic contrast. An air gap introduced between the object and image recorder can have an effect similar to that of a grid. As energetic scattered radiation emerges from the body, it continues to travel in its divergent fashion and, much of the time, will bypass the image recorder (see Fig. 12–38).

D. STRUCTURAL AND PATHOLOGIC CONDITIONS

Various tissue types and pathologic processes can alter tissue thickness and composition and thereby have a significant effect on radiographic contrast. Anatomic structures having high atomic numbers and pathologic conditions that increase tissue density will tend to produce a higher contrast.

The radiographer must be aware of the nature of pathology under investigation to make an intelligent and accurate selection of technical factors.

Summary

- ■ kVp selection determines the energy of x-ray photons and therefore degree of penetration of various tissues, thereby determining the contrast characteristics of the image.
- ■ Images of low subject contrast structures often benefit from the use of lower kVp, while high subject contrast structures

A

B

Figure 12–54. Note the striking improvement in radiographic quality in film **(A)** as beam restriction is increased in this lateral lumbar myelogram. Although a 50% increase in exposure was required to maintain appropriate density in film **(A)** (to compensate for less scattered radiation reaching the film), radiation protection is maintained because the volume of irradiated tissue is decreased. (From the American College of Radiology Learning File. Courtesy of the ACR.)

can be represented with a longer range of grays by using higher kVp.

■ The use of high kVp reduces patient dose and reduces the production of x-ray tube heat, but increases the production of scatter radiation fog.

■ Radiation that has scattered carries no useful information, but rather, adds noise that impairs visibility of image details.

■ The production of scatter radiation can be minimized by using optimum kVp techniques and by restricting the size of the x-ray beam as much as possible.

■ As the thickness and density of tissues increase, so does the production of scatter radiation; tissue thickness can sometimes be minimized with compression.

■ As normal tissues undergo pathologic change, their penetrability frequently also changes in ways characteristic of the disease process.

E. GRIDS

An image produced with a grid usually differs considerably from an image produced without a grid. Since thicker, denser parts can gen-

A   B

Figure 12–55. The volume of irradiated tissue is directly related to the quantity of scatter radiation generated. **(A)** AP film of knee. **(B)** AP film with paraffin absorbers *around* the knee. The loss of contrast exhibited in **(B)** is due to increased *volume* of irradiated material within the beam, resulting in increased scattered-radiation fog. Note that the part need not be *thicker* to generate significant scatter, just that the total irradiated *volume* be greater. (From the American College of Radiology Learning File. Courtesy of the ACR.)

erate significant amounts of scatter radiation, a grid should be used whenever a part measures 11 cm or greater in thickness. A possible exception to this rule is the chest, although much chest radiography performed today employs high kVp and grids.

Although collimation, optimum kVp, and compression may be used, a large amount of scatter radiation can still be generated within the part being radiographed and can have a severely degrading effect on image contrast. Without the use of a grid, scatter radiation can contribute 50% to 90% of the total image exposure. The function of a grid, then, is to remove scatter radiation exiting the patient *before* it reaches the image receptor thereby improving contrast (Fig. 12–56).

As discussed earlier in this part, two of a grid's physical characteristics that determine its degree of efficiency in the removal of scattered radiation are *grid ratio* (the height of the lead strips compared to the distance between them) and number of *lead strips per inch*. Other familiar ways of expressing and measuring grid efficiency include the *bucky factor* (grid conversion factor), *contrast improvement factor,* and *selectivity.*

The *bucky factor (B)* is the ratio of the total amount of radiation (primary and scattered) incident upon the surface of the grid to the amount of radiation transmitted through the grid.

$$B = \frac{\text{total incident}}{\text{total transmitted}}$$

Figure 12–56. Effect of grids on image contrast and radiographic quality. **(A)** Film made using 100 kVp and 12 mAs without a grid; scatter radiation fog obliterates recorded detail almost entirely. **(B)** Film made with 100 kVp, 60 mAs, and using a 12:1 grid, all other factors remaining constant; scatter radiation is "cleaned up" and image details are more readily perceptible. **(C)** Film made without a grid using 70 kVp and 4 mAs. **(D)** Film made with a 12:1 grid using 70 kVp and 20 mAs. Note the improved contrast and detail visibility. (From the American College of Radiology Learning File. Courtesy of the ACR.)

The *contrast improvement factor (CIF)* is the ratio of radiographic contrast obtained with a grid to that obtained without a grid.

$$CIF = \frac{\text{contrast with grid}}{\text{contrast without grid}}$$

Selectivity (S) is the ratio between the quantity of primary photons transmitted through the grid and the quantity of scattered photons transmitted.

$$S = \frac{\text{primary photon transmission}}{\text{scattered photon transmission}}$$

As previously discussed, the introduction of an air gap can have an effect similar to that obtained through the addition of a grid.

F. FILTRATION

The primary beam usually has a total filtration of 2.5 mm Al equivalent. Inherent filtration includes 0.5 mm Al from the glass envelope and 1.0 mm Al from the collimator. The manufacturer adds another 1.0 mm Al to meet the minimum requirements of 2.5 mm Al equivalent total filtration for radiographic tubes operated above 70 kVp.

Filtration serves to increase the overall average energy of the beam; it "hardens" the x-ray beam. The purpose of the 2.5 mm Al equivalent is to remove the diagnostically useless x-ray photons that simply contribute to patient dose. Since these photons do not have sufficient energy to reach the image receptor, the usual required filtration in the x-ray tube *has no significant effect on radiographic contrast* (Fig. 12–57).

The addition or removal of *compensating* filters (as discussed in section IIF) will impact the radiographic contrast unless exposure factors are adjusted to compensate for the change.

G. INTENSIFYING SCREENS

Radiographic images produced with intensifying screens possess higher contrast than those produced by direct exposure. In general, when comparing radiographs produced using different speed intensifying screens, the higher the screen speed the higher the contrast. That is, 400-speed screens will produce somewhat higher contrast than 200 and 100-speed screens, and 200 screens will produce higher contrast than 100 screens, and so on. Contrast differences among various speed screens, however, are rather slight.

Summary

- ■ **X-rays scattering within a part and having enough energy to exit the body and reach the image receptor produce scatter-radiation fog (noise) on the radiographic image.**
- ■ **Grids function to absorb scattered radiation before it reaches the image receptor.**
- ■ **Scattered radiation cleanup increases as grid ratio increases.**
- ■ **The higher the grid ratio, the higher (shorter-scale) the resulting contrast.**
- ■ **X-ray tube filtration ordinarily has little effect on contrast; it functions primarily for patient protection.**
- ■ **Compensating filters added or removed from the x-ray beam will affect contrast unless exposure adjustment is made.**

As Grid Ratio Increases

- • Scatter radiation clean-up increases
- • Contrast scale decreases (higher contrast produced)
- • Exposure factors (usually mAs) must increase

A

B

Figure 12–57. **(A)** and **(B).** The effect of filtration on image contrast. The contrast displayed in films **(A)** and **(B)** is very similar. An increase in filtration, however, results in a lower ESE and greater tube load (mAs). As filtration is increased above 2.5 mm Al, minimal dose reduction occurs and tube loading is significantly increased. (From the American College of Radiology Learning File. Courtesy of the ACR.)

 Chapter Review Questions

⭐ *Congratulations! You have completed a portion of this chapter. You may go on to the "Registry-type" multiple-choice questions that follow. For greatest success, be sure also to complete the short answer questions found at the end of this chapter.*

1. Which of the following contribute(s) to the radiographic contrast present on the finished radiograph?
    1. tissue density
    2. pathology
    3. muscle development
    (A) 1 and 2 only
    (B) 1 and 3 only
    (C) 2 and 3 only
    (D) 1, 2, and 3

2. In comparison to 60 kVp, 80 kVp will:
    1. permit greater exposure latitude
    2. produce longer scale contrast
    3. produce more scatter radiation
    (A) 1 only
    (B) 2 only
    (C) 1 and 2 only
    (D) 1, 2, and 3

3. A radiograph that exhibits many shades of gray from white to black may be described as having:
    (A) long-scale contrast
    (B) short-scale contrast
    (C) increased density
    (D) good recorded detail

4. Which of the following is NOT related to radiographic contrast?
    (A) photon energy
    (B) grid ratio
    (C) object-image distance
    (D) focal spot size

5. Which of the following groups of exposure factors will produce the longest scale of contrast?
    (A) 200 mA, 1/20 sec, 70 kVp, 12:1 grid
    (B) 500 mA, 0.02 sec, 80 kVp, 16:1 grid
    (C) 300 mA, 0.03 sec, 90 kVp, 8:1 grid
    (D) 600 mA, 0.015 sec, 70 kVp, 8:1 grid

6. Which of the following anatomic parts has the greatest subject contrast?
    (A) elbow
    (B) kidney
    (C) esophagus
    (D) lumbar spine

7. An increase in the kilovoltage applied to the x-ray tube increases the:
    1. x-ray wavelength
    2. exposure rate
    3. patient absorption
    (A) 1 only
    (B) 2 only
    (C) 2 and 3 only
    (D) 1, 2, and 3

8. The advantages of high-kilovoltage chest radiography include
    1. greater exposure latitude
    2. longer-scale contrast
    3. reduced patient dose
    (A) 1 only
    (B) 1 and 2 only
    (C) 1 and 3 only
    (D) 1, 2, and 3

9. Which of the following exposure factors is used to regulate radiographic contrast?
   (A) mA
   (B) exposure time
   (C) mAs
   (D) kVp

10. What are the effects of scattered radiation on the radiographic image?
   1. it produces fog
   2. it increases contrast
   3. it increases grid cut-off
   (A) 1 only
   (B) 2 only
   (C) 1 and 2 only
   (D) 1, 2, and 3

Answers and Explanations

1. (D) The radiographic subject, ie, the patient, is composed of many different tissue types of varying densities, resulting in varying degrees of photon attenuation and absorption. This *differential absorption* contributes to the various shades of gray (ie, scale of radiographic contrast) on the finished radiograph. Normal tissue density may be significantly altered in the presence of pathology. For example, destructive bone disease can cause a dramatic decrease in tissue density. Abnormal accumulation of fluid (as in ascites) will cause a significant increase in tissue density. Muscle atrophy, or highly developed muscles, will similarly decrease or increase tissue density.

2. (D) The higher the kVp range, the greater the exposure latitude (margin of error in exposure). Higher kVp is more penetrating and produces more grays on the radiograph, lengthening the scale of contrast. As kVp increases, the percentage of scatter radiation also increases.

3. (A) Radiographic contrast is described as the difference between the densities present on a radiograph. A radiograph possessing many shades of gray between black and white is said to exhibit long-scale, or low, contrast. A radiograph possessing only a few widely different shades of gray between black and white is said to exhibit short-scale, or high, contrast.

4. (D) As photon energy increases, more penetration and greater production of scatter radiation occurs, producing a longer scale of contrast. As grid ratio increases, more scatter radiation is absorbed, producing a higher contrast. As OID increases, the distance between the part and film acts as a grid and consequently less scatter radiation reaches the film, producing a higher contrast. Focal spot size is related only to recorded detail.

5. (C) Of the given factors, kilovoltage and grid ratio will have a significant effect on radiographic contrast. The mAs values are almost identical. Since an increased kilovoltage and low-ratio grid combination would allow the greatest amount of scatter radiation to reach the film, thereby producing more gray tones, C is the best answer. D also uses a low-ratio grid, but the kV is too low to produce as much gray as C.

6. (A) The greatest subject contrast is found in body parts made of a few widely differing tissue densities. The elbow has but bone, some muscle, and soft tissues—constituting high subject contrast. The abdomen, containing the kidneys, stomach, small and large intestines, and other viscera, is a heavy body part composed of many similar tissue densities, and thus, normally has very low subject contrast.

7. (B) As the kilovoltage is increased, a *greater number* of electrons are driven across to the anode with *greater force.* Therefore as energy conversion takes place at the anode, *more high-energy* (short-wavelength) photons are produced. However, because they are higher-energy photons, there will be *less* patient absorption.

8. (D) The chest is composed of widely differing tissue densities (bone and air). In an effort to "even out" these tissue densities and better visualize pulmonary vascular markings, high kV is generally used. This produces more uniform penetration and results in a longer scale of contrast with visualization of the pulmonary vascular markings as well as bone (which is better penetrated) and air densities. The increased kV also affords the advantage of greater exposure latitude (an error of a few kV will make little if any difference). The fact that the kV is increased means that the mAs is accordingly reduced and thus, patient dose is reduced as well.

9. (D) Kilovoltage regulates the energy, and therefore penetration, of the photons produced at the target. The greater the photon energy, the less the total absorption by dense tissues and the more that tissue densities will be "evened-out," ie, showing a longer scale of grays. Time and mA are the quantitative exposure factors controlling radiographic density.

10. (A) Scatter radiation is produced as x-ray photons travel through matter, interact with atoms, and are scattered (change direction). If these scattered rays are energetic enough to exit the body, they will strike the film from all different angles. They therefore do not carry useful information and merely produce a flat, gray (low-contrast) fog over the image. Grid cut-off increases contrast and is caused by improper relationship between the x-ray tube and grid.

IV. FILM, SCREEN, AND GRID OPTIONS

X-ray film may be described as being made of *silver bromide grains suspended in a gelatin emulsion and coated on a plastic base material.* X-ray film is an important means of recording and storing the radiographic image and so a brief overview of the process of x-ray film production is in order here.

First, gelatin is extracted from cattle hooves and hides and rendered into a very pure, uncontaminated state. Nitric acid is combined with pure silver to form silver nitrate. Then, *in total darkness,* silver nitrate is added to potassium bromide to form silver bromide. Silver bromide is then combined with the gelatin mixture to form the emulsion, which is coated onto one (single-emulsion film) or both sides *(duplitized)* of the *film base.*   ◀

The base material is a durable *polyester* plastic that will not tear and with a dimensional stability that will be unaffected as it travels through the processor roller system and various chemical temperatures. Film base is not absolutely clear; it has a measurable density, referred to as *base fog* or *base density.* Base fog or density is the sum of environmental exposure received during production and storage as well as the density resulting from the base material tint and dye. An additional, approximately equal, amount of fog results from proc-

► essing. The total ***base-plus-fog*** should not exceed 0.2 density as measured by a densitometer.

A *protective coat* of hard, clear gelatin is placed over the emulsion to help prevent damage in the form of scratches.

A. FILM CONTRAST AND LATITUDE

► Each type of x-ray-***film emulsion*** is manufactured with certain characteristics required for its particular use (eg, latitude film, mammography film), each having its own particular response to exposure (ie,

► ***film latitude***). Some film emulsion is manufactured especially to produce high contrast, eg, film used in mammography and vascular procedures. Others are produced to provide a long range of grays; this type of emulsion possesses more film *latitude,* ie, it is more "forgiving" of errors in technical factors (Fig. 12–58). The study of film emulsion response to exposure is called *sensitometry* and is illustrated by the characteristic (H&D) curve.

The characteristic curve (Fig. 12–59) illustrates the degree of film density as a result of exposure. Density is represented by the verti-

► cal axis, log exposure by the horizontal axis. The ***characteristic***

► ***curve*** has three portions: the ***toe*** (D_{min}), ***straight line portion,*** and

► ***shoulder*** (D_{max}). Exposures made in the toe and shoulder portions of the curve will be excessively under or overexposed. The useful diagnostic range of densities lies between 0.25 and 2.5, correspond-

Figure 12–58. **(A)** Film made using 80 kVp, 75 mAs, and regular film. **(B)** Film made under identical conditions and using the same factors, but with latitude (ie, low-contrast) film. (From the American College of Radiology Learning File. Courtesy of the ACR.)

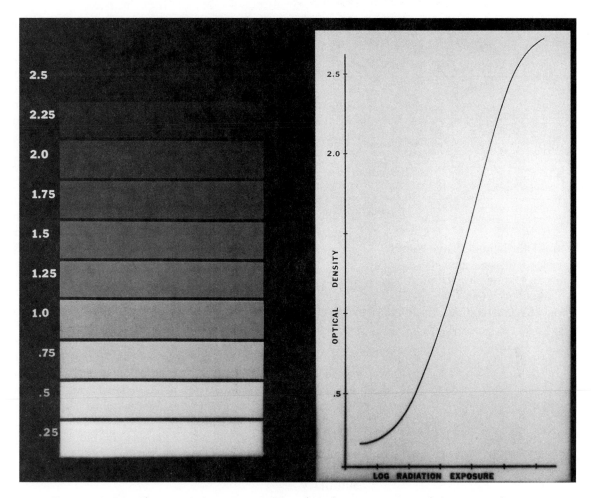

Figure 12–59. Characteristic curve. Notice that the toe portion of the curve does not begin at zero; this represents the slight exposure due to base fog. Total base-plus-fog should not exceed 0.2 density. (From the American College of Radiology Learning File. Courtesy of the ACR.)

ing to the *straight line portion* (average gradient) of the curve and is generally regarded as the *region of correct exposure*. Exposures made outside of this region do not record diagnostically useful information.

The highest point on the characteristic curve is where maximum density occurs, and is referred to as D_{max}. Just beyond D_{max}, the curve begins to descend again, representing a decrease in density. This is the *solarization point,* where additional exposure will actually cause a reversal of the image.

Have you noticed that an unexposed and processed duplicating film emerges from the processor black? If regular x-ray film were used for film duplication, a black/white reversed image would result. This is because, using regular film, the print box light will pass through the whiter areas causing exposure and darkening, while little light will pass through the darker areas, causing little or no exposure on the x-ray film: hence, a reversed image. Duplicating-film emulsion, however, has been chemically brought up to the solarization point so that further exposure will cause a reversal, thus remedying the problem of reversed images with regular film.

Higher/Shorter Scale Contrast Results When

Subject contrast increases
kVp decreases
Scattered radiation decreases
Grid ratio increases
Exposure latitude decreases

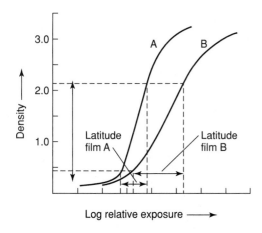

Figure 12–60. Film latitude. Note the differences in film latitude within the useful density range. Latitude and contrast are inversely related. **(A)** High-contrast, low-latitude film. **(B)** Low-contrast, high-latitude film.

A glance at the film's characteristic curve will tell you about its speed, latitude, and contrast. A curve having a steep slope (average gradient) is likely to be fast, having little latitude and producing high contrast. A fast film responds readily to fluorescent light or x-rays, and has the advantage of permitting a decrease in exposure factors, and ultimately, patient dose. When two or more curves are being compared, the curve farthest to the left represents the fastest emulsion.

The average gradient of a characteristic curve gives a good indication of that film's *contrast*. A steep characteristic curve (average gradient) is representative of high contrast, shorter scale, contrast. *Latitude* refers to the *range* of exposure that will provide densities within the diagnostically useful range; fast film generally offers less latitude (Fig. 12–60). Film and screen protocols are generally established at the radiographer's workplace; however he or she should be knowledgeable enough to use the types available to best advantage.

B. Exposure Latitude

▶ While *film latitude* is related to emulsion characteristics, **exposure latitude** is related to the technical factors selected. Exposure latitude is the leeway, or margin of error, one has with a given group of exposure factors; the degree of exposure latitude is generally determined by the kilovoltage. At higher kilovoltages, a difference of a few kVp, plus or minus, will make little, if any, difference radiographically (recall the 15% rule). At low kilovoltages, however, an error of just a few kVp can make a very noticeable difference in the radiographic image. While the radiographer has little control over film latitude, he or she has much control of exposure latitude.

Summary

- **X-ray film emulsion consists of silver-bromide grains suspended in gelatin.**
- **Film base is a tough polyester plastic.**
- **Base-plus-fog is a result of environmental factors, base tint, and processing.**
- **Base-plus-fog should not exceed 0.2 density.**
- **Various kinds of film emulsion are available from the manufacturer; emulsion characteristics differ according to their use and the desired radiographic requirements.**
- **Film emulsions are made to be of slow speed or high speed, low contrast or high contrast.**
- **Sensitometry is the study of film emulsion response to exposure.**
- **Characteristic curves are used to illustrate and compare film emulsion response to exposure.**
- **The typical characteristic curve has a toe (D_{min}), straight-line portion (average gradient), and shoulder (D_{max}).**
- **Diagnostically useful densities are within 0.25 to 2.5 on the vertical axis.**
- **A characteristic curve with a steep slope usually represents higher contrast emulsion.**
- **A characteristic curve with a gentle slope usually represents lower contrast emulsion.**
- **Exposure latitude is related to kVp level: as kVp increases, exposure latitude increases, and vice versa.**

C. Anatomic Factors

Consideration of patient habitus, tissue density, and ***pathology*** is ◄ important in the appropriate selection of radiographic accessories. For example, routine protocol may call for knee and shoulder examinations to be performed using the table or upright bucky. However, children, the elderly, and patients with degenerative conditions may not require the use of a grid. Small, thin parts and parts undergoing degenerative changes (such as in osteoporosis) can frequently be performed tabletop (ie, using intensifying screens without a grid), thereby significantly reducing patient dose.

Many radiology departments have two screen types available. Slower speed screens (eg, 100 speed) are generally used for extremities and other structures where better detail is desired. Faster screens (eg, 400 speed) are usually used for general radiography of larger, thicker, denser structures to reduce exposure while still maintaining reasonably good image detail.

The usual use of intensifying screens may be modified to suit the particular circumstances of the examination. With all other factors remaining the same, the use of faster screens results in less exposure dose to the patient. Faster screens permit the use of shorter exposure times, and therefore may be used for extremities of children and other examinations where motion may be a problem; they can also be helpful when the affected extremity is unusually large or casted. Slower screens may be used when improved detail of a small area is desired, keeping in mind that exposure dose will be increased.

D. Conversion Factors: Intensifying Screens and Grids

There are many variables associated with the practice of radiography. It is necessary that the radiographer be able to compensate for changes in imaging system components, such as intensifying screens and grids.

Intensifying screen speed is directly related to density and inversely related to mAs. As screen speed increases, all other factors remaining constant, radiographic density increases. As screen speed increases, therefore, mAs must be decreased in order to maintain the original density.

For example, if 200 speed screens (having a factor of 1) were used with 20 mAs for a particular examination, what mAs would be required using 400 screens?

$$\frac{\text{screen speed factor 1}}{\text{screen speed factor 2}} = \frac{\text{mAs 1}}{\text{mAs 2}}$$

$$\frac{1}{0.5} = \frac{20}{x}$$

$$x = 0.5\,(20)$$

$$x = 10 \text{ mAs using 400 speed screens}$$

Grid selection is dependent on the part being radiographed and the desired film characteristics. As grid ratio increases, scattered radiation cleanup increases and, as a result, contrast increases.

mAs Conversions for Screen Speed Changes

Screen Speed	mAs Conversion Factor
100	2
200	1
400	1/2 (.50)
800	1/4 (.25)

Relationship Between Grid Ratio and mAs

Grid Ratio	mAs Conversion Factor
No grid	1
5:1	2
6:1	3
8:1	4
10/12:1	5
16:1	6

Grid ratio is inversely related to radiographic density and directly related to mAs. As grid ratio increases, all other factors remaining constant, radiographic density decreases. As grid ratio increases, therefore, mAs must be increased to maintain the original radiographic density (Fig. 12–61). As discussed earlier in the chapter, conversion factors may be used when changing from nongrid to grid or from one grid ratio to another.

A

B

Figure 12–61. Grids are usually required for parts that generate large amounts of scattered radiation. **(A)** Film made without a grid, using 40 mAs. **(B)** Film with a 12:1 grid and 200 mAs. Although a significant increase in exposure is required, the use of grids enables the production of diagnostic radiographs. (From the American College of Radiography Learning File. Courtesy of the ACR.)

For example, 12 mAs was used with an 8 to 1 ratio grid for a particular exposure. It is desired to repeat the exposure using a 16 to 1 ratio grid. What new mAs factor will be required to maintain the original radiographic density?

$$\frac{mAs_1}{mAs_2} = \frac{conversion\ factor_1}{conversion\ factor_2}$$

$$4x = 6(12)$$

$$4x = 72$$

$$x = 18\ mAs\ using\ a\ 16{:}1\ grid$$

These conversion factors allow for mAs compensation from nongrid to moving grid, or for changing from one grid to another, all other technical factors remaining constant. Since stationary grids are somewhat less efficient in the cleanup of scatter radiation, their use may require slight modification of the correction factor.

Summary

- **When selecting technical factors and radiographic accessories, consideration must be given to the patient's age, habitus, and pathology.**
- **Screen speed choice is dependent upon patient-modifying factors (age, condition) and radiographic requirements (detail).**
- **The ratio of moving grids can differ from one radiographic room to another; stationary grids are usually low ratio.**

V. AUTOMATIC EXPOSURE CONTROLS

A. TYPES

Automatic exposure controls (AECs) are used in today's x-ray equipment and function to produce consistent and comparable radiographic results. AECs have sensors that signal to terminate the exposure once a predetermined (known correct) exposure has been made.

In one type of AEC there is an ***ionization chamber*** just ◀ beneath the tabletop, *above* the cassette (Fig. 12–62). The part to be examined is centered to the sensor and radiographed. When a predetermined quantity of ionization has occured (which equals the correct density), the exposure automatically terminates.

The other type of AEC is the *photomultiplier* type *(phototimer),* in which a small fluorescent screen is positioned *beneath* the cassette. When the exit radiation emerging from the patient exposes the film and exits the cassette, the fluorescent screen emits light and charges a photomultiplier tube. Once a predetermined charge has been reached, the exposure is automatically terminated.

In either case, the manual timer should always be used as a ***backup timer.*** In case of AEC malfunction, the exposure would ter- ◀ minate, thus avoiding patient overexposure and tube overload.

B. POSITIONING ACCURACY

In order to achieve the expected radiographic density, the appropriate sensor(s) must be selected and the part must be correctly positioned directly above the sensor(s) and photocell(s).

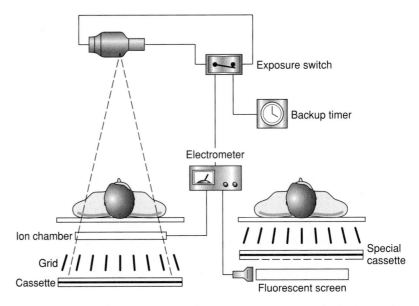

Figure 12–62. The two types of automatic exposure devices are the *ionization chamber* (left) and the *photomultiplier* (right). Note the *backup timer* that functions to terminate the exposure should the AEC fail to operate properly.

If a structure having less tissue density than the part of interest is positioned above the sensor, or if the sensor is not completely covered, the sensor will terminate the exposure sooner and the area of interest will be underexposed. Similarly, if the incorrect sensor for the anatomic part is selected, a density error will result.

On the other hand, if the sensor is positioned under a structure having greater tissue density than the part of interest (eg, if the center sensor is used for a PA chest film) the exposure will be greater than required and an overexposed radiograph will result.

Hence, although the exposure is "automatic," knowledge of anatomy and accurate positioning skills are essential to producing proper radiographic density.

C. PATHOLOGY

The presence of pathology often modifies tissue composition. Changes that occur are often spoken of as *additive* or *degenerative*. Additive pathology is that which makes tissues denser, requiring an increase in exposure factors (eg, ascites). Degenerative pathology involves deterioration of the part (eg, osteoporosis), and requires a decrease in exposure factors.

Since the function of an automatic exposure device is to "recognize" differences in tissue density and thickness, it will compensate for most pathologic changes by adjusting the mAs. In the event further compensation is necessary, most AEDs have a *master density control* that allows the radiographer to modify its output. The density control is frequently illustrated on the control panel as:

$$-1/2 \quad -1/4 \quad N \quad +1/4 \quad +1/2$$

Thus, the normal (N) exposure/density can be varied in increments of 25%, plus or minus. It must be noted that if a radiograph is overexposed because an exposure shorter than the ***minimum reaction time*** (shortest possible exposure) is required, a reduction in master density control will not resolve the situation. Rather, a lower mA station should be selected so that an exposure time within the machine's capability can be used.

Summary

- **The function of AECs is to produce consistent and comparable radiographic images.**
- **There are two types of AECs: ionization chamber and photomultiplier.**
  - **Ionization chambers are located between the x-ray table and cassette.**
  - **Photomultipliers are located beneath the cassette.**
- **Back-up timers are used in conjunction with AECs and function to terminate the exposure in case of AEC malfunction.**
- **Minimum reaction time is the shortest exposure time possible with a particular AEC.**
- **The successful use of AECs requires accurate patient positioning and proper photocell/chamber selection.**
- **Pathologic conditions may be either additive or degenerative; correct use of the AEC will usually compensate for pathologic conditions.**
- **AECs have a density control, usually adjustable in increments of 25%.**

VI. TECHNIQUE CHARTS

A. OPTIMAL AND FIXED kVP TECHNIQUE

A ***fixed kVp technique*** chart specifies a particular kVp for each body part or type of examination. A kVp is selected that will provide adequate penetration and the appropriate scale of contrast. mAs is used to compensate for variation of patient size and condition.

B. VARIABLE kVP TECHNIQUE

In a ***variable kVp technique*** chart, the mAs is fixed and the kVp is increased as part thickness increases. For each cm increase in thickness, the kVp is increased by two. Accurate measurement with calipers is required.

The variable kVp technique chart is not frequently used today because it is associated with increased scattered radiation production and inconsistent contrast and density.

C. VERSUS AECS

Fixed kVp techniques are generally used with AECs. An optimum kVp for each body part (hip, IVU, sinuses, etc) is selected and the exposure is automatically terminated once the predetermined correct exposure (mAs) has been reached.

Fixed kVp Technique Chart

	Fixed kVp[a]	Grid
Extremities	55	No grid
Skull	75	Grid
Abdomen	75	Grid
Lateral Lumbar Region	90	Grid
Barium Studies	120	Grid
Chest Examinations	120	Grid

[a]3φ equipment factors; single φ will require approximately 12% higher kVp.

D. Measurement of Part

Accurate measurement of the part to be radiographed is essential with the *variable* kVp technique chart, because the kVp increases by two for every 1-cm increase in part thickness. *Fixed* kVp charts may specify a specific kVp for the "small," "medium," or "large" patient, which corresponds to measurements within a particular range (eg, 10 cm to 12 cm = small; 13 cm to 15 cm = medium; 16 cm to 18 cm = large). Accurate measurement may be essential for the correct application of each method.

Structures radiographed using AECs do not require measurement, since the AEC automatically adjusts the exposure for tissue variations.

E. Other Considerations

Body position plays an important role in obtaining the expected radiographic results. For example, a well-exposed radiograph of a normal adult abdomen measuring 24 cm in the recumbent AP position cannot be duplicated using the same factors if the patient is turned prone or positioned decubitus or erect.

A particular chest properly exposed on inspiration using a 14 × 17 in cassette cannot be duplicated, without a change in factors, when the exposure is made on expiration or the field size is coned to an 8 × 10 in cassette.

A plain film of a particular abdomen requires different exposure factors from the same abdomen having a barium-filled stomach.

Different exposures will be required for extremities with and without casts.

Body parts undergoing additive or destructive pathologic changes can require substantial exposure changes in order to maintain the desired density and contrast.

AECs will compensate for thickness and density differences (including those caused by position and respiration), pathologic changes, and beam restriction. However, it should be emphasized that the radiographer's skill and accuracy in positioning and photocell selection play an important role in the proper function of AECs.

Summary

- **There are two types of technique charts: fixed kVp type and variable kVp type.**
- **The fixed kVp type chart uses an optimal kVp for each anatomic part.**
- **The advantage of the fixed kVp chart is consistency of radiographic contrast.**
- **The variable kVp type chart increases the kVp by two for each 1-cm increase in body thickness; thus accurate part measurement is necessary.**
- **AECs usually employ fixed kVp factors for consistent contrast, while varying the exposure/density.**
- **AECs will compensate for tissue thickness and density differences (including those caused by body position and respiration), pathologic changes, and beam restriction.**
- **The use of AECs requires accurate positioning and correct photocell selection.**

Chapter Exercises

1. Define the listed terms and/or correctly identify their definitions *(p. 287)*.

2. Define recorded detail; list other terms that can be used to refer to recorded detail *(pp. 287–290, 291)*.

3. To what does the term "resolution" refer; how is it measured and expressed *(pp. 287–290, 291)*?

4. Differentiate between *detail* and *distortion* *(pp. 249–291)*?

5. What are the geometric factors affecting recorded detail *(pp. 290–295)*?

6. What is the relationship among OID, recorded detail, and magnification *(pp. 290–291)*?

7. What is the relationship among SID, recorded detail, and magnification *(pp. 290–291)*?

8. What are the two types of shape distortion? How can shape distortion be avoided *(pp. 288–292)*?

9. How is object unsharpness, with respect to its three-dimensional shape and OID, an inherent part of every radiographic image *(pp. 290, 292, 293, 294)*?

10. Distinguish between actual and effective/projected/apparent focal spot size; what is the line focus principle *(pp. 294–297)*?

11. How is actual focal spot size related to recorded detail? How does the size of the projected focus vary along the length of the image receptor *(pp. 294–297)*?

12. How are focal spot size and anode angle related to x-ray tube heat-loading capacity *(pp. 295–296)*?

13. Distinguish between voluntary and involuntary motion and discuss the most effective means of avoiding each *(p. 298)*.

14. Why is motion intentionally introduced in some radiographic examinations? Give some examples *(pp. 299–302)*.

15. What is the relationship between the fluorescent light from intensifying screens and the total exposure received by the film emulsion *(p. 303)*?

16. What is the purpose of a thicker *rear* intensifying screen *(p. 303)?*

17. Discuss how phosphor type and size, active/phosphor layer thickness, and reflective backing affect the speed on intensifying screens *(pp. 303–304).*

18. What is lag or afterglow; how can it affect the radiographic image *(p. 304)?*

19. What are the three most commonly used rare earth phosphors *(p. 303–304)?*

20. What is the importance of spectral matching *(p. 304)?*

21. How is intensifying screen speed related to recorded detail? With what type of intensifying screens is quantum mottle usually associated *(pp. 305–308)?*

22. What is the importance of screen and film contact? How is its accuracy tested *(pp. 305–309)?*

23. Define radiographic density; describe optical density (OD) *(pp. 313–314).*

24. Describe how radiographic density and mAs are related to the intensity and exposure rate of the x-ray beam *(p. 315).*

25. What is the reciprocity law, and how is it related to radiographic density? Give examples *(p. 315).*

26. What change in mAs is required to make a perceptible change in radiographic density *(p. 317)?*

27. How is SID related to x-ray beam intensity and technical factors (specifically mAs)? What law expresses this relationship *(p. 318)?*

28. How is kVp related to x-ray beam intensity and radiographic density *(pp. 290–291, 317)?*

29. What is the 15% rule? Give examples *(p. 319–320).*

30. What is the relationship among radiographic density, mAs, and intensifying screen speed? Give examples *(pp. 319–320).*

31. What three factors determine the quantity of scatter radiation produced? How can each be modified to limit the production of SR *(pp. 321–322)?*

32. How do grids affect the amount of SR reaching the image recorder? How do they impact radiographic density *(p. 322–323)?*

33. What is a stationary grid? Give some examples of its use; what are its disadvantages *(p. 324)?*

34. What is a moving grid? How does its construction generally differ from the stationary grid? What is its advantage over a stationary grid *(p. 324)?*

35. Define convergence line; focusing distance; focal range; crossed grid *(pp. 323–324).*

36. Define grid cut-off; lateral decentering; focus-grid distance decentering *(pp. 324–325).*

37. Describe grid ratio, number of lead strips per inch, lead content; describe their relationship to *cleanup* and radiographic density *(pp. 325–327).*

38. Of what material(s) is grid interspace material usually made? How is each related to efficiency, patient dose, sturdiness *(pp. 326–327)?*

39. Describe contrast improvement factor and selectivity *(p. 327).*

40. Describe how the bucky factor, or grid-conversion factor, can be used to determine the required mAs adjustment *(pp. 327–328).*

41. How can an air gap influence radiographic density *(p. 329)?*

42. What is inherent filtration? Of what does it consist *(p. 330)?*

43. What is added filtration? Of what does it consist *(p. 330)?*

44. What is the primary purpose of total filtration? What effect does it have on radiographic density *(p. 330)?*

45. Describe why and how compensating filters are used, how they affect radiographic density; give examples of common usage *(pp. 330–331).*

46. Describe how body position, condition, and pathology affect radiographic density *(p. 332–333).*

47. Differentiate between and give examples of destructive and additive pathologic conditions *(p. 333).*

48. How are different types of x-ray generators related to changes in radiographic density? How is mAs (or kVp) changed when changing from single-phase equipment to 3ϕ 6P or 3ϕ 12P equipment? Which technical factor is it preferable to change *(pp. 332–335)?*

49. How can beam restriction affect radiographic density *(p. 336)?*

50. How can the anode heel effect impact radiographic density? Under what conditions is the heel effect most noticeable *(pp. 336–338)?*

51. How can automatic processing affect radiographic density *(pp. 336–339)?*

52. What is the function of radiographic contrast? What are its two components *(pp. 343–345)?*

53. Describe the difference between long-scale and short-scale contrast; what is the single most important technical factor regulating radiographic contrast *(pp. 343–345)?*

54. What is subject contrast and how is it related to beam quality *(pp. 343–345)?*

55. Describe the impact of scattered radiation on radiographic contrast; what is the most important way to limit the production of scattered radiation *(pp. 345–347)?*

56. What kinds of pathologic conditions impact radiographic contrast *(p. 349)?*

57. How does the use of grids affect radiographic contrast *(pp. 350–351, 353–354)?*

58. Of what material(s) are film base and film emulsion made *(p. 353)?*

59. To what three sources is base-plus-fog attributable? What is the maximum permissible base-plus-fog density *(p. 353)?*

60. Explain what is meant by film latitude; give examples of uses for high-contrast film and low-contrast (latitude) film *(p. 358).*

61. What do we call the study of film emulsion's response to exposure? How can this response be illustrated *(pp. 359–360)?*

62. Draw a simple characteristic curve and label its toe, straight-line portion, shoulder, D_{max}, and solarization point *(pp. 359–360).*

63. Explain what is meant by exposure latitude; what technical factor regulates exposure latitude *(pp. 359–360)?*

64. Describe the two types of AECs. Include in your description *(p. 363):*

    A. the location of each relative to the tabletop and cassette

    B. operation of each; how exposure is terminated

65. Explain the importance of a backup timer used in conjunction with an AEC *(p. 363).*

66. Explain the importance of proper AEC photocell selection; describe typical errors in photocell selection and the subsequent radiographic results *(pp. 363–366).*

67. Explain how to correct a radiographic image overexposed as a result of requiring an exposure shorter than the minimum reaction time *(pp. 363–366).*

68. Why are fixed kVp technique charts preferred over variable kVp technique charts *(p. 365)?*

69. Discuss why exposures made using an AEC do not require measurement of the part being examined *(p. 365–366).*

70. Discuss why positioning accuracy is essential to proper function of the AEC *(pp. 363–364).*

A&U Chapter Review Questions
REVIEW SERIES

⭐ *Congratulations! You have completed the entire chapter. If you are able to answer the following group of very comprehensive questions, you should feel confident that you have really mastered this section. You can refer back to the indicated pages to check your answers and/or review the subject matter.*

1. The use of optimum kVp for small, medium, and large body parts is the premise of:
   (A) fixed kVp, variable mAs technique chart
   (B) variable kVp, fixed mAs technique chart
   (C) fixed mAs, variable body part technique
   (D) fixed mAs, variable SID technique

2. The function(s) of automatic beam limitation devices include:
      1. reducing the production of scattered radiation
      2. absorption of scattered radiation
      3. changing the quality of the x-ray beam
   (A) 1 only
   (B) 2 only
   (C) 1 and 2 only
   (D) 1, 2, and 3

3. Base-plus-fog is a result of
      1. blue tinted base
      2. chemical development
      3. manufacturing
   (A) 1 only
   (B) 1 and 2 only
   (C) 1 and 3 only
   (D) 1, 2, and 3

4. The characteristic curve is used to illustrate the relationship between the:
   (A) source-to-image receptor distance and the resulting film density
   (B) exposure reaching the phosphors and the resulting fluorescence
   (C) exposure given the film and the resulting film density
   (D) kVp used and the resulting film density

5. That portion of a characteristic curve generally representative of the useful radiographic density range is the:
   (A) toe portion
   (B) straight line portion
   (C) shoulder portion
   (D) solarization point

6. Using the fixed mAs, variable kVp exposure factor technique, each centimeter increase in patient thickness requires what adjustment in technique?
   (A) increase 2 kVp
   (B) decrease 2 kVp
   (C) increase 4 kVp
   (D) decrease 4 kVp

7. Which of the following can be used to determine the sensitivity of a particular film emulsion?
   (A) characteristic curve
   (B) dose–response curve
   (C) reciprocity law
   (D) inverse square law

8. Film base is currently made of which of the following materials?
   (A) cellulose nitrate
   (B) cellulose acetate
   (C) polyester
   (D) glass

9. Which of the following chemicals is used in the production of radiographic film emulsion?
   (A) sodium sulfite
   (B) potassium bromide
   (C) silver halide
   (D) chrome alum

10. Which of the following pathologic conditions would require an increase in exposure factors?
    (A) pneumoperitoneum
    (B) obstructed bowel
    (C) renal colic
    (D) ascites

Answers and Explanations

1. (A) The optimum kVp (or fixed kVp) technique separates patients into small, medium, and large categories and assigns an optimum (or best) kVp for that particular body part. Patient thickness (cm measurement) determines mAs. This method of establishing exposure factors results in less variation in the scale of contrast than the variable kVp method of technique selection.

2. (A) Beam restrictors function to limit size of the irradiated field. In doing so, they limit the volume of tissue irradiated (thereby decreasing the percentage of scatter radiation built up in the part) and help reduce patient dose. Beam restrictors do not affect the quality (energy) of the x-ray beam—that is the function of kVp and filtration. Beam restrictors do not absorb scatter radiation—that is a function of grids.

3. (D) Every film emulsion has a particular base-plus-fog which should not exceed 0.2. Base density is a result of the manufacturing process (ie, environmental radiation) and the blue tint added to the base to reduce glare. The remaining fog density is a result of the chemical development process, when exposed silver bromide grains are converted to black metallic silver.

4. (C) The characteristic (or H&D) curve is used to illustrate the relationship between the exposure given the film and the resulting density. The relationship between the source-to-image receptor distance and resulting density is expressed in the inverse square law of radiation. The effect of kVp on contrast can be illustrated using a penetrometer (aluminum step wedge).

5. (B) A characteristic curve is the representation of a film emulsion's response to exposure by light or x-rays. Upon observation, it is seen that a characteristic curve does not begin at zero density. That is because an "unexposed" and processed film has a small base-plus fog density (which should not exceed 0.2) due to base dye, environmental radiation fog during production, transportation and storage, and chemical fog from high processing temperatures. The initial ascent of the curve is called the "toe," and represents minimal density. The straight line portion of the curve represents the useful radiographic density range, lying approximately between densities 0.25 and 2.0. The characteristic curve levels off again at the "shoulder" portion of the curve, which represents maximum radiographic density (D_{max}). Past the shoulder is the solarization point, where further exposure would actually reverse image densities.

6. (A) Using the variable kVp method, a particular mAs is assigned to each body part. As part thickness increases, the kVp (penetration) is also increased. The body part being radiographed must be carefully measured and for each centimeter increase in thickness, 2 kVp is added to the exposure.

7. (A) The characteristic curve is used to show the relationship between the exposure given the film and the resulting film density. It can therefore be used to evaluate a particular film emulsion's response (speed, sensitivity) by determining how long it takes to record a particular density. A dose–response curve is used in radiation protection and illustrates the quantity of dose required to produce a particular effect. The reciprocity law states that a particular mAs, regardless of the combination of mA and time, should produce the same degree of blackening. The inverse square law illustrates the relationship between distance and radiation intensity.

8. (C) Film base functions to support the silver halide emulsion. Today's film base is made of tough, nonflammable polyester. Cellulose nitrate was used in the past, but was highly flammable. Cellulose acetate was not flammable, but was not as durable as polyester. The earliest supports for emulsion were plates of glass (hence the term "flat *plate*").

9. (C) Film emulsion consists of silver halide crystals suspended in gelatin. Sodium sulfite is a film processing preservative and potassium bromide is a developer restrainer. Potassium and chrome alum are emulsion hardeners used in fixer solution.

10. (D) Because pneumoperitoneum is an abnormal accumulation of air or gas in the peritoneal cavity, it would require a decrease in exposure factors. Obstructed bowel usually involves distended, air or gas-filled bowel loops, again requiring a decrease in exposure factors. With ascites, there is an abnormal accumulation of fluid in the abdominal cavity, necessitating an increase in exposure factors. Renal colic is the pain associated with the passage of renal calculi; no change from the normal exposure factors is usually required.

Automatic Processing and Quality Assurance

KEY TERMS ◀

ACTIVATOR	FILM IDENTIFICATION	RECEIVING BIN
AGITATION	FIXER	RECIRCULATION SYSTEM
ARCHIVAL QUALITY	GUIDE-SHOE MARKS	REDUCING AGENT
ARTIFACT	HARDENER	REPLENISHMENT
CASSETTE	HUMIDITY	SAFELIGHT
CHEMICAL FOG	LATENT IMAGE	SAFELIGHT FILTER
CLEARING AGENT	MANIFEST IMAGE	SENSITOMETER
CROSSOVER ROLLERS	MEDICOLEGAL	SILVER RECOVERY
DEEP RACKS	METALLIC DISPLACEMENT	SQUEEGEE
DENSITOMETER	PRECIPITATE METHOD	STATIC ELECTRICITY
DEVELOPER	PRESERVATIVE	TRANSPORT SYSTEM
ELECTROLYTIC METHOD	PRESSURE MARKS	TURNAROUND ASSEMBLY
FEED TRAY	PREVENTIVE MAINTENANCE	WIRE-MESH TEST
FILM BIN	QUALITY ASSURANCE	

I. FILM STORAGE CONSIDERATIONS

A. STORAGE CONDITIONS

The conditions under which x-ray film is stored can have considerable impact on the final radiographic image. The most common result of improper film storage is fog, which has a severely degrading effect on image quality.

1. Temperature and Humidity. Films should be stored at a temperature no greater than 70°F. Temperatures greater than 70°F can accelerate the deterioration process and cause film fog. Atmospheric
► **humidity** should be kept between 40% and 60%. Excessively low
► humidity is conducive to the production of **static electricity** discharge (Fig. 13–1). High humidity levels encourage the production of fog. An unopened (ie, hermetically sealed) bag of film protects the film from humidity but not excessive temperatures.

2. Chemicals and Radiation. Boxes of film must also be stored away from chemicals with fumes that can fog film emulsion. Film can be fogged if stored too close to radiographic rooms or radionuclides.

3. Expiration Dates. Each box of x-ray film is identified with an expiration date before which the film must be used in order to avoid age fog. When replenishing film supply, film boxes should be rotated so that the oldest film is used first. (Use the "fifo" system: first in, first out.)

4. Position of Film Boxes. Film boxes, should be stored in the upright position. If film boxes are stacked on one another, the sen-

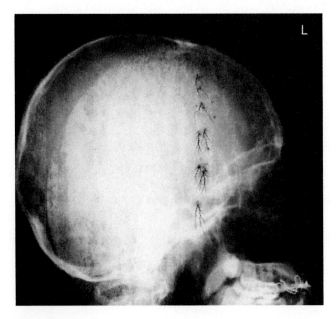

Figure 13–1. Plus-density artifact resulting from static electric discharge. (From Saia, DA. *Appleton & Lange's Review For The Radiography Examination* (3rd ed). East Norwalk, CT: Appleton & Lange, 1997.)

sitive emulsion (especially in the central portion) will be affected by pressure from the boxes above. ***Pressure marks*** (ie, areas of fog) ◄ are produced and result in loss of contrast in that area of the radiographic image. Larger size film boxes are particularly susceptible to this problem.

5. Film Bin. The ***film bin*** is a light-tight storage area where ◄ opened boxes of film are available for reloading empty cassettes. If a single door separates the darkroom from exterior white light, it is wise to have an automatic interlock system in place that prevents opening of the darkroom door while the film bin is open.

B. Safelight Illumination

Adequate and safe darkroom lighting is an essential part of ensuring quality radiographic images. A source of white light is required for cleaning and routine maintenance. The white light often has a safety device to help prevent accidental film exposure. ***Safelight*** illumina- ◄ tion must be appropriate for the type film used and bright enough to provide adequate illumination and still not expose the sensitive emulsions (exposed film emulsion is about eight times more sensitive than unexposed emulsion).

1. Types. A frequently used *safelight* is the Kodak Wratten Series 6B, a brownish ***safelight filter,*** with a 7.5 to 15-watt frosted light ◄ bulb placed 4 feet above the work surface. Another available safelight, which is somewhat brighter, is the Kodak GBX all-purpose filter, which provides a more reddish illumination. This type of filter is often placed in the darkroom so that its light is directed upward toward the ceiling and reflected back down, thus reducing the chance of safelight fog.

2. White Light Leaks. Routine darkroom maintenance includes regular cleaning of all surfaces and walls and checks for white light leaks. When checking for light leaks, all darkroom lights must be turned off, adequate time given for eyes to adjust to the darkness, then a careful visual inspection made for white light leaks.

Summary

- **Film should be stored in a cool and dry environment, under 70°F and between 40% and 60% humidity.**
- **Excessive temperatures cause film fog.**
- **Excessively low humidity encourages buildup of static electricity.**
- **Film should be stored away from radiation and chemicals.**
- **The film-box expiration date should be noted, and oldest film used first.**
- **Film boxes should be stored upright to avoid production of pressure marks.**
- **Kodak Wratten Series 6B and GBX darkroom filters are the most frequently used.**
- **Safelights should be placed 4 feet from the work surface with 7.5 to 15-watt light bulbs.**

Common Artifacts and Their Causes

Crescent (Kink) Marks Bending film sharply over finger
Minus Density, Pinhole Marks Dust on intensifying screens (Fig. 13–2)
Static Electricity Low humidity, improper handling (Fig. 13–1)
Fingerprints Body oils, other material on skin
Scratches Pressing film down on feed tray
Fog Damaged cassette; cracked safelight; bulb too bright; exposure to radiation; chemical fumes; illuminated clock or watch face; turning on white light before film is in processor; darkroom light leak

Figure 13–2. Dirty and dusty screens. Small particles of dust, or other foreign objects, on intensifying screens keep the fluorescent light from reaching the film emulsion, hence a clear (unexposed) area corresponds to each foreign particle. (From the American College of Radiology Learning File. Courtesy of the ACR.)

II. CASSETTES

A. ROUTINE CARE

Routine documented care of all imaging system components is part of an efficient ***quality assurance*** program.

 Cassettes require care and maintenance inside and out. They should be stored upright, according to size (ie, 14″ × 17″, 10″ × 12″, etc) and speed (ie, 100, 400). Stacking cassettes on top of each other or stuffed in a passbox renders the cassettes more susceptible to damage. Cassettes should be inspected visually for damage and cleanliness. The inside of cassettes should be cleaned regularly to keep them lint and dust-free; screens should be cleaned with special antistatic cleaner appropriate for the type screen used; incorrect cleaner can affect the speed of screens.

Screens must also be tested periodically for screen-film contact with a ***wire-mesh test.*** The cassette to be tested is placed on the x-ray table, the wire-mesh device on *top* of the cassette, and an exposure made of about 5 mAs and 40 kVp. The processed film should be viewed at a distance of at least 6 feet. Any blurry areas are indicative of poor screen–film contact and representative of diminished image detail. The areas of poor contact will also exhibit an increase in density and loss of contrast.

B. ARTIFACTS

 Radiographically speaking, an ***artifact*** is a fault, blemish, or aberration in an x-ray image. It can be the result of improper handling, automatic processing, or use of defective radiographic accessories.

Cassettes, screens, and film must be handled carefully to avoid leaving fingerprints or producing other film artifacts. Hands should be kept clean and dry, free from residue-leaving creams and powder from gloves. Film should be handled carefully by the corners when loading and unloading cassettes. The technologist should not *slide* film into or out of the cassette, as the friction can cause static electricity build-up. Cassettes should be numbered or otherwise identified so that artifact-causing problems can be located and removed (Fig. 13–2).

Summary
- Cassettes should be stored upright according to size and speed.
- Cassettes should be tested periodically for adequate screen–film contact.
- Intensifying screens must be cleaned periodically with antistatic screen cleaner.
- Inadequate cleaning can result in white pinhole-type film artifacts.
- Rough, improper handling or storage of cassettes can lead to damage resulting in poor screen–film contact.
- Film must be handled carefully and properly to avoid artifacts such as static electricity, scratches, fog, or crescent marks.

III. IDENTIFICATION OF RADIOGRAPHS

A. ESSENTIAL INFORMATION

Every radiograph *must* (for ***medicolegal*** reasons) include certain ◄ specific patient information.

- Patient's name or identification number
- The side marker, right or left
- The examination date
- Name of the institution

Other pertinent information *may* be included.

- Patient's age or birthdate
- Attending physician
- Time of day

When multiple films are taken of a patient on the same day, it is important that the time the radiographs were taken be included on the film. This permits the physician to chronologically follow the patient's progess.

B. TYPES OF SYSTEMS

There are a number of ***film-identification*** systems. Cassettes are ◄ purchased with a lead blocker in a specified corner to shield the underlying film from x-ray exposure. This unexposed corner of the film is then "flashed" with essential patient information. Some identification devices are used only in the darkroom because the film is removed from the cassette before the information is flashed onto it. Another type of film-identification device allows recording of patient information in normal lighted conditions with the film inside the specially designed cassette.

Summary

- Medicolegal implications require that every radiograph include the patient's name or identification number, left or right side marker, examination date, and name of institution.
- When multiple films are taken of a patient the same day, the time of day should be indicated on the radiographs.
- Some film-identification systems can be used only in a darkroom.
- Other film-identification systems use special cassettes and are used in daylight conditions.

IV. AUTOMATIC FILM PROCESSING

Film emulsion consists of silver bromide (halide) crystals suspended in gelatin. Sensitization specks are added to increase the sensitivity of the silver salts. Positive silver ions form the inner portion of the emulsion, while the negative bromine ions form the outer layer. At the time of exposure, the outer, negative bromine ions are energized, and their valence electrons ejected and absorbed by the (now nega-

Advantages of Automatic Over Manual Processing

- Speed
- Convenience
- Consistency
- Reduced labor
- Improved archival quality

tively charged) sensitivity speck. The inner, positive silver ions migrate to the negative charges and become metallic silver. Thus, the ▶ *latent* (exposed but invisible) *image* is formed. This is referred to as the Gurney–Mott theory of latent image formation. The development ▶ process transforms the latent image to a *manifest* (visible) black ▶ metallic silver *image.*

Automatic film processing is carried out by a machine that *transports* the x-ray film through the necessary chemical solutions, at ▶ the same time providing *agitation, temperature regulation,* and ▶ *chemical replenishment.* Within the processor are the *developer, fixer,* and wash tanks, followed by the dryer.

Rapid processing is accomplished by the use of increased solu- ▶ tion temperatures, which requires that a *hardener* be added to the developer to control excessive emulsion swelling.

Each of the processor systems accomplishes specific functions; a basic understanding of these systems is required so that the processor can be used correctly and efficiently. A properly maintained and monitored processor will ensure consistent radiographs that will retain their quality images over a long period of time (archival quality).

A. CHEMISTRY OVERVIEW

1. Developer. The developer functions to convert the latent (invisible) image into the manifest (visible) silver image by *reducing* the exposed silver bromide crystals to black metallic silver. Important factors affecting the development process are *time* (length of development), *temperature* (of the developer solution), and solution *activity* (strength, concentration).

The developer solution has an *alkaline* nature for optimal func- ▶ tion of the *reducing agents. Sodium* or *potassium carbonate* pro- ▶ vides the necessary alkalinity and serves as an *activator* (or accelerator) by swelling the gelatin emulsion so that the reducing agents are better able to penetrate the emulsion and reach the exposed silver bromide crystals.

The *reducing agents* are *hydroquinone,* which works slowly to build up blacks in the film areas of greater exposure, and *phenidone,* which quickly produces the gray tones in areas of lesser exposure. With respect to sensitometry, hydroquinone controls the shoulder (D_{max}) of the characteristic curve, and phenidone controls the toe (D_{min}) area.

The developer solution, particularly the hydroquinone, is especially sensitive to oxygen. If the developer oxidizes, it becomes ▶ weaker and less effective. The *preservative, sodium sulfite,* or *cycon,* is added to the developer to prevent its rapid oxidation. A hood always covers the developer tank and replenisher solution. The *solvent* for the concentrated chemicals is water, used to dilute the concentrate to the proper strength.

Rapid processing is achieved through the use of high temperatures that accelerate the development process; however, high temperatures can cause excessive emulsion swelling. Since excessive swelling can result in roller transportation problems a hardener, traditionally *glutaraldehyde,* is added to the developer to control the amount of emulsion swelling.

A *restrainer,* or antifog agent, is added to the developer to limit its activity to only the exposed silver crystals. The typical restrainer

Developer Reduces Exposed Silver Crystals to Black Metallic Silver

Sodium and Potassium Carbonate Activator and accelerator: swells gelatin; provides alkaline medium.
Hydroquinone Reducing agent: works slowly; builds up black areas.
Phenidone Reducing agent: works quickly; produces gray tones.
Sodium Sulfite and Cycon Preservative: prevents oxidation of developer.
Potassium Bromide Restrainer: antifog agent.
Glutaraldehyde Hardener: controls emulsion swelling.
Water Solvent.

is *potassium bromide*. Without the restrainer the developing agents would attack the *unexposed* crystals, creating **chemical fog.** Potassium bromide is frequently referred to as "starter solution" because it is added only to fresh, new developer. As films are developed, bromine ions are released from the emulsion into solution; thus, potassium bromide is not found in replenisher solution.

2. Fixer. The function of the fixer *(hypo)* is to clear the film of the unexposed, undeveloped silver bromide crystals. This process serves to protect the film from further exposure. The *fixing* or **clearing agent** is *ammonium thiosulfate.*

The fixer is an acidic solution that functions to neutralize any residual developer carried over and provide the required acid medium for the hardener. *Acetic acid* provides the required acidic medium.

The fixer contains a hardener whose function it is to shrink and re-harden the gelatin emulsion, thus protecting it from abrasion and promoting **archival quality.** The most commonly used hardeners are *potassium alum* or *aluminum chloride*. Fixer preservative is the same as that found in the developer, ie, sodium sulfite.

3. Wash. The function of the wash is to rid the film of residual chemicals. Should chemicals remain in the emulsion (eg, as a result of defective wash cycle), the film will discolor with age. Since radiographic records are kept for a number of years, it is important that they have sufficient archival quality.

Cold water processors are, in general, less efficient in removing chemicals than warm water processors. Agitation during the wash process and large quantities of water help to rid the emulsion of chemical residue.

> ### Fixer Clears Film of Unexposed and Undeveloped Silver Bromide Crystals
>
> ***Acetic Acid*** Activator: provides acid medium. Neutralizes any residual developer.
> ***Ammonium Thiosulfate*** Fixing or clearing agent: removes unexposed and undeveloped silver.
> ***Potassium Alum*** or ***Aluminum Chloride*** Hardening agent: shrinks, rehardens emulsion for protection and archival purposes.
> ***Sodium Sulfite*** Preservative: prolongs the effective life of the solution.
> ***Water*** Solvent.

Summary

- **Developer solution reduces the exposed silver bromide crystals to black metallic silver.**
- **The development process is greatly affected by development time and solution temperature and activity.**
- **Sodium or potassium carbonate provides the necessary alkalinity and functions as the solution activator by swelling the gelatin emulsion.**
- **Reducing agents are phenidone and hydroquinone.**
- **Sodium sulfite or cycon preserves the developer solution from excessive oxidation.**
- **Glutaraldehyde is a hardener, added to developer solution to control excessive swelling.**
- **Potassium bromide serves as an antifog agent and restrains the developer from attacking the unexposed silver bromide crystals.**
- **Potassium bromide is starter solution, and is not required in replenisher solution.**
- **The fixing or clearing agent (ammonium thiosulfate) removes unexposed silver bromide crystals from the emulsion, preventing further exposure.**
- **Acetic acid provides the necessary acid medium for the fixer solution.**

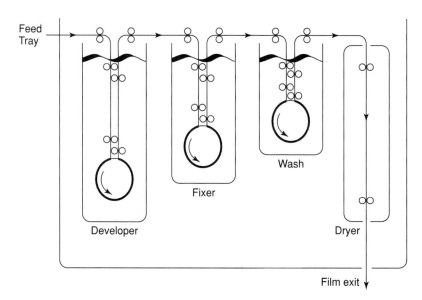

Figure 13–3. Major components of an automatic processor. A series of rollers conveys film through each processor section. (From Wolbarst, AB. *Physics of Radiology.* East Norwalk, CT: Appleton & Lange, 1993.)

Figure 13–4. Because adjacent rollers are positioned closer together at their periphery, roller pressure on film emulsion is greater at film edges. This can cause a plus-density mottled appearance *(wet-pressure sensitization marks)* along film edges. If developer hardener or replenisher is insufficient, allowing excessive emulsion swelling, this artifact can occur across the length of the film. (From the American College of Radiology Learning File. Courtesy of the ACR.)

■ **Potassium alum or aluminum chloride serves to harden the film emulsion.**
■ **The fixer preservative is sodium sulfite.**
■ **Adequate washing of residual chemicals from the film emulsion is essential for good archival quality.**

B. TRANSPORT SYSTEM

▶ The **transport system** functions to convey the film through the different processor sections by means of a series of rollers (Fig. 13–3) driven by gears, chains, and sprockets. This is accomplished without damage to the film and at a prescribed speed, which determines the length of time film spends in each solution. The roller system also provides constant, vigorous agitation of the solution at the film surface.

▶ The entire conveyance system consists of the **feed tray, crossover**
▶ **rollers, deep racks, turnaround assemblies,** and **receiving bin.**

Film is aligned against one side of the feed tray as it is introduced into the processor. A sensor initiates solution replenishment as the film enters, and replenishment continues as the length of the film passes the sensor. Films should be fed into the processor along their short edge; feeding the film in "the long way" leads to over-replenishment and increased radiographic density.

Crossover racks are out of solution and bridge the gaps between developer and fixer, fixer and wash, and wash and dry sections of the processor. Crossover rollers must be kept free of crystallized solutions that can cause film artifacts as the soft emulsion passes by (Fig. 13–4). The last set of rollers in each solution section has a

▶ **squeegee** action on film emulsion, thus removing excess solution before film enters the next tank.

When the processor is not in use for a period of time, it is advisable to leave the lid open so that moisture can escape. Since the crossover rollers are out of solution, chemicals carried onto them by film can crystallize and should be cleaned off before the processor is used again.

Turnaround assemblies are located at the bottom of the deep racks and serve to change the film direction as it changes from downward to upward motion. Guide shoes, or deflector plates, are also located where film must change direction. They will occasionally scratch film, leaving characteristic **guide-shoe marks,** when ◀ they require adjustment.

When returning rollers to the processor after cleaning, care must be taken to seat them securely in their proper position. Transport problems (processor jam-up) will result if racks are misaligned.

C. REPLENISHMENT SYSTEM

As films travel from one processor solution section to another, chemical solution is carried away in the swollen film emulsion. It is the function of the processor **replenishment** system to keep solution ◀ tanks full. If solution level is allowed to lower, film-immersion time decreases and radiographic density and contrast changes will occur. Transport problems can also arise from inadequate replenishment, ie, if insufficient developer replenisher, the inadequate addition of hardener will result in excessive emulsion swelling. The essentially "thicker" film has difficulty transporting between the closely distanced rollers.

As film travels through the fixer, it accumulates residual developer solution; fixer solution also accumulates unexposed silver cleared from the emulsion. Wash water accumulates fixer. In these ways, the activity of each solution is depleted through continual use. Diminished solution activity can have the same effects as low solution levels. The replenishment system assures that proper solution concentration is maintained.

D. TEMPERATURE REGULATION

The temperature-regulation system functions to control the temperature of each section of the automatic processor. Developer is the most important solution temperature to regulate; in a 90-sec processor, developer temperature is usually maintained at 92° to 95°F. Once the correct developer temperature is established, it must be constantly maintained. Even a minor fluctuation (ie, 0.5°) in developer temperature can cause a visible change in radiographic density and contrast.

Developer temperature is thermostatically controlled and developer solution is circulated through a heat exchanger under the fixer tank. Thus, the fixer temperature is regulated (in cold water processors) by heat conducted from the developer solution. In older processors having stainless steel tanks, fixer temperature is regulated by heat convection from the neighboring developer solution.

E. RECIRCULATION SYSTEM

As replenishment chemicals are added to solution, the **recirculation** ◀ **system** provides agitation necessary for uniform solution concentration. As temperature adjustments are made, the recirculation system agitates solution to promote temperature uniformity. *Agitation* provided by the system also functions to keep fresh solution in contact

Transport System Functions

Conveys film through processor.
Establishes processing time (via roller speed).
Activates replenishment.
Agitates solution over film surface.
Provides squeegee action on film emulsion.

Replenishment System Functions

Maintain solution level.
Maintain solution activity and concentration.

Temperature Regulation

Especially important for developer solution.
Developer heated by thermostat.
Fixer/wash warmed by heat exchangers.

Recirculation System Functions

Maintain uniform solution activity through agitation.
Maintain uniform temperature through agitation.
Keep fresh solution in contact with film emulsion.
Provide filtration of processor debris.

Wash Functions

Remove chemicals from emulsion.
Contribute to archival quality.

Dryer Functions

Air recirculation.
Dry film.

Daily Monitoring and Maintenance Procedures

At Start-Up Time
Clean crossover and other out-of-solution rollers.
Check solution levels in processor tanks and replenisher tanks.
Process two to four *un*exposed 14″ × 17″ films to clean rollers.
Clean feed tray, receiver tray, and darkroom work surfaces.
Perform sensitometric tests.
At Shut-Down Time
Another sensitometric test may be done.
Clean crossover and other out-of-solution rollers.
Leave lid open 1″ to allow escape of moisture.

with film emulsion. The recirculation system also functions to filter debris, such as gelatin particles, from the solutions.

F. WASH AND DRYER SYSTEMS

Thorough removal of chemical solutions from the film emulsion is required for good *archival film quality* and is provided by the wash section of the automatic processor. Agitation of the water makes the process more efficient. Any residual chemicals will eventually result in film stain. *Residual fixer* will eventually stain the film a yellowish brown that ultimately obscures the image and diminishes the archival quality. Films can be tested (usually by the film manufacturer or distributor) to determine their degree of fixer retention.

The dryer section functions to remove water from the film by blowing warm, dry air over the film surface. Dryer temperature is usually 120° to 130°F, sufficient to shrink and dry the emulsion without being excessive. Excessive heat and overdrying can cause film damage. If films emerging from a properly heated dryer are damp, the problem may be excessive emulsion swelling and water retention as a result of inadequate developer or fixer replenisher (hardener).

G. SILVER RECOVERY

X-ray film is expensive and represents a large part of a radiology department annual budget. About half of the film's silver remains in the emulsion after exposure and processing. The other half (unexposed silver) is removed from the film during the fixing process and
▶ most of it is recoverable through **silver recovery** methods. A drain is connected to the fixer tank and fixer is allowed to flow directly into a silver recovery unit or to a large centrally located receptacle.

Silver recovery is desirable for financial and ecological reasons. Fixer silver is toxic to the public water supply and environmental legislation makes persons responsible for its direct passage into sewer lines, or other means of improper disposal, subject to severe fines and penalties.

There are three types of silver recovery methods. Used fixer
▶ enters a **metallic displacement** (or metallic replacement) cartridge and metallic silver is precipitated onto the steel wool within. This method of silver recovery is most useful for low volume locations.
▶ **Electrolytic** silver recovery units (cells) pass an electric current through the fixer solution, causing silver to be plated onto the cathode cylinder of the unit. The silver is periodically removed by scraping it from the stainless-steel cathode. Electrolytic cells are best used in locations having medium to high volume.
▶ There are a number of chemicals that will **precipitate** metallic silver. In the presence of one of these chemicals (eg, sodium borohydride), metallic silver falls to the bottom of the tank and forms a sludge. This method of silver recovery is generally used only by large institutions having large, centralized receptacles or by professional silver dealers, who employ special techniques for separating the sludge or removing the entire tank.

H. PROCESSOR MAINTENANCE

The biggest advantage of automatic processors is their contribution to radiographic consistency. Testing and monitoring procedures serve to indicate potential problems before they arise. Developer, fixer, and wash temperature should be checked twice a day. ***Preventive maintenance*** is frequently provided for by a commercial cleaning and parts-replacement service.

Sensitometry is the measure of film response to exposure and processing. A particular box of film is designated for testing purposes only, and a special device ***(sensitometer)*** is used to precisely and consistently expose the film. Once the film is processed and its densities read (with a ***densitometer***) and compared to known correct readings, any variation in film density must be due to processor variation.

If solution levels in processor and replenisher tanks are frequently low, a bigger problem may exist and should be brought to the attention of the processor service company. *Preprocessed* films should *not* be used to clean rollers, because they may contain residual fixer which will contaminate the developer solution.

The more effective the processor quality control program, the less troubleshooting will be required. Nevertheless, it is important that the radiographer be able to recognize and resolve some common processor problems.

COMMON PROCESSOR PROBLEMS AND THEIR CAUSES

Transport Problems (Jam-Ups)
Inadequately maintained (dirty) rollers
Too rapid film feeding, overlapping
Misaligned crossover or other racks
Inadequate developer replenisher (hardener)

Excessive Density (Processor Related)
Developer temperature elevated
Insufficient dilution of developer

Inadequate Density (Processor Related)
Developer temperature too low
Excessive dilution of developer

Damp Films
Dryer temperature too low
Faulty dryer blower
Inadequate fixing
Inadequate developer replenisher (hardener)

Fog (Darkroom Related)
Unsafe safelight
Contaminated developer
Outdated film
Improper film storage conditions
Darkroom light leak

Chapter Exercises

 Congratulations! *You have completed the entire chapter. If you are able to answer the following group of very comprehensive questions, you should feel confident that you have really mastered this section. You can refer back to the indicated pages to check your answers and/or review the subject matter.*

1. Define the key terms listed on pages xxx and xxx and/or correctly identify their definitions *(pp. 375)*.

2. What are the ideal conditions for x-ray film storage *(p. 376)*.

3. Describe the possible effect of excessive temperature; of very low humidity *(p. 376)*.

4. Describe how each of the following can affect radiographic film *(pp. 376–377)*:

    A. chemical fumes

    B. radiation

    C. storage past the expiration date

    D. stacking boxes of film upon each other

    E. film bin or darkroom with light leaks

    F. safelight too close to work bench

    G. too high wattage safelight

5. Explain correct care of cassettes; intensifying screens *(p. 378)*.

6. How can suspected flaws in film-screen contact be detected *(p. 378)?*

7. List at least five radiographic artifacts and identify their cause *(p. 378)*.

8. What information *must* every radiographic image include? Describe two types of film identification systems *(p. 379)*.

9. Define latent image; manifest image *(p. 380)*.

10. List five advantages of automatic processing over manual processing; what modification of manual processing helps achieve rapid processing *(p. 380)?*

11. What is the main function of the developer solution? What are the three important factors in the development process *(pp. 380–381)?*

12. Identify the chemical associated with each of the following developer constituents and describe its function(s) *(pp. 380–381):*

    A. reducing agents (two)

    B. preservative

    C. activator and accelerator

    D. restrainer

    E. hardener

    F. solvent

13. What are the main functions of the fixer solution *(p. 381)?*

14. Identify the chemical associated with each of the following fixer constituents and describe its function(s) *(p. 381):*

    A. fixing and clearing agent

    B. activator

    C. hardener

    D. preservative

    E. solvent

15. List the order in which film travels through each of the four sections of the automatic processor *(p. 382).*

16. List five functions of the transport system; what can result from transport problems *(pp. 382–383)?*

17. Describe the appropriate care of crossover racks *(pp. 384–385).*

18. Describe the location of the rollers having squeegee action, and explain their purpose *(p. 383).*

19. What is the usual cause of wet-pressure sensitization marks occasionally found along film edges *(p. 383)?*

20. Name and describe the location of the structures that function to guide film in the proper direction through the processor roller systems *(p. 382)*.

21. What are the two functions of the processor replenishment system? What can be the result of inadequate replenishment *(p. 383)?*

22. Describe the importance of temperature-regulation systems in automatic processing *(p. 383)*.

23. List four functions of the processor recirculation system *(pp. 383–384)*.

24. What are the functions of the processor wash and dry sections? What can result from an inadequate wash process? Inadequate drying *(p. 384)?*

25. Explain the economic and ecologic importance of silver recovery *(p. 384)*.

26. Describe the three types of silver recovery methods *(p. 384)*.

27. Describe the start-up and shut-down procedures recommended for daily processor maintenance *(pp. 384–385)*.

28. List at least ten common radiographic problems associated with processing and identify their cause *(pp. 384–385)*.

A&U Chapter Review Questions

1. The developer temperature in a 90-second automatic processor is usually about:
   - (A) 75 to 80°F
   - (B) 80 to 85°F
   - (C) 85 to 90°F
   - (D) 90 to 95°F

2. Conditions contributing to poor radiographic archival quality include:
     1. fixer retention
     2. insufficient developer replenishment
     3. poor storage conditions
   - (A) 1 only
   - (B) 3 only
   - (C) 2 and 3 only
   - (D) 1, 2, and 3

3. The amount of replenishment solution added to the automatic processor is determined by:

    1. size of the film

    2. position of film on tray feeding into processor

    3. length of time required for film to enter processor

(A) 1 only

(B) 1 and 2 only

(C) 1 and 3 only

(D) 1, 2, and 3

4. The device used to give a predetermined exposure to a film to test its response to processing is called the:

(A) sensitometer

(B) densitometer

(C) step wedge

(D) spinning top

5. The cause of films coming from the automatic processor still damp can be:

(A) air velocity too high

(B) unbalanced processing temperatures

(C) insufficient hardening action

(D) excessive hardening action

6. Some of the causes of static electric discharge in the x-ray darkroom include:

    1. low humidity

    2. sliding films from cassette

    3. use of rubber-soled shoes

(A) 1 only

(B) 1 and 2 only

(C) 2 and 3 only

(D) 1, 2, and 3

7. The conversion of the invisible latent image into a visible manifest image takes place in the:

(A) developer

(B) stop bath

(C) first half of the fixer process

(D) second half of the fixer process

8. Which of the following can result from poor storage or handling practices?

    1. film fog from outdated film

    2. film fog from exposure to excessive temperatures

    3. film fog from exposure to chemical fumes

(A) 1 only

(B) 1 and 2 only

(C) 2 and 3 only

(D) 1, 2, and 3

9. Which of the following will result if developer replenisher is inadequate?
   (A) films with excessively high contrast
   (B) films with excessively low contrast
   (C) films with excessively high density
   (D) dry, brittle films

10. Crescent-shaped crinkle mark artifacts on a film are due to:
    (A) improper film storage
    (B) improper film handling
    (C) exposure to white light
    (D) exposure to excessive humidity

Answers and Explanations

1. (D) The advantages of automatic processors are quicker, more efficient operation and consistent results. Quicker operation is attained with increased solution temperatures. The usual temperature of a 90 second developer is 90 to 95°F. Excessively high developer temperature can cause chemical fog.

2. (D) The archival quality of a film refers to its ability to retain its image for a long period of time. Many states have laws governing how long a patient's medical records, including films, must be retained. Very importantly, they must be retained in their original condition. Archival quality is poor if radiographic films begin to show evidence of stain after being stored for only a short time. Probably the most common cause of stain, and hence poor archival quality, is retained fixer within the emulsion. Fixer may be retained due to poor washing, or because there was insufficient hardener (under-replenishment) in the developer, thus permitting fixer to be retained by the swollen emulsion. A test for quantity of retained fixer in film emulsion is often included as part of a quality control program. Stain may also be caused by poor storage conditions. Storage in a hot, humid place will cause even the smallest amount of retained fixer to react with silver, causing stain.

3. (D) When a film first enters the processor from the feed tray, a microswitch signals the replenishment pump to begin sending replenisher solution into the processor. Replenishment continues until the microswitch senses the end (edge) of the film and terminates pump action. So, as long as film is being fed into the processor, replenishment solution will be added. There is therefore more replenisher added with larger-size films. There is also more replenisher added when rectangular films are fed into the processor "the long way" because the processor is sensing, for example, 17 inches of film rather than 14 inches of film. Film should be put through the processor consistently according to the particular department's preference/routine. A change in film direction can lead to over/under replenishment and hence, a change in film density.

4. (A) To test a film's response to processing, the film must first be given a predetermined exposure with a *sensitometer*. The film is then processed and the densities are read using a *densitometer*. Any significant variation from the expected densities is further investigated. A step wedge is used to evaluate the effect of kVp on contrast, and a spinning top test is used to check timer accuracy.

5. (C) If the fixer fails to sufficiently re-harden the gelatin emulsion, water will remain within the still swollen emulsion. The dryer mechanism will be unable to completely rid the emulsion of wash water, and the film will emerge from the processor damp and tacky. On the other hand, excessive hardening action may produce brittle radiographs. High air velocity usually encourages more complete drying. Unbalanced processing temperatures can result in blistering of the emulsion.

6. (D) Static electricity builds up in non-conductive materials, such as plastic and synthetic fibers, until it reaches a point where it discharges the electricity in the form of a spark. Since gelatin is semiconductive, it will accept the electric discharge, and static electricity artifacts will appear on the radiographic image. Darkroom personnel should be instructed to wear leather-soled shoes and non-synthetic clothing (eg, cotton). Polyesters and nylons will encourage the production of static electricity. Low humidity also encourages static electric build-up. Sliding films in and out of cassettes causes friction and is another means of creating a static electrical build-up.

7. (A) The invisible silver halide image is composed of exposed silver grains. These are "reduced" to a visible black metallic silver image in the developer solution. The fixer solution functions to remove unexposed silver halide crystals from the film.

8. (D) All of those effects listed can result from poor storage practices. Film should be rotated with the oldest being used first to avoid fog from outdated film. By protecting film from chemical fumes and from excessive temperatures, fogging of the sensitive emulsion is prevented.

9. (B) As films are developed, the developer solution becomes weaker and oxidation products are produced in solution. If sufficient replenishment of new developer solution does not take place, and the older solution activity decreases, chemical fog is produced. Films lack contrast, and have a flat, gray appearance.

10. (B) An *artifact* is an unnatural feature on a radiograph. Several kinds of artifacts can be produced from careless handling during production of a radiographic image. A crinkle mark appears as a crescent shaped artifact and is a result of bending the film sharply, as over one's finger when removing from the cassette. Improper storage conditions, exposure to light, and excessive humidity are also harmful to film emulsion and can cause fogging of the film.

Evaluating Radiographs

I. EVALUATION STANDARDS AND IMAGE CHARACTERISTICS

A. OVERVIEW

It is important to look at radiographic images with a critical eye, evaluating each of the components that contribute to their overall quality. The goal is to have as much information as possible transferred as accurately as possible from the part being radiographed to the image recorder.

B. RECORDED DETAIL AND DISTORTION

The radiograph should illustrate maximum transference of information without visible loss of *image detail* as a result of patient ◀ motion, excessive OID, insufficient SID, inappropriate screen and film combination or focal spot size. There should not be evidence of shape *distortion* as a result of improper *alignment* of x-ray tube, ◀ part, and film.

C. RADIOGRAPHIC DENSITY AND CONTRAST

There should be adequate *background density* and a *scale of* ◀ *grays* sufficient to make various *tissue densities* visible. ◀

D. GRID SELECTION AND USE

A grid ratio should be used that is appropriate for the kVp level employed. X-ray-tube centering, angulation, and SID should be suitable for the particular type grid used.

E. FILM IDENTIFICATION

All essential medicolegal information should be visible on each radiograph: patient name or identification number, side marker, date, and institution.

F. COLLIMATION AND SHIELDING

▶ To ensure patient protection, there must be visible evidence of **collimation. Shielding** should be evident when the reproductive organs are in the primary beam, or within 5 cm of it, when the patient has reproductive potential, and when diagnostic objectives permit.

G. DEMONSTRATION OF STRUCTURES

The radiograph must include the anatomic areas of interest in the desired position and projection.

II. IDENTIFYING AND CORRECTING ERRORS

It is essential that the radiographer recognize the impact each of the imaging components has on the finished radiographic image. The radiographer must be able to identify and correct imaging errors.

Each radiograph should be evaluated according to the standards addressed above. If the image is suboptimal in any category, steps must be taken to determine the cause, correct the error, and ensure that the error will not be repeated.

It is impossible to address and illustrate here all possible errors in technical factor selection, equipment use and positioning, patient variables, artifacts, and processing. Some have been illustrated in earlier portions of this volume and others will be illustrated here. Patient-positioning errors are addressed in Part II. Try to identify the illustrated error, then check your answer with that given in the caption.

A. TECHNICAL FACTOR SELECTION
(SEE FIGS. 14–1 THROUGH 14–4)

A   **B**

Figure 14–1. Excessive density; improper selection of mAs. Both films were made at 100-cm SID using 75 kVp. **(A)** Film correctly exposed at 80 mAs. **(B)** Film exposed at 160 mAs demonstrates excessive density. (From the American College of Radiology Learning File. Courtesy of the ACR.)

Figure 14–2. High contrast; insufficient kVp. (From the American College of Radiology Learning File. Courtesy of the ACR.)

A   B

Figure 14–3. **(A)** X-ray beam intensity at a given point is dependent upon the distance from its source. Radiographic density increases in film **(B)** as a result of decreased SID. (From the American College of Radiology Learning File. Courtesy of the ACR.)

A   B

Figure 14–4. Quantum mottle. Compare images **(A)** and **(B)**. **(A)** The graininess of the film demonstrates quantum noise produced by a fast imaging system requiring very low mAs factors. **(B)** Film obtained using a slower imaging system resolves the quantum-noise problem. (From the American College of Radiology Learning File. Courtesy of the ACR.)

B. EQUIPMENT USE AND POSITIONING (SEE FIGS. 14–5 THROUGH 14–10)

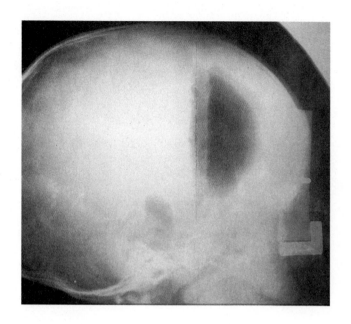

Figure 14–5. A defective grid; probably a wafer grid or grid cassette. Lead strips in grids are exceedingly thin and fragile. If grids are handled carelessly, lead strips can become damaged and/or misaligned and they can create uneven bands of density. (From the American College of Radiology Learning File. Courtesy of the ACR.)

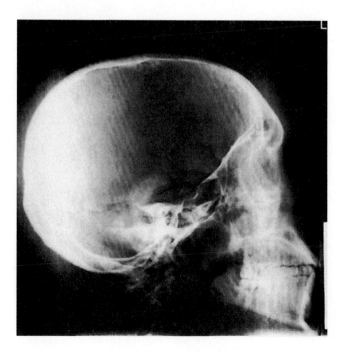

Figure 14–6. Inverted focused grid. If a focused grid is placed upside down, the divergent x-ray-beam will be absorbed by the grid's lead strips (everywhere but the grid's central portion, where grid lines are vertical; see density versus grids section of Chapter 12). (From Saia, DA. *Appleton & Lange's Review for the Radiography Examination* (2nd ed). East Norwalk, CT: Appleton & Lange, 1997.)

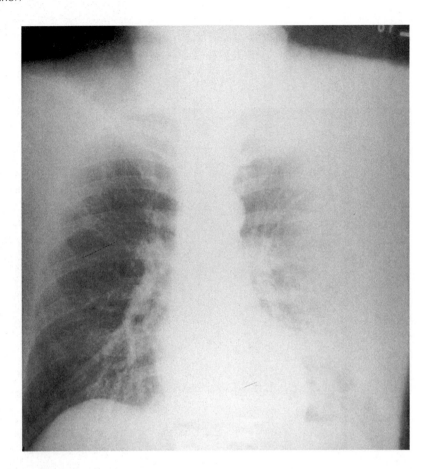

Figure 14–7. Off-focus and lateral-decentering errors. Notice the asymmetric cut-off from right to left (see density versus grids section of Chapter 12). (From the American College of Radiology Learning File. Courtesy of the ACR.)

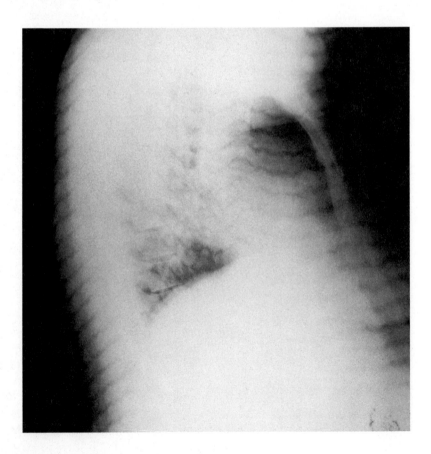

Figure 14–8. Moiré effect. This is a classic example of the effect of superimposing two linear grids, that is, a grid cassette placed in a bucky tray. When the lead strips are aligned in the same direction, yet not exactly superimposed, this unmistakable moiré pattern occurs. (From the American College of Radiology Learning File. Courtesy of the ACR.)

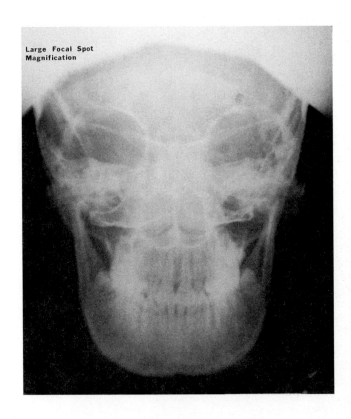

Figure 14–9. Magnification film performed using large focal spot. Magnification studies can yield useful information about tiny details *only* if a fractional (0.3 mm or smaller) focal spot is used. Use of a larger focal-spot size causes loss of recorded detail as a result of increased visualization of penumbra. (From the American College of Radiology Learning File. Courtesy of the ACR.)

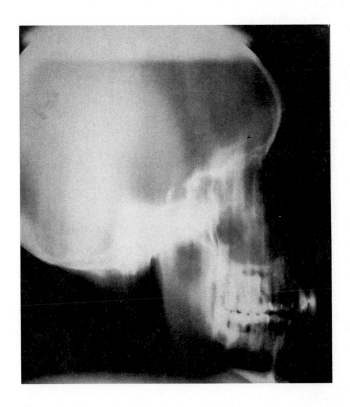

Figure 14–10. Tomographic streaking. Longitudinal streaking can be very pronounced in linear tomography when the dominant anatomic lines parallel tube motion. Placing the x-ray tube motion and dominant lines at right angles to each other, or using an appropriate tube motion (with pluridirectional tomographic equipment), can remedy the situation. (From the American College of Radiology Learning File. Courtesy of the ACR.)

C. PATIENT VARIABLES
(SEE FIGS. 14–11 THROUGH 14–17)

Figure 14–11. Involuntary motion on right (ureter) due to obstruction. Use of the shortest possible time is the best way to avoid loss of detail due to involuntary motion. (From the American College of Radiology Learning File. Courtesy of the ACR.)

Figure 14–12. Osteoporotic bone as a result of thalassemia (Cooley's or Mediterranean anemia) requires reduction of technical factors. (From the American College of Radiology Learning File. Courtesy of the ACR.)

Figure 14–13. Pathologic fractures of distal tibia and fibula as a result of osteoporotic changes in patient shown in Figure 14–12 (thalassemia). (From the American College of Radiology Learning File. Courtesy of the ACR.)

Figure 14–14. Paget's disease (osteitis deformans) is characterized by bone thickening, and therefore requires an increase in technical factors. (From the American College of Radiology Learning File. Courtesy of the ACR.)

A

B

Figure 14–15. Osteopetrosis (Albers-Schönberg, or marble-bone, disease) is characterized by increased bone density, requiring an appropriate increase in technical factors. (From the American College of Radiology Learning File. Courtesy of the ACR.)

Figure 14–16. Pathology such as increased amounts of air can require decrease in technical factors. (From the American College of Radiology Learning File. Courtesy of the ACR.)

Figure 14–17. A change in body position from recumbent to erect will require an increase in technical factors. (From the American College of Radiology Learning File. Courtesy of the ACR.)

D. Identification of Artifacts

▶ Many **artifacts** are produced by misuse of imaging equipment, as discussed in section B. Several others, having various origins, are illustrated in Figures 14–18 through 14–28. Artifacts can be classified as *exposure* artifacts (ring on finger, hair braids, etc), *handling* artifacts (crinkle or crescent marks, fingerprints, etc), or *processor* artifacts (guide-shoe marks, pi lines, etc.)

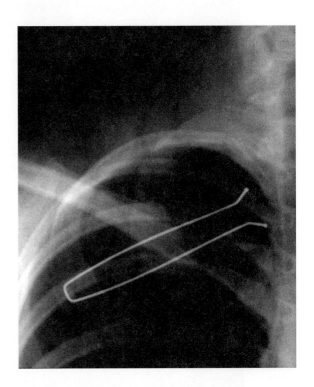

Figure 14–18. Hairpin and braid artifacts. (From the American College of Radiology Learning File. Courtesy of the ACR.)

Figure 14–19. The suspicious "coin lesion" seen in the mid-left lung field was discovered to be a wad of chewing gum placed there for safekeeping during the radiographic examination!! (From the American College of Radiology Learning File. Courtesy of the ACR.)

Figure 14–20. Light leak. Fogging from exposure to white light, such as film-bin exposure resulted in exposed upper edge of film. (From the American College of Radiology Learning File. Courtesy of the ACR.)

Figure 14–21. Safelight fog. Notice the fingers imaged in the soft tissues of the right thorax. This was probably caused by an unsafe safelight over the processor feed tray. The safelight wattage may be too great, or the safelight may be positioned too close to the feed tray. (From the American College of Radiology Learning File. Courtesy of the ACR.)

Figure 14–22. Fingerprints. Notice that the fingerprints are black (mid-right edge of film). If developer solution is on fingers while handling film, silver grains will be overdeveloped (black). If oils from the skin are deposited on the film during handling, developer will be prevented from reaching the silver grains and the fingerprints will be white (undeveloped). (From the American College of Radiology Learning File. Courtesy of the ACR.)

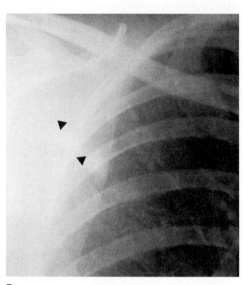

B

A

Figure 14–23. Sensitized and desensitized marks. **(A)** Typical, obvious *sensitized* (plus-density) crescent (kink) mark caused by bending the film sharply *after* exposure. **(B)** Less-obvious *desensitized diffuse* (minus-density) area (near the axillary border of the fourth and fifth ribs) is caused by bending the film *before* exposure. Both of these artifacts are caused by pressure on the film emulsion. (From the American College of Radiology Learning File. Courtesy of the ACR.)

Figure 14–24. Scratches. Notice that the scratches are varied and irregular, unlike processor scratches, which are usually uniform and regularly spaced. These scratches were probably made by sliding one film from a box of tightly packed films. (From the American College of Radiology Learning File. Courtesy of the ACR.)

A

B

C

Figure 14–25. Static electrical discharge. **(A)** *Tree* static. **(B)** *Crown* static. **(C)** *Smudge* static. Static electricity artifacts are caused by low humidity and improper handling of films, and can obscure diagnostic information. Darkroom personnel should avoid clothing made of synthetic materials and screens should be cleaned with special antistatic screen cleaner. Most importantly, since friction between film and screen causes static buildup, it is essential not to slide film in and out of cassettes. (From the American College of Radiology Learning File. Courtesy of the ACR.)

Figure 14–26. Dentures artifact. (From the American College of Radiology Learning File. Courtesy of the ACR.)

Figure 14–27. Neck chain held in patient's mouth, but IV pole left between patient and x-ray tube!! (From the American College of Radiology Learning File. Courtesy of the ACR.)

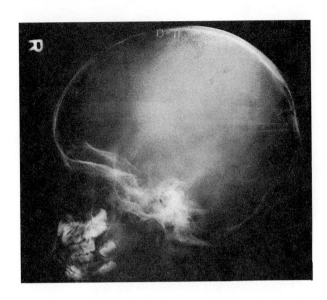

Figure 14–28. Tape used for immobilization is often imaged and can obscure bony detail. (From the American College of Radiology Learning File. Courtesy of the ACR.)

E. PROCESSING ERRORS AND MALFUNCTION (SEE FIGS. 14–29 THROUGH 14–37)

A

B

Figure 14–29. **(A)** Film received adequate development at 95°F and exhibits satisfactory density. **(B)** Film received insufficient development at 90°F and exhibits inadequate density caused by underdevelopment. Developer activity is retarded by too low a temperature. (From the American College of Radiology Learning File. Courtesy of the ACR.)

A

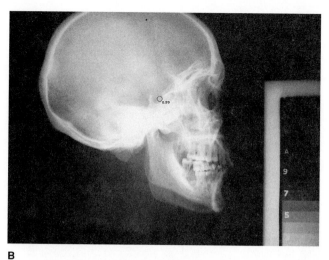

B

Figure 14–30. Underreplenishment. The only differences between films **(A)** and **(B)** are replenishment rate and mAs. Notice the difference in exposure factors required to reproduce identical density: film **(A)** at 37 mAs; film **(B)** at 50 mAs. While film **(A)** replenishment rate was 150 cc per 14″ × 17″ film, film **(B)** replenishment rate was 30 cc per 14″ × 17″. Underreplenishment leading to underdevelopment (and a "light" film) was compensated for by an increase in mAs. This problem was common before automatic processing. Today's quality control measures make this an unlikely occurrence. (From the American College of Radiology Learning File. Courtesy of the ACR.)

Figure 14–31. Minus-density artifacts (scratches), running in the direction of film travel, caused by misaligned guide shoes. (From Saia, DA. *Appleton and Lange's Review For The Radiography Examination* (2nd ed). East Norwalk, CT: Appleton & Lange, 1997.)

B

A

Figure 14–32. Chemicals splashed on film before development. **(A)** Film (across mid-thorax: anterior chest wall, in heart, soft-tissue posterior chest) illustrates *fixer* splash. **(B)** *Developer* splash. (From the American College of Radiology Learning File. Courtesy of the ACR.)

Figure 14–33. Underdeveloped areas caused by fixer spill on processor feed tray. (From the American College of Radiology Learning File. Courtesy of the ACR.)

Figure 14–34. Spots and runs (to left of ilium) frequently seen in manual processing but eliminated with automatic processing. (From the American College of Radiology Learning File. Courtesy of the ACR.)

Figure 14–35. Dirty-roller artifact. Notice that the artifact is most apparent on the leading edge of the film (anterior chest) and diminishes with the film travel (as the film "cleans" the roller). (From the American College of Radiology Learning File. Courtesy of the ACR.)

Figure 14–36. A "pi line" is a plus-density artifact occurring 3.14 in from the film edge. (From the American College of Radiology Learning File. Courtesy of the ACR.)

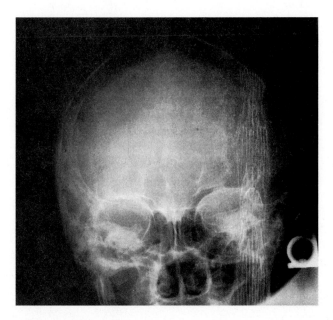

Figure 14–37. Artifact was caused by partially crystallized fixer on the edge of the developer-fixer crossover roller. (From the American College of Radiology Learning File. Courtesy of the ACR.)

Chapter Exercises

 Congratulations! *You have completed this chapter. If you are able to answer the following group of very comprehensive questions, you should feel confident that you have really mastered this section.*

1. Define the key terms listed on page xxx and/or correctly identify their definitions. ***(p. 393).***

2. Evaluate radiographs, assessing them for:

    A. recorded detail and distortion ***(p. 393)***

    B. radiographic density and contrast, including structural considerations ***(p. 393)***

    C. film and screen combinations ***(p. 396)***

    D. grid selection and use ***(pp. 394, 397, 398)***

    E. film identification ***(p. 394)***

    F. beam restriction ***(p. 394)***

    G. patient shielding ***(p. 394)***

    H. proper use of AEC ***(p. 394)***

    I. positioning accuracy, including structural considerations ***(p. 397)***

    J. evidence of artifacts ***(pp. 404–407)***

    K. processing malfunctions or errors ***(pp. 409–413)***

3. Determine the cause(s) of any problem(s) your evaluation has uncovered and discuss recommendations for corrective action. ***(p. 394).***

p a r t

V

Equipment Operation and Maintenance

Radiographic and Fluoroscopic Equipment

I. TYPES OF EQUIPMENT

The various kinds of x-ray machines are generally named according to the x-ray energy they produce or the specific purpose(s) for which they are designed, eg, mammographic unit, head stand, tomographic equipment, mobile unit, 150 kVp chest unit, and 1200 mA general diagnostic unit.

A. FIXED

Most x-ray equipment is *fixed,* or stationary, that is, it is installed in a particular place and cannot be moved. Most general radiographic and fluoroscopic equipment in the radiology department is fixed.

B. MOBILE

Mobile x-ray equipment is designed for patients who are unable to travel to the radiology department, for example, the very ill, incapacitated patients, and patients in surgery. Mobile equipment is available for radiographic and/or fluoroscopic x-ray procedures.

C. DEDICATED

X-ray equipment that is designed for a specific purpose or type of examination is referred to as **dedicated equipment.** Examples of ◄ dedicated equipment are head units, mammography equipment, chest units, and tomographic equipment.

II. X-RAY TRANSFORMERS AND RECTIFIERS

KEY TERMS ◄

ALTERNATING CURRENT	AUTOTRANSFORMER LAW	ELECTROMAGNET
AMPLITUDE	DEDICATED EQUIPMENT	HELIX
AUTOTRANSFORMER	DIRECT CURRENT	KILOVOLTAGE

(continued) **417**

KEY TERMS *CONTINUED* ◀

MAGNETIC FIELD	SEMICONDUCTIVE MATERIALS	TRANSFORMER
MUTUAL INDUCTION	SINGLE-PHASE RECTIFICATION	TRANSFORMER LAW
RECTIFICATION	SOLENOID	TURNS RATIO
SELF INDUCTION	THREE-PHASE RECTIFICATION	

Alternating Current Amplitude and Polarity Vary Periodically

- Amplitude and polarity vary periodically.
- *Wavelength:* Distance between 2 consecutive crests; one positive and one negative half curve.
- *Crest:* Positive half cycle peak.
- *Trough:* Negative half cycle peak.
- *Amplitude:* Maximum height of the wave.
- *Frequency:* Number of cycles per second.
- *Hertz:* Unit of frequency.

Fundamental to the study of x-ray equipment is a basic understanding of magnetism and electricity. The relationship between magnetism and electricity is central to the operation of many x-ray circuit components; therefore, it is important to review these concepts prior to reviewing x-ray circuit components.

Generators function to change mechanical energy to *electrical energy* (whereas motors convert electrical energy to mechanical energy). Electrical current flowing through a conductor in only one ▶ direction and with constant magnitude, is called **direct current** (DC). A familiar source of direct current is the battery.

Electricity is more efficiently transported over long distances at low current and high voltage values to avoid excessive power loss (according to the power, or heat, loss formula: $P = I^2R$). Most appli- ▶ cations of electricity require the use of **alternating current** (AC), in which the amplitude and polarity of the current vary periodically with time (Fig. 15–1). AC consists of sinusoidal waves. One *wavelength* consists of two half-cycles: a *positive half-cycle* and a *negative half-cycle*. A wavelength is defined as the distance between two consecutive *crests*. A crest is the positive half-cycle peak and a *trough* is the negative half-cycle peak. The maximum height of the wave/impulse ▶ is referred to as its **amplitude,** and represents electrical potential, or voltage. *AC is therefore characterized by varying amplitude and periodic reversal of polarity.* The number of cycles per unit of time (eg, second) is called *frequency* (Fig. 15–1) and its unit of measure is the *hertz* (Hz). In the United States, AC is generated at 60 Hz or cps (cycles per second) ie, 60 cycles (60 positive half-cycles and 60 negative half-cycles) occur each second. One-half second, therefore, would include 30 cycles ($1/2 \times 60 = 30$); 4 cycles, then, represent a 4/60 or 1/15-sec time interval.

X-rays are produced when high-speed electrons are suddenly decelerated upon encountering the tungsten atoms of the anode. To produce x-rays of diagnostic value, high voltage must be available. To produce high quality radiographs, a selection of x-ray energy levels (kVp) must be available. The use of alternating current and electromagnetic principles are fundamental to the operation of the high-voltage transformer and the autotransformer—the x-ray circuit devices respectively responsible for producing the required high voltage and permitting a selection of kilovoltages.

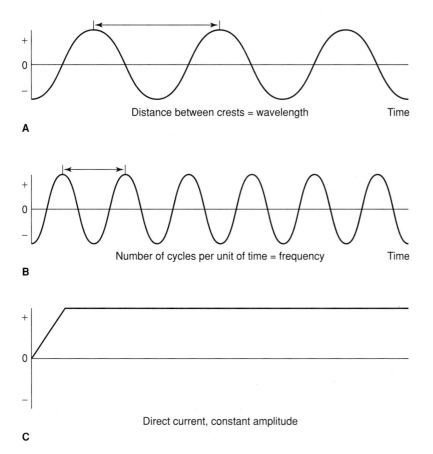

A

Distance between crests = wavelength   Time

B

Number of cycles per unit of time = frequency   Time

C

Direct current, constant amplitude

Figure 15–1. Alternating and direct current waveforms. **(A)** Alternating current (AC), low frequency. **(B)** High-frequency AC. Compare the distance between crests and troughs in **(B)** with those in **(A)**. **(C)** Direct current, like that supplied by a battery, is characterized by constant amplitude (peak potential).

It has long been known that there is an important relationship between magnetism and electricity. Famous scientists such as Volta, Oersted, Lenz, and Faraday worked various experiments demonstrating the relationship, making important observations, and formulating principles that explain the operation of electromagnetic devices.

Faraday's observation that a ***magnetic field*** will induce an electric current in a conductor if there is motion of either the magnetic field or the conductor (Fig. 15–2), is the fundamental principle of operation of the high voltage ***transformer.*** If a coiled conductor is supplied with an alternating current, a magnetic field expands and collapses around the coil, accompanying the peaks and valleys of the AC waveform. If a second coiled conductor is placed near, but not touching, the first (primary) coil, the moving magnetic field will interact similarly with the second coil and an electric current will be induced in it. Thus, the moving magnetic field from the primary coil can be used to induce a current in another circuit with whom it has no physical connection; this is called ***mutual induction.*** An alternating current, producing a continuously moving magnetic field, is necessary for mutual induction to occur.

Figure 15–2. Electromagnetic induction. An electric current will be induced in a conductor whenever there is relative motion between a conductor and magnetic field, ie, if a conductor moves through a magnetic field, if a magnetic field moves across a conductor, or if the magnetic field is constantly changing (as in AC). (From Wolbarst, AB. *Physics of Radiology.* East Norwalk, CT: Appleton & Lange, 1993.)

▶   A conductive wire shaped into a coil is called a **helix,** a helix
▶ supplied with a current is a **solenoid.** If an iron core is inserted
▶ within the coil, a simple **electromagnet** is formed and the magnetic
lines of force are intensified. Thus, a transformer's conductor is frequently coiled around an iron core to increase its efficiency.

Summary

- **X-ray equipment may be described as either *fixed* or *mobile*.**
- **X-ray equipment designed for a particular purpose (eg, mammographic, head, chest units) is called *dedicated*.**
- **A generator converts mechanical to electrical energy; a motor converts electrical to mechanical energy.**
- **Electricity is transported over long distances at high voltage and low current values to minimize energy loss, according to the heat-loss formula: $P = I^2R$.**
- **Alternating current is characterized by constantly changing polarity and amplitude.**
- **A coil of wire is a *helix;* supplied with current it is a *solenoid;* with an iron core it is the simplest type of *electromagnet*.**
- **X-ray transformers operate on the principle of *mutual induction*.**

A. High-Voltage Transformers

X-ray transformers are used to increase the incoming voltage to the
▶ more useful **kilovoltage** required for x-ray production. Transformers
that increase voltage are called *step-up transformers* or high-voltage
transformers. The degree to which transformers increase voltage is
▶ determined by their **turns ratio,** that is, the number of turns in the
secondary (high-voltage) coil compared to the number of turns in
the primary (low-voltage) coil; the higher the ratio, the greater the
voltage increase. As voltage increases, however, current decreases
▶ proportionally according to the **(transformer law)** equations that
follow.

$$\frac{V_S}{V_P} = \frac{N_S}{N_P} \qquad \frac{N_S}{N_P} = \frac{I_P}{I_S}$$

Notice that the relationship between the turns ratio and the *volt-age* is a *direct one,* while there is an *inverse* relationship between the
turns ratio and *current.*

For example, if a particular x-ray transformer has a turns ratio of
500 to 1 and is supplied with 50 amps and 220 volts, what is its kVp
and mA output?

$$\frac{x}{200} = \frac{500}{1} \qquad\qquad \frac{500}{1} = \frac{50}{x}$$

$$x = (500)(220) \qquad\qquad 500x = 50$$

$$x = 110,000 \text{ volts} = 110 \text{ kVp} \qquad x = 0.1 \text{ amp} = 100 \text{ mA}$$

Transformers can also be the *step-down* type, like that found in
the x-ray filament circuit.

Although transformers operate at about 95% efficiency, energy
loss varies according to transformer design. An *open core* transformer

Types of Energy Loss Inherent in All Transformers

- **Copper losses** are caused by the resistance to current flow that is characteristic of all conductors and are reduced by using larger *diameter* conductive wire.
- **Hysteresis losses** are a result of the continually changing magnetic domains of the core material (as a result of changing polarity of AC) and can be reduced by using core material of greater *permeability* (eg, silicon).
- **Eddy-current losses** are a result of small currents (eddy currents) built up in the core material as a result of the continually changing magnetic fields. Eddy-current losses are reduced by *laminating* the core material; any currents generated can travel only the small distance between lamina-tions and, therefore, represent a smaller energy loss.

consists of two parallel iron cores with conductive windings; however, a loss or leaking away of magnetic flux occurs at the ends of the iron cores. A *closed core* transformer (Fig. 15–3) consists of a ring-shaped core of iron that serves to reduce leakage flux energy loss. A *shell* type transformer has a central partition, effectively dividing it into two halves. The transformer primary and secondary coil are wound around the center bar (but not touching each other) and this arrangement serves to reduce energy loss still further.

B. AUTOTRANSFORMERS

The x-ray circuit transformer is a *fixed*-ratio transformer, that is, the turns relationship is constant. How, then, are we able to have a selection of kilovoltages from which to choose? It is through the use of an **autotransformer,** which sends the correct amount of voltage ◄ to the primary of the high voltage transformer to be stepped-up to the required level.

The autotransformer consists of an iron core with a single coil wrapped around it (that serves as its primary and secondary winding) and operates on the principle of **self induction.** Each coil turn ◄ has a contact or tap. A movable contact (corresponding to the kV-selector dial on the control panel) makes connection with the appropriate tap on the autotransformer. The voltage sent to the primary coil of the high-voltage transformer depends upon the number of coils "tapped." For example, a particular autotransformer has 2,000 windings and is supplied with 220 volts. If 500 windings are tapped, what voltage is sent to the primary of the step-up transformer? The solution can be determined by using the **autotransformer law** ◄ (which is the same as the transformer law).

$$\frac{V_S}{V_P} = \frac{N_S}{N_P}$$

$$\frac{x}{220} = \frac{500}{2000}$$

$$2000x = (500)(220)$$

$$2000x = 110,000$$

$$x = 55 \text{ volts sent to primary coil of step-up transformer}$$

Figure 15–3. The *closed core* transformer reduces loss of magnetic flux. Note the *laminated* silicon steel that serves to reduce *eddy-current* losses. (Modified from Wolbarst, AB. *Physics of Radiology.* East Norwalk, CT: Appleton & Lange, 1993.)

Summary

- **High-voltage (step-up) transformers function to provide the necessary kilovoltage for x-ray production.**
- **As the high-voltage transformer steps up voltage to kilovoltage, it proportionally steps down current according to the primary to secondary turns ratio and the transformer law.**
- **The transformer and autotransformer laws are expressed by the following equations.**

$$\frac{V_S}{V_P} = \frac{N_S}{N_P} \qquad \frac{N_S}{N_P} = \frac{I_P}{I_S}$$

- **Step-down transformers are also called filament transformers; they function on the same principles as step-up transformers, and are placed in the filament circuit.**
- **Transformers can be designed as open core, closed core, or shell type.**

- **Transformers are about 95% efficient.**
  - **Types of transformer losses include copper losses, eddy-current losses, and hysteresis losses.**
- **The autotransformer, operating on the principle of self-induction, functions to provide a selection of kilovoltages.**
- **Both the transformer and autotransformer require AC for operation.**

C. RECTIFICATION

Some x-ray circuit devices, such as the transformer and autotransformer, will operate only on AC. The efficient operation of the x-ray tube, however, requires the use of unidirectional current, so current must be *rectified* before it gets to the x-ray tube. The process of full-wave ▶ **rectification** changes the negative half-cycle to a useful positive half-cycle.

An x-ray circuit rectification system is located between the secondary coil of the high-voltage transformer and the x-ray tube. Rec-▶ tifiers are solid-state diodes made of ***semiconductive materials*** such as silicon, selenium, or germanium that conduct electricity in only one direction. Thus, a series of rectifiers placed between the transformer and x-ray tube function to change alternating current to a more useful unidirectional current.

Although rectification remedies the changing polarity problem of single-phase AC, the problem of constantly varying amplitude remains. The continually changing voltage from zero to maximum potential and back to zero produces a pulsating beam of x-rays hav-▶ ing a wide range of energies. ***Three-phase rectification*** superimposes three AC waveforms, each separated from the other two by 120° and resulting in a nearly constant potential waveform. Whereas ▶ ***single-phase rectification*** produces a waveform having 100% "ripple" (ie, 100% drop in potential between pulses), the three-phase waveform exhibits only a slight drop between pulses (Fig. 15–4).

Figure 15–4. **(A)** Single-phase, full-wave rectified wave form. Note the 100% voltage ripple as each pulse starts at 0 potential, makes its way to 100%, and returns to 0 potential. **(B)** The three-phase/six-pulse waveform exhibits a 13% voltage drop between peak potentials. **(C)** Three-phase/12-pulse has only a 4% voltage drop between peak potentials. **(D)** High frequency generators are most efficient and produce a less than 1% voltage ripple. (From Wolbarst, AB. *Physics of Radiology.* East Norwalk, CT: Appleton & Lange, 1993.)

Three-phase/six-pulse rectification presents a 13% ripple; three-phase/12-pulse presents only a 4% ripple. The average beam energy therefore increases. For example:

1φ 2p − 100 kVp − approximately 70 keV beam

3φ 6p − 100 kVp − approximately 95 keV beam

3φ 12p − 100 kVp − approximately 98 keV beam

Three-phase rectification requires the use of *three autotransformers* (one for each incoming current) and *one transformer* having three windings. A transformer winding can be arranged in either *star* (wye) or *delta* configuration (Fig. 15–5).

Remember that a change in technical factors is required when changing among Sφ to 3φ 6p to 3φ 12p rectified equipment.

Summary

- **The x-ray tube operates most efficiently on unidirectional current.**
- **The rectification system changes AC to unidirectional current and is located between the secondary coil of the high-voltage transformer and the x-ray tube.**
- **Rectifiers are solid-state diodes made of semiconductive materials such as silicon, selenium, or germanium that permit the flow of electricity in only one direction.**
- **3φ rectification uses three alternating currents out of phase with each other by 120°.**
  - **In 3φ rectification, only the peak values of the waveform are utilized, thus creating a nearly constant potential current.**
  - **3φ rectification may be 6 pulse (13% ripple) or 12 pulse (4% ripple), depending on the number of rectifiers employed.**
  - **3φ rectified equipment requires three autotransformers and one high-voltage transformer.**
  - **3φ high-voltage transformer windings are arranged in either star (wye) or delta formation.**

Comparison of Technical Factors Required		
Single φ	3φ 6p	3φ 12p
x mAs	2/3x mAs	1/2x mAs

Figure 15–5. A simplified diagram of the secondary (high-voltage) side of a 3φ 6p rectified x-ray circuit. 3φ equipment requires the use of three autotransformers (not shown) and one transformer having three windings arranged in *delta* and *star* (or wye) configuration. (From Wolbarst, AB. *Physics of Radiology.* East Norwalk, CT: Appleton & Lange, 1993.)

III. THE X-RAY TUBE

KEY TERMS ◀

ANODE	FOCUSING CUP	LINE-FOCUS PRINCIPLE
ANODE COOLING CURVE	GLASS ENVELOPE	PITTING
CATHODE	HEAT UNITS	THERMIONIC EMISSION
FILAMENT	HEEL EFFECT	TUBE RATING CHART
FOCAL TRACK	INDUCTION MOTOR	VAPORIZED

X-rays are produced when high-speed electrons emitted from the cathode filament are suddenly decelerated as they encounter tungsten atoms of the x-ray-tube anode/target:

1) *Bremsstrahlung* ("brems") or "braking" *radiation:*

A high speed electron, passing through a tungsten atom is attracted ("braked") by the positively charged nucleus, and therefore is deflected from its course with a resulting loss of energy. This energy loss is given up in the form of an x-ray photon (figure 8–4). The electron may not give up all its kinetic energy in one such interaction; it may go on to have several more interactions deeper in the target, each time giving up an x-ray photon having less and less energy. This is one reason the x-ray beam is heterogeneous (ie, has a spectrum of energies). Brems radiation comprises 70–90% of the x-ray beam.

2) *Characteristic radiation:*

In this case, a high speed electron encounters the tungsten atom and ejects a K-shell electron (figure 8–5 a), leaving a vacancy in the K shell (figure 8–5 b). An electron from the shell above (that is, the L shell) fills the vacancy and in doing so emits a K characteristic ray (figure 8–5 c). The energy of the characteristic ray is equal to the difference in energy between the K and L shell.

A. COMPONENT PARTS

X-ray tubes are used for both radiographic and fluoroscopic pur-
▶ poses. Their basic components are the **anode** (positive electrode)
▶ and **cathode** assembly (negative electrode), enclosed within an evacuated glass envelope (Fig. 15–6).

▶   The **glass envelope** enclosure creates a diode tube somewhat reminiscent of early radio and television tubes. The x-ray tube glass enclosure, however, is made of glass that is extremely heat resistant to maintain the necessary *vacuum* for the production of x-rays. Should the vacuum begin to deteriorate, air molecules within the tube would collide with, and decelerate, the high-speed electrons traveling to the anode, thus diminishing the production of x-rays. Air within the glass envelope is referred to as a "gassy tube," and will eventually cause oxidation and burnout of the cathode filament.

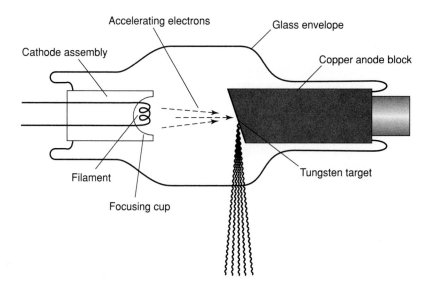

Figure 15–6. A simplified illustration of a *stationary* anode x-ray tube. The tungsten target is embedded in a solid block of copper that serves to conduct heat away from the tungsten and into the oil coolant that surrounds the glass envelope. Most x-ray tubes today utilize *rotating* anodes as a means of more even heat distribution. (From Wolbarst, AB. *Physics of Radiology.* East Norwalk, CT: Appleton & Lange, 1993.)

The cathode assembly consists of one or more **filaments,** their ◀ supporting wires, and a **focusing cup.** The filament is a fine (about ◀ 0.2-mm diameter), 1 to 2-cm coil of tungsten wire that, when heated to incandescence by about 4 amps of current, boils off (ie, liberates) outer-shell tungsten electrons. This event is called **thermionic emis-** ◀ **sion.** Most x-ray tubes actually have two or more filaments and are called double-focus tubes. The typical x-ray tube has two filaments, one small and one large, to direct electrons to either the small or large anode focal spot. Each filament is closely embraced by a negatively charged molybdenum focusing cup that serves to direct the electrons toward the anode.

As the filament boils off electrons, small quantities of tungsten can be vaporized and deposited on the inner surface of the glass envelope. If tungsten is deposited on the port window, it acts as a filter and reduces the intensity of the x-ray beam; it can also affect the tube vacuum and ultimately lead to tube failure.

The filament is heated with the required 3 to 5 amps and 10 to 12 volts by the *filament circuit.* The filament current is kept at a standby quantity until the rotor is activated; at that time the *filament booster circuit* brings it up to the level required for exposure. The rotor switch should not be activated for extended periods because the filament current is at maximum potential and tungsten vaporization can increase. Extended activation can also result in bearing damage and decreased tube life.

The anode is a 2″ to 5″ diameter molybdenum or graphite disc with a beveled edge. The beveled surface has a **focal track** of tung- ◀ sten and rhenium alloy. The anode rotates at about 3500 rpm (high-speed anode rotation is about 10,000 rpm), so that heat generated

Characteristics of Tungsten (W) as Target Material

- High atomic number (74) increases x-ray production.
- High melting point (3410°C) to resist pitting and cracking.
- Thermal conductivity for heat dissipation.

during x-ray production is evenly distributed over the entire track. *Rotating anodes* can withstand delivery of a greater amount of heat for a longer period of time than *stationary anodes*.

The anode is made to rotate through the use of an ***induction motor.*** An induction motor has two main parts, a *stator* and a *rotor*. The stator is the part located outside the glass envelope and consists of a series of electromagnets occupying positions around the stem of the anode. The stator's electromagnets are supplied with current and the associated magnetic fields function to exert a drag or pull on the rotor within (Fig. 15–7).

Tungsten (W) is usually chosen as target material because of its *high atomic number* (Z 74), *high melting point* (3410°C), and *thermal conductivity* (equal to that of copper). The high atomic number serves to increase the efficiency of x-ray production; its high melting point makes it resistant to pitting and cracking; its thermal conductivity helps it dissipate the heat produced during x-ray production. Rhenium is added to further resist anode pitting at high temperatures (Fig. 15–8).

Summary

- X-rays (brems and characteristic) are produced by the abrupt deceleration of high-speed electrons by tungsten atoms within the target (anode).
- The x-ray tube is a *diode,* ie, it has a negative electrode (cathode) and a positive electrode (anode).
- The x-ray tube's electrodes are enclosed within a vacuum glass envelope; a "gassy" tube produces x-rays less efficiently and results in filament oxidation, or burnout.
- The cathode assembly consists of tungsten filament(s) with supporting wires and a (negatively charged) molybdenum focusing cup.

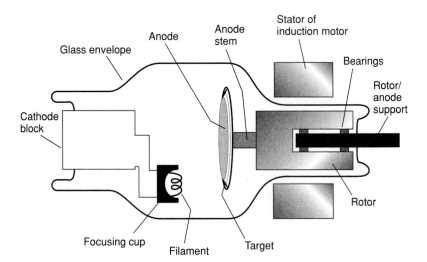

Figure 15–7. The component parts of a rotating anode x-ray tube. Note the position of the stator and rotor. Note the beveled edge of the anode, forming the focal track, and the position of the filament directly across from the rotating focal track. (Modified from Wolbarst, AB. *Physics of Radiology.* East Norwalk, CT: Appleton & Lange, 1993.)

- **Most x-ray tubes have at least two filaments, one for each focal spot.**
- **Heating of the filament to *incandescence* (with 3 to 5 amps, 10 to 12 volts) and subsequent "boiling off" of electrons is called *thermionic emission.***
- **The anode is a 2″ to 5″ molybdenum or graphite disc with a peripheral *focal track* of tungsten and rhenium alloy.**
- **Tungsten is the target material of choice because of its high atomic number, high melting point, and thermal conductivity; rhenium helps prevent pitting.**
- **An induction motor, consisting of stator and rotor, rotates the anode approximately 3500 rpm.**

The production of x-rays involves the generation of significant amounts of heat; less than 1% (ie, 0.2%) of the kinetic energy of the electron stream is converted to x-rays; the rest of the energy is converted to *heat*. Since heat can be very damaging to the x-ray tube and its efficient operation, several features are incorporated to expedite its dissipation. The *thermal conductivity* of tungsten is one feature; however, most cooling is a result of heat diffusion to the oil that surrounds the x-ray tube. If large quantities of heat were continually directed to a single stationary small spot, that spot would be subjected to all the heat generated and would suffer more abuse and subsequent damage. The focal track of the rotating anode serves to spread generated heat over a large area. The width of the focal track on the anode's beveled edge is about 6 mm. Rotating anodes having a diameter of 2 to 5 inches will, therefore, provide significant surface area for the production and dissipation of heat.

The width of the beveled focal track is referred to as the *actual* focal spot size. A distinction is made between the actual focal spot and the *effective,* projected, or apparent focal spot size. The actual focal spot size is the width of the finite area on the tungsten target that is actually bombarded by electrons from the filament. The effective, projected, or apparent focal spot is the *foreshortened* size of the focus as it is projected down toward the image receptor, ie, as it would be seen looking up into the x-ray tube (Fig. 15–9). This is called line focusing or the ***line-focus principle.*** The effective focal ◄ spot size is also affected by the degree of focal track bevel, or anode angle. Anode angles are usually 5° to 20°. Anode angle also has a significant effect on the severity of the ***heel effect.*** The line focus ◄ principle and the heel effect, and their effects on radiographic quality, are discussed more fully in Part IV. When specifying focal spot size, it is the effective focal spot size that is quoted. We often speak of "double-focus" x-ray tubes, meaning that a small (eg, 0.6 mm) and a large (1.2 mm) focal spot is available to choose from. These x-ray tubes actually have only one focal track, a portion of it is used for the small focus setting. It is more accurate to say that these are *double filament* tubes, for there are two filaments—the smaller one is activated when the small focal spot is selected, and the large one is activated for the large focal spot.

The amount of heat produced at the target is expressed in terms of ***heat units*** (HU). Exposure-factor selection has a signifi- ◄ cant effect on the production of heat as expressed in the following equation.

Area = (6 mm)(2π · 50 mm) = 1900 mm²

Figure 15–8. A typical rotating anode. The anode disc is usually made of molybdenum and has a beveled edge containing a "band" of tungsten/rhenium alloy that forms the focal track. (Modified from Wolbarst, AB. *Physics of Radiology.* East Norwalk, CT: Appleton & Lange, 1993.)

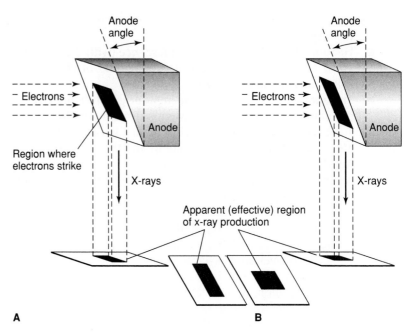

Figure 15–9. Line-focus principle. Note how foreshortening of the actual focal spot impacts the effective (projected or apparent) focal spot. **(A)** A square actual focal spot produces a rectangular effective focal spot. **(B)** An elongated actual focal spot produces a square effective focal spot. As the anode *angle* is made smaller, the actual focal spot may be made larger while a small effective focal spot is still maintained. (From Wolbarst, AB. *Physics of Radiology.* East Norwalk, CT: Appleton & Lange, 1993.)

$$HU = mA \times s \times kVp \text{ (single phase)}$$

For example:

$$300 \text{ mA, } 0.4 \text{ second, } 80 \text{ kVp} = 9600 \text{ HU}$$

$$300 \text{ mA, } 0.2 \text{ second, } 92 \text{ kVp} = 5520 \text{ HU}$$

Thus, a greater number of heat units are produced with higher mAs and lower kVp exposure factors. A *correction factor* is added to the equation when using three-phase equipment.

$$HU = mA \times s \times kVp \times 1.35 \ (3\phi \ 6p)$$

$$HU = mA \times s \times kVp \times 1.41 \ (3\phi \ 12p)$$

For example:

$$300 \text{ mA, } 0.4 \text{ second, } 80 \text{ kVp } (3\phi \ 6p) = 12,960 \text{ HU}$$

$$300 \text{ mA, } 0.4 \text{ second, } 80 \text{ kVp } (3\phi \ 12p) = 13,536 \text{ HU}$$

B. OPERATION

▶ Each x-ray tube has its own ***tube rating chart*** and ***anode cooling curve*** that illustrate safe tube-heat limits and the particular cooling characteristics of the anode. It is essential that the radiographer know how to use these charts in order to use the x-ray tube properly and safely, and to prolong its useful life (Fig. 15–10).

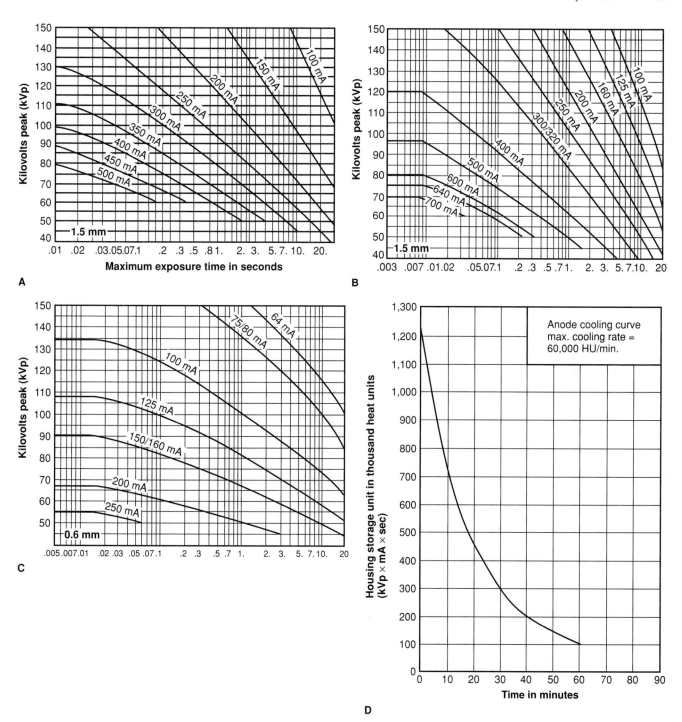

Figure 15–10. Three radiographic tube-rating charts. **(A)** A Sφ 60 Hz tube with 1.5 mm focal spot. **(B)** A 3φ 60 Hz tube with 1.5 mm focal spot. **(C)** A 3φ 60 Hz tube with 0.6 mm focal spot. **(D)** An anode-cooling curve illustrates the cooling characteristics of the x-ray tube. (Reproduced with permission of General Electric Company.)

For example: What is the maximum safe kVp that may be used with each of the three x-ray tubes using 200 mA and 0.2 second exposure?

Find the exposure time on the horizontal axis, follow it up until it meets the 200 mA line, then follow that across to the vertical axis and read the kVp.

A = about 147 kVp; B = greater than 150 kVp (off the chart); C = about 57 kVp.

Comparing these answers with the information provided in the legend for Figure 15–10, it can be seen that the *size of the focal spot* and the *type of rectification* significantly impact heat loading characteristics of the x-ray tube.

Next, refer to the anode cooling curve. For example, if the x-ray tube were saturated with 1,300,000 HU, it would take 30 min to cool down to 300,000 HU. How long would it take to cool from 700,000 HU to 450,000 HU? (about 10 minutes).

C. CARE

Careless treatment or abuse of the x-ray tube, as well as normal wear and tear, will lead to its ultimate demise.

SOME CAUSES OF X-RAY TUBE FAILURE

Vaporized Tungsten
As a result of thermionic emission, quantities of tungsten can be vaporized and deposited on the inner surface of the glass envelope. When deposited on the port window, tungsten acts as a filter and reduces the intensity of the beam; it can also alter the tube vacuum and finally lead to tube failure.

Pitted Anode
Exposures made exceeding the tube rating create enough excessive heat to produce many small melts, or pits, over the surface of the focal track. X-ray photons are absorbed by these surface irregularities and, consequently, x-ray intensity is reduced. Extensive ***pitting*** also results in ***vaporized*** tungsten deposited on the inner surface of the tube window that acts as an additional filter and further reduces beam intensity. Arcing can occur between the filament and tungsten deposit, resulting in a cracked glass envelope.

Cracked Anode
A single large excessive exposure to a cold anode can be severe enough to crack the anode: the large dose of heat creates sudden expansion of the cold anode. It is therefore advisable to practice tube *warm-up procedures,* as suggested by the manufacturer, prior to starting the day's examinations.

Gassy Tube
If the tube vacuum begins to deteriorate, air molecules collide with and decelerate the high-speed electrons, thus decreasing the efficiency of x-ray production. The condition is referred to as a "gassy tube," and eventually causes oxidation and burnout of the cathode filament.

Summary

- **Most of the energy used to produce x-rays is converted to heat; only 0.2% is converted to x-rays.**
- **Heat is damaging to x-ray tubes; x-ray tubes are surrounded with oil to carry heat away from the anode (also for insulating purposes).**

- The width of the focal track is identified as the *actual focal spot;* its bevel (angle) projects a smaller, *effective focal spot* to the image receptor according to the line-focus principle.
- The degree of anode bevel (angle) influences the degree of *heel effect;* the smaller the angle, the more pronounced the heel effect.
- Heat units (HU) are used to express the degree of accumulation of anode heat and are determined by mA × time × kVp; the correction factor for 3φ 6p is 1.35; for 3φ 12p it is 1.41.
- Excessive heat-loading will cause accelerated tube-aging and failure as a result of conditions such as pitted or cracked anode, gassy tube, or vaporized tungsten.
- Tube-rating charts and anode-cooling curves must be used to determine safe exposures and heat loading.

IV. THE RADIOGRAPHIC CIRCUIT

Key Terms ◀

Automatic Exposure Control	Secondary Circuit	Synchronous Spinning Top
Filament Circuit	Spinning-Top Test	Timer
Primary Circuit	Step-Down Transformer	Variable Resistor
Rectification		

The x-ray circuit can be divided into three portions.

1. The *low voltage,* or **primary circuit** contains most of   ◀
   the devices found on the control console.
2. The **filament circuit** varies the current sent to the fila-   ◀
   ment in order to provide the required mA value.
3. The *high-voltage,* **or secondary circuit** includes the   ◀
   high-voltage transformer, rectification system, and x-ray
   tube.

A. Primary Circuit Components

PRIMARY OR LOW-VOLTAGE CIRCUIT DEVICES

Main Switch and Circuit Breakers
These are usually located on a wall in or near the x-ray room (Fig. 15–11).
   Circuit-breaker switches must be closed to energize the equipment.

Autotransformer
The autotransformer is a variable transformer that operates on AC and
   enables the radiographer to select kilovoltage. The function and operation
   of the autotransformer has been discussed earlier in this section.

Figure 15–11. Simplified x-ray circuit. High-voltage current from the secondary transformer coil is rectified before it reaches the x-ray tube.

kV Selector

This is used by the radiographer to choose the kilovoltage, often as kV major (in increments of ten) and kV minor (in increments of two). In doing so, the appropriate number of coils (representing volts) on the autotransformer are selected by the movable contact.

Line-Voltage Compensator

This functions to automatically adjust for any fluctuations in incoming voltage supply. A uniformly consistent and accurate voltage supply is required for predictable radiographic results. A small variation in voltage entering the primary transformer coil voltage represents a much larger variation as it leaves the secondary coil. The control consoles of some older x-ray units were equipped with line-voltage compensators that were adjustable by the radiographer, but in equipment manufactured today, the process takes place automatically within the machine.

Timer

▶ *Timers* function to regulate the length of x-ray exposure. Very simple timers such as the mechanical, synchronous, and impulse timers are rarely used in x-ray equipment manufactured today because they do not permit very fast, accurate exposures. *Mechanical timers* are capable of exposures only as short as 1/4 sec; *synchronous timers* as short as 1/60 sec. *Impulse timers* are more accurate and capable of exposures as short as 1/120 sec.

The *electronic timer* used in x-ray equipment manufactured today, is somewhat complex and based on a capacitor-resistor circuit. Electronic timers are very accurate and capable of rapid exposures as short as 1 millisecond (ie, 1/1000 or 0.001 sec).

The *milliampere-second timer* (mAs timer) monitors the product of mA and time and terminates the exposure when the desired mAs

Types of X-Ray Timers

- Mechanical
- Synchronous
- Impulse
- Electronic
- mAs
- AEC (photomultiplier or ionization chamber)

has been reached. Milliampere-second timers are found on some mobile x-ray units. They are also found on some older fixed x-ray units and display the mAs exposure value when exposure time is too short to permit the actual mA to register on the mA meter.

Another type of timer is the automatic-exposure device (AED), or **automatic exposure control** (AEC), which functions to produce ◀ consistent radiographic results (Fig. 15–12). AECs have sensors that signal to terminate the exposure once a predetermined, known-correct, exposure has been reached.

One type of AEC, the *ionization chamber,* is located just beneath the tabletop, above the x-ray cassette. The part being radiographed is centered to the sensor and exposed. When the predetermined quantity of air ionization has occurred within the chamber, as measured and determined by an electrometer, the exposure is automatically terminated.

Another type of AEC is the *photomultiplier (phototimer),* located behind the cassette. The phototimer consists of a special fluorescent screen that, when activated by x-ray, produces light and charges a photomultiplier tube. When the correct charge has been reached, as determined by the electrometer, the exposure is automatically terminated. Special cassettes, having little foil backing, are often used with phototimers.

A *backup timer* (the manual timer) is used to protect the patient from excessive exposure and x-ray tube from damage should the AEC fail to operate properly. Additional discussion of AECs can be found in Part IV.

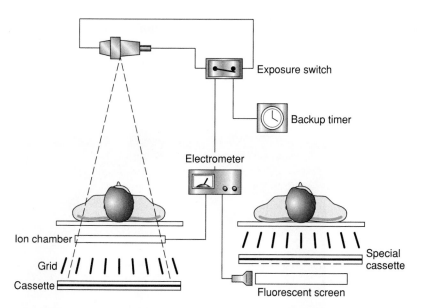

Figure 15–12. Two types of automatic exposure controls. The AEC on the *left* consists of an *ionization chamber* located *under the x-ray tabletop.* The electrometer measures the number of ionizations and terminates the exposure once a predetermined quantity has been reached. The AEC on the *right* consists of a *photomultiplier* tube located *behind the cassette.* Note that a backup timer is in place to terminate the exposure, should the AEC fail to do so. (Modified from Wolbarst, AB. *Physics of Radiology.* East Norwalk, CT: Appleton & Lange, 1993.)

X-ray timer malfunction can cause undesirable fluctuation in radiographic density. If the timer terminates the exposure too soon, the radiograph will be underexposed; if the exposure is delayed in terminating, the radiograph will be overexposed. The radiographer

▶ should be able to perform a ***spinning-top test*** to evaluate timer accuracy (Figs. 15–13 and 15–14).

A simple spinning top consists of a circular steel or lead disc with a small hole in its periphery. The disc is mounted on a base that allows the disk to revolve freely. The device is placed on a cassette, the spinning top is set in motion, and an exposure made using the exposure time station to be evaluated.

Recall that with single phase equipment there are 120 x-ray impulses per second using *single-phase full-wave rectified* current. If the x-ray timer is set to use some portion of the impulses, eg, 1/4 sec, then one fourth of the 120 impulses should be recorded on film if that time station is accurate. Thus, the film should show 30 dots. A minor discrepancy usually indicates a timer malfunction; exactly one half the correct number of dots indicates a rectifier problem. If an exposure of 1/10 second is made, 12 dots should be recorded, and so on. Simply multiply the number of impulses per second (120 in the case of Sϕ full-wave rectified equipment) by the exposure time. In the unlikely event that *half wave rectified* equipment is being tested, the exposure time is multiplied by 60 (useful impulses/second).

Since most x-ray equipment manufactured today is three phase, a slightly different approach must be taken when evaluating these timers. Since *three-phase full-wave rectified* equipment produces a ripple wave, ie, almost constant potential, the standard spinning-top test does not demonstrate impulses; rather, a solid arc is recorded.

▶ The use of a ***synchronous*** (motorized) ***spinning top*** is required. The exposure is made at the time station to be evaluated and the resulting radiograph demonstrates a solid arc. If the exposure time made was 1 sec, an entire circle (360°) should be demonstrated. For

Figure 15–13. The spinning-top test was made using 1/20 (0.05) sec exposure and correctly produced 6 dots. (Courtesy of The Stamford Hospital.)

Figure 15–14. Synchronous spinning-top test. An exposure was made using 1/12 sec (0.083 sec). The resulting image correctly demonstrates a 30° arc. (From Saia, DA. *Appleton & Lange's Review for the Radiography Examination* (3rd ed). East Norwalk, CT: Appleton & Lange, 1997.)

exposure times less than 1 sec, the corresponding portion of a circle should be recorded. For example, an exposure made at 1/4 sec should record a 90° arc (ie, 1/4 of a 360° circle); at an exposure of 1/10 sec, a 36° arc should be recorded.

Primary Coil of the High Voltage Transformer
The primary coil of high voltage transformer is the final component of the primary, or low voltage, circuit. The low voltage entering the primary coil is stepped up to high kilovoltage in the secondary coil by means of mutual induction.

Exposure Switch
The exposure switch is a remote-control switch that functions to start the x-ray exposure (the timer terminates the exposure).

B. FILAMENT CIRCUIT COMPONENTS

The filament circuit is responsible for supplying low-voltage current (3 to 5 amps, 10 to 12 volts) to the filament of the x-ray tube. Since the incoming voltage (110 to 220 volts) is greater than that required, a **step-down transformer** is placed in the filament circuit to make ◄ the required voltage adjustment. A *rheostat,* or other type of **variable resistor,** is placed in the filament circuit to adjust amperage and corresponds to the *mA selector* on the control console.

C. SECONDARY CIRCUIT COMPONENTS

SECONDARY OR HIGH-VOLTAGE CIRCUIT DEVICES

Secondary Coil of High-Voltage Transformer
This carries the required high voltage for x-ray production (and proportionally smaller current value).

mA Meter
This is located at the midpoint of the secondary transformer coil. Since it is grounded, it can be safely placed in the operator's console. The mA meter displays the tube current value.

Rectifiers
The **rectification** system of diodes is located between the secondary coil of ◄ the high voltage transformer and the x-ray tube. Recall from earlier

discussion that it functions to change alternating current to unidirectional pulsating current. Current pulsations decrease with solid-state three-phase rectification (3ϕ 6p rectification has a 13% ripple; 3ϕ 12p has a 4% ripple).

X-ray Tube

The x-ray tube is the final device in the secondary circuit. The filament of its negative electrode, the cathode, is heated by its own circuit to produce *thermionic emission*. As high voltage is applied, the thermionic electron cloud is driven to the anode target. The rapid deceleration of electrons, and their interaction with tungsten atoms of the target, result in an energy conversion to heat and x-rays (99.8% heat, 0.2% x-rays).

D. CIRCUITRY OVERVIEW OF A SINGLE EXPOSURE

1. X-ray machine is turned on. This activates the filament circuit and heats the x-ray tube filament (10–12 volts; 3–5 amps).

2. If the machine has been off overnight warm-up exposures are made to warm the anode throughout (anode cracking can occur when surface heat is applied to a cold anode).

3. Appropriate exposure factors are chosen on the control panel (machines having a line voltage compensator on the control panel should be adjusted to compensate for any incoming voltage fluctuation).

4. The rotor/exposure switch is a two-step button and should be depressed completely in one motion; the first click heard after partial depression is the induction motor bringing anode rotation up to speed. At this time the filament is heated to maximum (thermionic emission) and produces an electron cloud.

5. Upon complete depression of the rotor/exposure switch, the exposure is made. The moment the exposure button is depressed the voltage selected by the autotransformer is sent to the step-up transformer where it is converted to the high voltage (kV) and low amperage (mA) required. This high voltage current then passes through the rectification system which changes AC to pulsating DC.

6. The applied high voltage (potential difference) propels the electron cloud to the anode where interactions between the high speed electrons and tungsten target atoms converts electron kinetic energy to (99.8%) heat energy and (0.2%) x-ray photon energy (see *x-ray production* details in Chapter 8).

Summary

- **The x-ray circuit has three major portions: 'the primary, or low-voltage, side; the filament circuit, and the secondary, or high-voltage, side.**
- **Most of the control console devices are in the primary circuit.**
- **Primary-circuit devices include the main switch and circuit breaker, the autotransformer and kV selector, line voltage compensator, timer, primary coil of the high-voltage transformer, and exposure switch.**
- **The line-voltage compensator automatically adjusts for any fluctuations in the incoming electrical supply.**

- The timer regulates the length of the x-ray exposure; types of timers include mechanical, impulse, synchronous, mAs timer, electronic timer, and AEC.
- There are two types of AECs: the photomultiplier (phototimer), located behind the cassette; and the ionization chamber, located above the cassette.
- A back-up timer terminates the exposure should the AEC fail, thereby functioning to protect the patient and x-ray tube from excessive exposure.
- Timer accuracy can be tested with a spinning-top test: a simple spinning top for single-phase equipment, and a synchronous spinning top for three-phase equipment.
    - Single-phase spinning-top tests show a series of dots, each representing an x-ray impulse.
    - Three-phase spinning-top tests show a solid arc exposure: a portion of a circle (measured in degrees) representative of a portion of a second.
- A step-down transformer and rheostat are placed in the filament circuit to supply the x-ray tube with low-voltage current.
- Secondary circuit devices include the secondary coil of the high-voltage transformer, mA meter, rectifiers, and x-ray tube.
- The grounded mA meter displays the tube current value on the control console.
- Rectifiers are located between the transformer's secondary coil and the x-ray tube; they function to change AC to unidirectional current.

V. THE FLUOROSCOPIC SYSTEM

KEY TERMS ◀

AUTOMATIC BRIGHTNESS CONTROL	INPUT SCREEN	PLUMBICON
BRIGHTNESS GAIN	MATRIX	RAM
CENTRAL PROCESSING UNIT	MEMORY	ROM
CESIUM IODIDE	MINIFICATION GAIN	SOFTWARE
CINEFLUOROGRAPHY	ORTHOCHROMATIC	VAXEL
COUPLING	OUTPUT SCREEN	VIDICON
ELECTROSTATIC FOCUSING LENS	PANCHROMATIC	VIGNETTING
FLUX GAIN	PHOTOCATHODE	WINDOWING
HARDWARE	PIXEL	ZINC CADMIUM SULFIDE
IMAGE INTENSIFIER		

Fluoroscopic x-ray examinations are used to study the dynamics of various parts in *motion*. Fluoroscopy was performed almost exclusively in the very early days of radiology, due to the lack of dependable x-ray tubes and image-recording systems. In the late 40s and early 50s, image intensification was developed and served to provide much brighter images at lower exposures. Present day ***image-intensifiers*** (II) brighten (intensify) the conventional, or "dark," fluoroscopic image 5,000 to 20,000 times. Today's fluoroscopic procedures are much safer (lower exposure) and brighter; the fluoroscopic image can be photographed still or moving (cine), or viewed with a television camera and projected onto a nearby or remote television monitor.

A fluoroscope has two principle components, an x-ray tube and a fluorescent screen, attached at opposite ends of a C-shaped arm.

Fluoroscopic x-ray tubes are standard rotating anode tubes, usually installed under the x-ray table, but operated at much lower tube currents than radiographic tubes. Instead of the 50 mA to 1200 mA used in radiography, fluoroscopic tubes are operated at currents that range from *0.5 mA to 5.0 mA* (averaging 1–3 mA). For radiation protection purposes, *all* fluoroscopic equipment must provide *at least 12″* (30 cm), and preferably 15″ (38 cm), between the x-ray source (focal spot) and the x-ray tabletop, according to NCRP Report no. 102. The tabletop exposure rate must not exceed *10R/min*. Patient dose is much higher in fluoroscopic than radiographic procedures because of the significantly shorter source-to-object distance (SOD); remember also that entrance exposure is significantly greater than exit exposure as a result of attenuation processes within the patient.

A *five-minute timer* is used to measure accumulated fluoroscopic examination time and make an audible sound or interrupt exposure after five minutes of fluoroscopy. X-ray production is usually activated by a footswitch *(dead-man switch),* thus leaving the fluoroscopist's hands free to handle the carriage and position and palpate the patient. The fluoroscopic tube is usually equipped with electrically driven collimating *shutters*. Leaded glass provides shielding from radiation passing through the intensifying screen and the image intensifier is lead-lined. A *Bucky-slot cover* and *protective curtain* also help reduce exposure to the fluoroscopist.

Most fluoroscopes are equipped with a *spot film* device to record fluoroscopic images. To expose a spot film, a motor is activated that brings a cassette from a lead-lined compartment within the carriage over into the fluoroscopic field between the intensifying screen and grid (Fig. 15–15). The fluoroscopic x-ray-tube current then automatically increases to a conventional radiographic level of about 300 mA or more for the cassette exposure. The lead shutters usually adjust automatically but may be operated manually.

Summary

■ **Fluoroscopes are used to examine moving parts and are usually equipped with a device to take cassette-loaded spot films.**

■ **A fluoroscope has two major parts: an x-ray tube and a fluorescent screen, attached at opposite ends of a C-shaped arm.**

■ **The fluoroscopic tube is usually located (at least 12″) under the x-ray table and operated at 1 mA to 3 mA; mA automatically increases for cassette-loaded spot films.**

Some Radiation Safety Features of Fluoroscopic Equipment

- Maximum of 5 mA
- 12″ minimum between focal spot and table top
- 10 R/min maximum tabletop exposure
- 5 min cumulative timer
- Dead-man switch
- Automatic collimation
- Bucky-slot cover
- Protective curtain

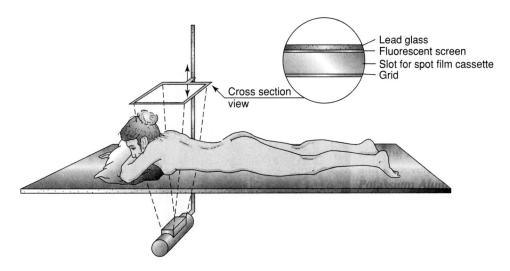

Figure 15–15. Basic early fluoroscope.

- **Many guidelines regulate the operation of fluoroscopic equipment because of the unavoidably high patient-dose inherent in fluoroscopic procedures (due to the short focus-to-patient distance).**
- **Image intensifiers brighten the conventional, dark fluoroscopic image 5,000 to 20,000 times.**

A. THE IMAGE INTENSIFIER

The fluorescent layer of early conventional (or "dark") fluoroscopic screens was made of ***zinc cadmium sulfide*** (Patterson B-2 screen). ◄ The ***input screen*** of today's image-intensifier tube is made of a thin ◄ layer of ***cesium iodide,*** is 5″ to 12″ in diameter, and slightly convex ◄ in shape.

Cesium iodide is much more efficient than zinc cadmium sulfide because it absorbs, and converts to fluorescent light, a greater number of the x-ray photons striking it. For each absorbed x-ray photon, about 5,000 light photons are emitted. This fluorescent light strikes a ***photocathode*** made of a photoemissive metal. A number of elec- ◄ trons are subsequently released from the photocathode and focused toward the output side of the image tube. Although this step actually represents a *deamplification,* it has very little effect on the end result. A thin (0.2 mm) layer of glass or other transparent material is placed between the input screen and photocathode to prevent chemical reaction between the two; otherwise, the two must be as close as possible for maximum transfer of accurate information.

The electrons emitted from the photocathode are focused toward the output end of the tube by negatively charged ***electro-*** ◄ ***static focusing lenses.*** They then pass through the neck of the tube where they are accelerated through a potential difference of 25,000 to 35,000 volts and strike the small (0.5″–1″) fluorescent ***out-*** ◄ ***put screen*** that is mounted on a flat glass support (Fig. 15–16).

The entire assembly is enclosed within a 2-mm to 4-mm thick vacuum-glass envelope. The glass is then coated to prevent the entry of light. The glass tube is enclosed within a metal housing that

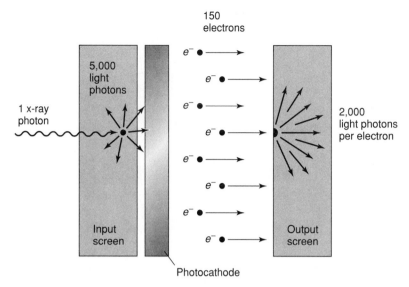

Figure 15–16. Conceptualization of relationship and function of an image intensifier input screen, photocathode, and output screen. For every one x-ray photon interacting with the input screen, 5000 fluorescent-light photons are emitted. Note the close (but not touching) relationship between the input screen and photocathode for maintenance of resolution. The light photons interact with the photocathode and about 150 electrons are emitted by the photoemissive metal. The photoelectrons then interact with the output screen and 2000 fluorescent-light photons are emitted for every electron. (Modified from Wolbarst, AB. *Physics of Radiology.* East Norwalk, CT: Appleton & Lange, 1993.)

functions to attenuate magnetic fields from outside the tube that would distort the electron paths within.

For there to be undistorted focusing of electrons onto the output screen, each electron must travel the same distance; thus the slight curvature of the input screen.

There are several occasions of information transfer within the image intensifier: from x-ray beam to input screen, from input screen to photocathode, from photocathode to electron beam, from electron beam to output screen, and from output screen to the human eye (Fig. 15–17). Thus, an electrical image is transformed to a light image, then back to an electron image, and finally back to a light image. Because a degree of image distortion unavoidably occurs at each point of information transfer, conventional "dark" fluoroscopy actually has greater resolution than image-intensified fluoroscopy. The much brighter image provided by the image intensification process, however, permits the use of physiologically superior photopic (cone) vision, so that anatomic details can be seen more readily and accurately. The greater resolution offered by conventional fluoroscopy cannot be appreciated by the inferior scotopic (rod) vision.

Electrons from the photocathode are accelerated as they travel toward the output screen. The gain in brightness achieved by the image intensifier is the result of this *electron acceleration (flux gain)* and *image minification.* **Flux gain** is defined as the ratio of light photons at the output phosphor to the number at the input phosphor. A typical image intensifier has a flux gain of about 50.

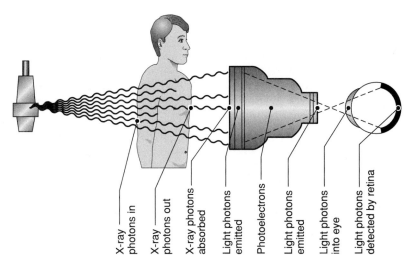

Figure 15–17. Transition of x-ray photons emerging from x-ray tube, through part under study, into image intensifier, to human eye. (Modified from Wolbarst, AB. *Physics of Radiology.* East Norwalk, CT: Appleton & Lange, 1993.)

The image produced on the input screen of the image intensifier is reproduced as a minified image on the output screen. Since the output screen is much smaller than the input screen, the amount of fluorescent light emitted from it per unit area is significantly greater than the quantity of light emitted from the input screen. This process is referred to as ***minification gain,*** and is equal to the ratio ◀ of the diameters of the input and output screens squared.

$$\text{minification gain} = \left(\frac{\text{input screen diameter}}{\text{output screen diameter}} \right)^2$$

For example, the minification gain for an image intensifier with an input screen of 11 in and output screen of 1 in is 121.

$$\text{minification gain} = \left(\frac{11''}{1''} \right)^2$$

$$\text{minification gain} = 121$$

The total ***brightness gain*** of an image intensifier is the product ◀ of flux gain and minification gain.

$$\text{total brightness gain} = \text{flux gain} \times \text{minification gain}$$

For example, the total brightness gain for an image intensifier with a flux gain of 50 and minification gain of 121 is 6050.

$$\text{total brightness gain} = 50(121)$$

$$\text{total brightness gain} = 6050$$

The brightness, resolution, and contrast of an intensified image are greatest in the center of the image. Since the exposure rate is reduced at the periphery of the input screen, and because there is less than exact peripheral electron focusing from the photocathode, brightness, resolution, and contrast are reduced (up to 25%) toward the periphery; this characteristic of image intensifiers is called ***vignetting.*** ◀

Comparisons Between Large and Small Fields of View and Modes

Larger Field of View
- More minification
- Focal point closer to output screen
- Less magnification of perceived image
- Brighter image and less exposure required

Smaller Field of View
- Less minification
- Focal point farther from output screen
- More magnification of perceived image
- Less brightness and more exposure required.

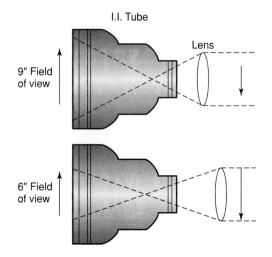

I.I. Tube

Lens

9" Field of view

6" Field of view

Figure 15–18. As field of view (patient area) decreases, magnification of the output screen image increases and contrast and resolution improve. Note that the focal point on the 6" field, or mode, is further away from the output phosphor; therefore the output image appears magnified. Since less minification takes place in this instance, the image is not as bright. Exposure factors are automatically increased to compensate for the loss in brightness. (Modified from Wolbarst, AB. *Physics of Radiology.* East Norwalk, CT: Appleton & Lange, 1993.)

Input-screen diameters of 5" to 12" are available. Although smaller diameter input screens improve resolution, they do not permit viewing of large patient areas.

A type of image distortion, called *pincushion distortion,* is common to intensified images and is caused by the curvature of the input screen and diminished electron focusing precision at the image periphery.

There will always be some degree of magnification in image intensification (just as in radiography); the degree depends on the distance of the image intensifier from the patient.

Dual and triple field image intensifiers are available that permit magnified viewing of fluoroscopic images. Magnified images are reduced in brightness unless the mA is automatically increased when the image intensifier is switched to the magnification mode (Fig. 15–18).

Summary

- **The basic parts of the image intensifier are the input screen, photocathode, electrostatic focusing lenses, accelerating anode, and output screen, within a vacuum glass envelope.**
- **The process of energy conversion within the image intensifier is from electrical to light, to electrical, and back to light.**
- **Cesium iodide is the preferred phosphor for the image intensifier's input screen; for each x-ray photon it absorbs, it emits about 5,000 light photons.**
- **Light photons strike the photocathode, which releases a number of electrons that are directed toward the neck of the image intensifier by the negatively charged focusing lenses.**
- **The input screen and photocathode are slightly curved so that each electron travels the same distance to the output phosphor, to prevent distortion.**
- **Electrons are accelerated by the anode's 25 to 30-kV potential, thus making the output image brighter (flux gain).**
- **The electrons strike the output screen and are converted to a much brighter, smaller (minification gain), and inverted fluorescent image.**
- **Minification gain is determined by dividing the input screen diameter by the output screen diameter and squaring the result.**
- **Total brightness gain is equal to the product of flux gain and minification gain.**
- **Diminished resolution and contrast at the image periphery is called vignetting.**
- **Magnification results in some loss of brightness and mA is automatically increased to compensate.**

B. Viewing Systems

The optical system of the image intensifier can transfer the output screen image to a mirror-viewing apparatus. Mirror viewing offers good resolution, but its disadvantages include limited viewing by one person at a time and limited fluoroscopist movement. In comparison, closed circuit television fluoroscopy is far more convenient, allows the fluoroscopist freedom of movement, and permits simultaneous viewing by a number of people.

As body areas of different thicknesses and density are scanned with the image intensifier, image brightness and contrast require adjustment. The ***automatic brightness control*** (ABC) functions to ◀ maintain constant brightness and contrast of the output screen image, correcting for fluctuations in x-ray beam attenuation with adjustments in kVp and/or mA. There are also brightness and contrast controls on the monitor that the radiographer can regulate.

The image on the output screen can be transferred via a television camera to a display *monitor*. The ***vidicon*** and ***plumbicon*** are ◀ currently the most frequently used television cameras. They are about 6″ long and 1″ in diameter.

Transfer of the output screen fluoroscopic image to the television camera is accomplished by one of two possible means. Fiberoptic ***coupling*** of the output screen to the television camera is the sim- ◀ pler method, involving only a thin layer of fiberoptics between the two devices. The only disadvantage, but a significant one, is that fiberoptic coupling does not permit the use of other imaging accessories such as a cine or spot-film camera; only cassette-loaded spot films can be made with this type of coupling.

The other coupling method is more complex and involves the use of precisely adjusted lenses and mirror. An *objective lens* intercepts the output screen image and transfers it to the *beam-splitter* mirror. Thus, only a small portion of the light image from the output screen is sent (via lenses) to the television camera (and on to the monitor), while the larger portion of light image is transmitted (also via lenses) to the *cine* or *spot-film camera*. The transmitting lenses are critically positioned, delicate structures and, as such, require that the image intensifier be handled with care.

C. Recording Systems

In addition to being transmitted to nearby or remote monitors, the image can be recorded on *video tape* or *cine* film. Television monitors do not offer the very good image resolution obtained from the image intensifier, so film-recording systems such as spot-film cameras and cine cameras are used to record high-resolution images directly from the image intensifier (Fig. 15–19).

1. Cinefluorography. The fluorescent image on the image intensifier's output screen can be photographed with a 16-mm or 35-mm movie camera. About 85% to 95% of the light from the image intensifier's output screen is transmitted to the cine camera when it is in use. The rest of the light is used for television-monitor viewing. During ***cinefluorography,*** x-ray exposure is on only when the film is ◀ in proper position for exposure (ie, no exposure during film movement between frames). *Grid-controlled x-ray tubes* are used to synchronize x-ray exposure with proper film position. Cine "flickering" is noticeable only with frame rates below 30 frames per second.

Film used in cine cameras must be sensitive to the fluorescent light emitted by the output screen. ***Panchromatic*** film is sensitive ◀ to all wavelengths (ie, colors) of visible light; ***orthochromatic*** film ◀ is sensitive to all but red light. These are the two film types most often used in cine cameras. Higher-quality images are obtained with

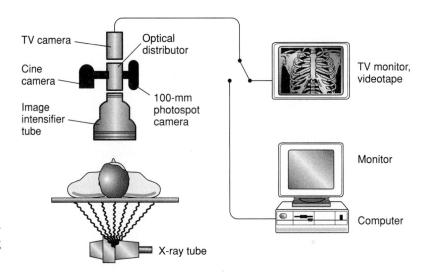

Figure 15–19. Image-intensified fluoroscopic unit with several ancillary imaging devices.

35-mm film (rather than 16-mm) because the film size is four times greater than 16-mm frames; however, for that same reason, 35-mm film requires greater patient exposure and is more expensive. Another reason patient dose is significantly greater in cinefluorography than in routine image-intensified fluoroscopy is because the output screen image must be bright enough to expose the cine film (hence, increased mA). Typical doses measured at the image intensifier input phosphor are approximately 10 microR/frame.

2. Spot Films. Spot films in 70-mm, 90-mm, and 105-mm sizes can be made from the image on the output screen of the image intensifier. This type of spot filming has gained wide acceptance over the cassette-loaded spot filming procedures (taken from the input screen of the image intensifier). The film used for spot-film cameras is less expensive, easier to store, can be exposed in rapid succession, and requires less patient exposure (because of its small size). Typical doses measured at the image intensifier input phosphor are approximately 50 to 100 microR/spot film. Image quality is slightly less than cassette-loaded spot films (9″ × 9″ cassette), whose typical doses measured at the image intensifier input phosphor are approximately 300 to 400 microR/film.

3. Video Recording. Fluoroscopic procedures can also be recorded on videotape. The most significant advantage of videotape recordings is that it allows *immediate* playback (eliminating film processing). Other advantages include the availability of sound, and capability of playing at slower speeds and viewing single frames. Its biggest disadvantage is loss of some resolution. New video-disc recorders are similar to videotape machines, sharing all their advantages and having the added advantage of improved image quality (resolution).

4. Computed Radiography

▶ *l. Computer System.* The computer system consists of the ***hardware,*** which is any physical component of the computer, and the ▶ ***software,*** which is a set of instructions or program to operate the computer.

The hardware consists of input and output devices. These devices allow information to be put into a computer and allow information to be directed outside the computer. The ***central processing unit*** is the primary control center for the computer consisting of a control unit, arithmetic unit, and memory. The speed is measured in "millions of instructions per second" (MIPS). Most desktop computer speeds are given in MHz. The ***memory*** is solid state. It is used by the computer during execution of a program. There are two types of memory. The first is ***RAM,*** or random access memory. This memory is volatile and will lose all information when the computer is turned off unless previously saved. Read only memory, or ***ROM,*** is memory that is hard wired into the computer, which means it stays in the computer even when the computer is turned off. ROM usually contains the booting instructions.

The software is a set of instructions the computer uses to function effectively, known as a program. Computer programmer languages include, but are not limited to:

- Fortran: Formula translation. Used mainly in science and engineering applications.
- Basic: A beginners all-purpose language with symbolic instructions and code.
- Cobol: Common business oriented language.
- Pascal: High level mathematics.

II. Binary Numbers. The computer hardware interprets all information as a simple "yes" or "no" decision. Current "on" implies "yes" and current "off" implies "no." This is symbolically represented with digits 1 and 0. A bit in computer terminology refers to an individual one or zero and is a single bit of information. A byte is equal to eight bits, and a word is equal to 16 bits or 2 bytes.

Image Storage. Image storage is located in a ***pixel*** (Fig. 15–20), which is a two dimensional "picture element." Pixels are measured in the "XY" direction.

The third dimension in the matrix of pixels is the depth which together with the pixel is referred to as the ***voxel*** (Fig. 15–21). The voxels are measured in the "Z" direction. The depth of the block is the number of bits required to describe the gray level that each pixel can take on. This is known as the bit depth.

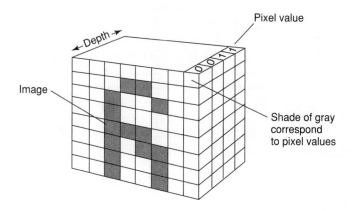

Figure 15–20. A digital image may be likened to a three dimensional object made up of many small cubes, each containing a binary digit or bit. The image is seen on one surface of the block, whose depth is the number of bits required to describe each pixel's gray level.

Figure 15–21. The third dimension in the matrix of pixels is the depth, which together with the pixel is referred to as the voxel (volume element).

The **matrix** is the number of pixels in the XY direction. The ◄ larger the matrix size, the better the image resolution (Fig. 15–22).

Typical image matrix sizes used in radiography are:

- Nuclear medicine   128 × 128
- DSA (Fig. 15–23)   512 × 512
- CT   512 × 512
- Chest radiography   2048 × 2048

One of the most important factors to consider in computed radiography is the ability to transmit images over distances, known as *teleradiography.* The amount of information transferred per unit time is known as the baud rate and is in units of bits per second.

Example: A network is capable of transmitting data at a rate of 9600 baud. If each pixel has a bit depth of 8 bits how long will it take to transmit a 512 × 512 image?

Solution:

(512 × 512 pixels)(8 bits/pixel)/9600 bits/second = 128 seconds.

There are three possible means of image transmission. Telephone wires offer low transmission speed while using a modem. Coaxial cable will transmit at approximately 100 MBaud. Finally, there are fiber optic cables.

Figure 15–22. The matrix is the number of pixels in the XY direction. The larger the matrix size the better the image resolution.

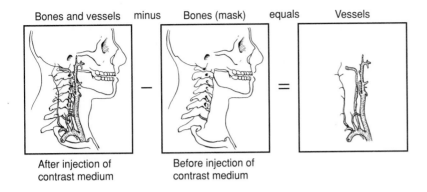

Figure 15–23. Digital Subtraction Angiography (DSA). Image details not required for diagnosis can be subtracted from an image. Only vessels containing contrast medium are visualized in the final image.

Another advantage of computed radiography is the ability to manipulate the image after exposure. Image post-processing can be used for noise reduction, contrast modification, image subtraction (Fig. 15–23), and windowing. Image subtraction is used primarily in angiography to remove superimposed bone structures on contrast filled vessels.

Windowing is a process of changing the contrast and density ◄ setting on the finished image. The window width controls the number of shades of gray in the image, while the window level (center) controls the density, or where on the contrast scale you begin.

Example: Window width = 100

Window level = 0

All pixels with values greater than the upper window limit are displayed as white. All pixel values below the lower window limit are displayed as black. Pixel values between the two limits are spread over the full scale of gray. Therefore, in this example, gray scales with pixel values ranging from −50 to +50 will be displayed. The −50 pixels will be black and +50 pixels will be white.

Applications for computed radiography include the following.

- CT scanning
- Nuclear medicine
- Magnetic resonance imaging
- Ultrasound
- Digital subtraction radiography (DSA) (Fig. 15–23)

Summary

- ■ **The optical system transfers the output screen image to either mirror viewing or television monitor (via plumbicon or vidicon camera).**
- ■ **Television monitor viewing is more practical and convenient, though it involves some loss of image quality.**
- ■ **Automatic brightness control automatically adjusts kVp or mA; brightness and contrast controls are also available for adjustment on the TV monitor.**
- ■ **The output screen image is usually coupled to the television camera via a series of complex and precisely adjusted lenses and mirror.**

- When used in conjunction with cine and spot-film cameras, the largest portion of the output screen light is diverted to the spot film or cine camera; the remainder goes to the television monitor.
- Cineradiographic film is either 16-mm or 35-mm panchromatic or orthochromatic film.
- Better quality images are obtained with 35 mm, but patient exposure dose is greater.
- Spot-film cameras use 70-mm, 90-mm, or 105-mm film.
- Spot-film cameras are preferable to cassette-loaded spot films because the film is more economical (smaller size), easier to store, and requires less patient exposure.
- Videotape recordings, permitting immediate playback, may be made of the fluoroscopic procedure, although there is some loss of image resolution.
- There are 2 types of memory: RAM and ROM.
- A two-dimensional picture element is a pixel; a three-dimensional picture element is a voxel.
- Computed radiography enables image manipulation after exposure.
- Windowing is the process of changing contrast and density on the finished image.

Chapter Exercises

⭐ *Congratulations! You have completed your review of the entire chapter. If you are able to answer the following group of very comprehensive questions, you should feel confident that you have really mastered this section. You can refer back to the indicated pages to check your answers and/or review the subject matter.*

1. Define and give examples of dedicated x-ray equipment *(p. 417).*

2. Distinguish between an AC and DC waveform *(p. 418).*

3. Discuss the following characteristics of AC: amplitude, polarity, wavelength, and frequency *(pp. 418–419).*

4. Define helix, solenoid, electromagnet *(p. 419).*

5. Describe the function of the transformer and identify the principle on which it operates *(p. 420).*

6. Using the transformer law, determine the voltage and current delivered to the x-ray tube *(p. 420).*

7. Identify four types of x-ray transformer construction *(pp. 420–421).*

8. Describe three types of transformer energy losses and methods by which they can be reduced *(pp. 421–422).*

9. Describe the function of the autotransformer and identify the principle on which it operates *(p. 421).*

10. Using the autotransformer law, determine the voltage sent to the transformer primary *(pp. 421–423).*

11. Identify the type current required for operation of the transformer and autotransformer *(pp. 421–423).*

12. Define the function of the generator; motor *(p. 420).*

13. Describe the rectification process *(p. 422).*

14. Identify and give examples of the type of material of which solid state diodes are made *(p. 423).*

15. Differentiate among single-phase, three-phase/six-pulse, and three-phase/twelve-pulse waveforms *(p. 422)*.

16. Identify the pulse ripple for single-phase, three-phase/six-pulse, and three-phase/twelve-pulse rectification *(p. 423)*.

17. Identify the number of autotransformers and transformers required for three-phase rectification *(p. 423)*.

18. Identify the two types of transformer winding configurations *(p. 423)*.

19. List the three basic component parts of the x-ray tube *(p. 424)*.

20. Discuss the importance of the evacuated-glass envelope *(p. 424)*.

21. Identify the component parts of the cathode assembly *(p. 424)*.

22. Describe thermionic emission *(p. 425)*.

23. Describe how a double or dual-focus tube differs from a single-focus tube *(pp. 425–427)*.

24. Explain why x-ray tube inherent filtration increases as the x-ray tube ages *(p. 425)*.

25. Identify the current and voltage required by the filament circuit *(p. 425)*.

26. Discuss why prolonged periods of rotor activation should be avoided *(p. 426)*.

27. Describe the construction of the anode *(p. 427)*.

28. Discuss the composition and function of the anode focal track *(p. 427)*.

29. Discuss the value of anode rotation (versus stationary anode) *(pp. 425–427)*.

30. Identify the device responsible for anode rotation and its two major parts *(p. 426)*.

31. Identify two characteristics of tungsten that make it a desirable target material *(p. 426)*.

32. Describe the line focus principle; distinguish between actual and effective focal spot *(p. 427)*.

33. Describe the anode heel effect; relate it to focal-track bevel (anode angle) *(p. 427)*.

34. Discuss why heat removal mechanisms are important in x-ray tube construction; give examples of heat reduction features *(p. 427)*.

35. Determine heat units for Sφ, 3φ 6p, and 3φ 12p x-ray equipment *(p. 427)*.

36. Determine safe exposure limits using tube-rating charts and anode-cooling curves *(pp. 428–429)*.

37. Discuss at least three causes of x-ray tube failure *(p. 430)*.

38. Identify the three portions of the x-ray circuit *(p. 431)*.

39. Identify the components of the primary, or low-voltage, circuit *(pp. 431–432)*.

40. Describe the various types of x-ray timers and identify their accuracy *(pp. 432–433.*

41. Describe the two types of AECs and identify the location of each *(pp. 433)*.

42. Discuss the importance of a back-up timer *(p. 433)*.

43. Describe the tests used to evaluate Sφ and 3φ timers *(pp. 434–435)*.

44. Evaluate Sφ and 3φ timer tests for accuracy *(pp. 434–435)*.

45. Identify the function of the rheostat and transformer in the filament circuit *(p. 435)*.

46. Identify and describe the components of the secondary, or high-voltage, circuit *(pp. 435–436)*.

47. Explain the function of fluoroscopy *(p. 438)*.

48. Identify the usual location of the fluoroscopy tube *(p. 438)*.

49. Identify the fluoroscopic mA range of operation *(p. 438)*.

50. List at least six fluoroscopic equipment features designed to reduce patient and personnel exposure *(p. 438)*.

51. Explain why fluoroscopic exposure dose is greater than radiographic dose *(p. 438)*.

52. Identify, with respect to the image intensifier (II), the:

   A. composition of the input screen, and its characteristics and advantages *(p. 439)*

   B. action of the photocathode *(p. 439)*

   C. function of the electrostatic focusing lenses *(p. 439)*

   D. function and potential difference of the accelerating anode *(p. 440)*

   E. function and size of the output screen *(p. 441)*

   F. two components of total brightness gain *(p. 441)*

53. Determine minification gain *(pp. 441–442)*.

54. Define vignetting *(p. 441)*.

55. Discuss advantages and disadvantages of magnified images *(p. 442)*.

56. Identify ways in which the fluoroscopic image can be recorded *(pp. 444–445)*.

57. Identify by what means the image intensifier compensates for varying body thicknesses *(p. 443)*.

58. Define what is meant by coupling *(p. 443)*.

59. Identify the monitor controls regulatable by the radiographer *(p. 443)*.

60. Compare television monitor resolution with that of spot films *(p. 444)*.

61. Identify the sizes of cine film available and compare each with regard to patient dose and image quality *(p. 443)*.

62. Differentiate between panchromatic and orthochromatic film *(p. 443)*.

63. Identify the spot-film sizes available and relate each to patient dose and image quality *(p. 444)*.

64. Describe the advantages and disadvantages of videotape image recording *(p. 444)*.

Chapter Review Questions

1. Advantages of digital radiography (computed radiography) include all of the following, EXCEPT the ability to:
   - (A) compensate for exposure factors
   - (B) make changes in contrast characteristics
   - (C) improve geometric detail
   - (D) store images in binary form

2. The device used to ensure reproducible radiographs, regardless of tissue density variations, is the:
   - (A) phototimer
   - (B) penetrometer
   - (C) grid
   - (D) rare earth screen

3. Which of the following circuit devices operate(s) on the principle of self induction?
   1. autotransformer
   2. choke coil
   3. high-voltage transformer
   (A) 1 only
   (B) 1 and 2 only
   (C) 2 and 3 only
   (D) 1, 2, and 3

4. Which of the following will occur as a result of decreasing the anode target angle?
   1. anode heel effect will be less pronounced
   2. effective focal spot size will decrease
   3. greater photon intensity toward the cathode side of the x-ray tube
   (A) 1 only
   (B) 1 and 2 only
   (C) 2 and 3 only
   (D) 1, 2, and 3

5. The source of electrons within the x-ray tube is a result of which of the following processes?
   (A) electrolysis
   (B) thermionic emission
   (C) rectification
   (D) photosynthesis

6. A three-phase timer can be tested for accuracy using a synchronous spinning top. The resulting image looks like a:
   (A) series of dots or dashes, each representative of a radiation pulse
   (B) solid arc, the angle (in degrees) representative of the exposure time
   (C) series of gray tones, from white to black
   (D) multitude of small mesh-like squares of uniform sharpness

7. Which of the following statements regarding transformer laws is (are) correct?
   1. the voltage and current values are increased with a step-up transformer
   2. the voltage is directly related to the number of turns in the two coils
   3. the product of voltage and current in the two circuits must be equal
   (A) 1 only
   (B) 1 and 2 only
   (C) 2 and 3 only
   (D) 1, 2, and 3

8. If the primary coil of the high-voltage transformer is supplied by 220 volts and has 150 turns, and the secondary coil has 75,000 turns; what is the voltage induced in the secondary coil?
   (A) 75 kilovolts
   (B) 110 kilovolts
   (C) 75 volts
   (D) 110 volts

9. In the production of bremsstrahlung radiation, the incident electron:
   (A) ejects an inner-shell tungsten electron
   (B) ejects an outer-shell tungsten electron
   (C) is deflected with resulting energy loss
   (D) is deflected with resulting energy increase

10. In which of the following portions of the x-ray circuit is a step down transformer located?
    (A) high-voltage side
    (B) filament circuit
    (C) rectification system
    (D) secondary side

Answers and Explanations

1. (C) All other factors can be changed in the computer to manipulate the image. Geometric detail is only controlled by SID, OID, and focal spot size. These factors are fixed during the x-ray exposure.

2. (A) Radiographic reproducibility is an important concept in producing high-quality diagnostic films. Radiographic results should be consistent and predictable, not only in positioning accuracy but with respect to exposure factors as well. Automatic exposure devices (phototimers and ionization chambers) automatically terminate the x-ray exposure once a predetermined quantity of x-ray has penetrated the patient, thus ensuring consistent results.

3. (B) The principle of self induction is an example of the second law of electromagnetics (Lenz's Law) which states that an induced current within a conductive coil will oppose the direction of the current that induced it. It is important to note that self induction is a characteristic of alternating current *only.* The fact that alternating current is constantly changing direction accounts for opposing currents set-up in the coil. Two x-ray circuit devices operate on the principle of self induction: The *autotransformer* operates on the principle of self induction and enables the radiographer to vary the kilovoltage. The *choke coil* also operates on the principle of self-induction; it is a type of variable resistor that may be used to regulate filament current. The high-voltage transformer operates on the principle of mutual induction.

4. (C) Target angle has a pronounced geometric effect on the effective, or projected, focal spot size. As target angle *decreases* (ie, gets steeper or smaller), the effective (projected) focal spot becomes smaller. This is advantageous because it will improve radiographic detail without creating a heat-loading crisis at the anode (as would be the case if the actual focal spot size were reduced to produce a similar detail improvement). There are disadvantages, however. With a smaller target angle the anode heel effect increases; photons are more noticeably absorbed by the "heel" of the anode, resulting in a smaller percentage of x-ray photons at the anode end of the x-ray beam and a concentration of x-ray photons at the cathode end of the radiograph.

5. (B) The thoriated tungsten filament of the cathode is heated by its own filament circuit. The x-ray tube filament is made of thoriated tungsten and is part of the cathode assembly. Its circuit provides current and voltage to heat it to incandescence, at which time it undergoes *thermionic emission*—the liberation of valence electrons from the filament atoms. *Electrolysis* describes the chemical ionization effects of an electric current. *Rectification* is the process of changing AC to unidirectional current. Photosynthesis is the process by which plants take in carbon dioxide and release oxygen as a byproduct.

6. (B) Using a spinning top to test the efficiency of a single-phase timer, the result is a *series of dots* or dashes, with each representing a pulse of radiation. With full-wave rectified current, and a possible 1/20 dots (pulses) available per second, one should visualize 12 dots at 1/10 sec, 24 dots at 1/5 sec, 6 dots at 1/20 sec, and so on. But since three-phase equipment is almost constant potential, a synchronous spinning top must be used, and the result is a *solid arc* (rather than dots). The number of degrees formed by the arc is measured and equated to a particular exposure time. A multitude of small mesh-like squares describes a screen contact test. An aluminum step wedge (penetrometer) may be used to demonstrate the effect of kVp on contrast (demonstrating a series of gray tones from white to black), with a greater number of grays demonstrated at higher kVp levels.

7. (C) Transformers are used in the x-ray circuit to change the value of the supplied voltage to a value appropriate for the production of x-rays. Although the incoming voltage supply may be 220 volts, thousands of volts are required for the production of x-rays. A step-up transformer consists of two coils, a primary and a secondary, in close proximity to each other (eg, side by side). As the primary coil is supplied with AC, a magnetic field rises up around the coil and proceeds to "cut" the secondary coil. Because the current supply is AC, the magnetic field is constantly expanding and contracting (rising and falling) and continuously "cutting" the secondary coil. This interaction between magnetic field and conductive coils induces a current in the secondary coil *proportional to* the number of turns in the secondary coil. As the number of turns in the secondary coil increases, so does the induced voltage. However, because we cannot just create energy, only change its form, *the amperage in the second coil is proportionally less.* For example, if the voltage in the secondary coil increased 10 times, the current would decrease by a factor of 10. Therefore, in keeping with the law of conservation of energy, the product of the voltage and current in one coil must equal the product of voltage and current in the second coil.

8. (B) The high-voltage, or step-up, transformer functions to *increase voltage* to the necessary kilovoltage. It *decreases the amperage* to milliamperage. The amount of increase or decrease *depends on the transformer ratio,* ie, the number of turns in the primary coil to the number of turns in the secondary coil. The transformer law is as follows:

To Determine Secondary V   **To Determine Secondary I**

$$\frac{V_S}{V_P} = \frac{N_S}{N_P}$$ $$\frac{I_S}{I_P} = \frac{V_P}{V_S}$$

Substituting known values:

$$\frac{x}{220} = \frac{75{,}000}{150}$$

$$150\,x = 16{,}500{,}000$$

$$x = 110{,}000 \text{ volts } (= 110 \text{ kV})$$

9. (C) Bremsstrahlung (or brems) radiation is one of the two kinds of x-rays produced at the tungsten target of the x-ray tube. The incident high-speed electron, passing through a tungsten atom, is attracted by the positively charged nucleus; therefore it is *deflected from its course with a resulting loss of energy.* This energy loss is given up in the form of an x-ray photon.

10. (B) Transformers are used to change the value of alternating current, and operate on the principle of mutual induction. The secondary coil of the step-up transformer is located in the high-voltage (secondary) side of the x-ray circuit. The step-down transformer, or filament transformer, is located in the filament circuit and serves to regulate the voltage and current provided to heat the x-ray tube filament. The rectification system is also located on the high-voltage, or secondary, side of the x-ray circuit.

Standards of Performance and Equipment Evaluation

16

NCRP Report no. 102 serves as a guide to good medical radiation practices by describing the federal regulations on equipment design, performance, and use. Manufacturers of x-ray equipment must follow guidelines that state maximum x-ray output at specific distances, total quantities of filtration, positive beam limitation, and other guidelines. Radiographers must practice safe principles of operation; ***preventive*** ◀ ***maintenance*** and ***quality control*** checks must be performed at ◀ specific intervals to ensure continued safe equipment performance.

Radiologic quality control involves monitoring and regulating the variables associated with image production and patient care. Every radiologic facility today must establish *quality control* (QC) guidelines and conduct quality control programs to provide a consistent standard of care. A properly documented, ongoing, and effective QC program is required by hospital accrediting agencies and state departments of health.

The rationale behind QC is that a radiographic imaging system performing in an erratic and undependable manner results in repeat exposures, thus contributing to unnecessary patient dose and uneconomical use of time, equipment, and supplies. *Radiographic quality control* is an organized and methodical evaluation of imaging components from the x-ray tube to the automatic film processor, with

457

Elements of a Typical Quality Control Program

- Timer accuracy testing
- mA linearity testing
- kVp accuracy testing
- HVL testing
- Exposure reproducibility testing
- Focal-spot size test
- X-ray beam/light field/Bucky-tray alignment evaluation
- Intensifying screen cleaning and testing
- Illuminator cleaning and evaluation
- Automatic processor maintenance and control
- X-ray evaluation of lead aprons and gloves

the purpose of decreasing repeat exposures, thereby decreasing patient radiation exposure and increasing cost-effectiveness. The frequency of testing ranges from daily processor checks to quarterly, semiannual, and annual equipment performance testing. Processor QC was discussed in Part IV.

The position of QC technologist is an increasingly important one requiring advanced knowledge and skills. In recognition of this, the ARRT has implemented an advanced certification examination in QC.

The QC program requires the combined efforts of the radiographer, QC technologist, service engineers, and medical physicist. The radiographer must be alert to any equipment malfunctions or unusual occurrences and report them to the QC technologist without delay. The QC technologist, service engineer, and medical physicist are responsible for equipment testing, correlation of test results, any necessary corrections or modifications, and accurate documentation of their activities.

I. EQUIPMENT CALIBRATION

A. *kVp*

Kilovoltage accuracy is essential to achieve the desired radiographic contrast. ***Calibration*** of kVp was formerly evaluated using a Wisconsin test tool and cassette. The digital kVp test meters used today are more convenient and simple to use. When various kilovoltages are tested in the normal diagnostic range (40 kVp to 150 kVp), the selected kV and actual kV value should not differ by more than 5 kVp or 10% for general diagnostic equipment and by 1 kVp or 5% for mammography equipment (Fig. 16–1).

B. *mA*

The accuracy of individual mA stations is related to patient dose and is essential for production of expected radiographic density levels. An aluminum step wedge ***(penetrometer)*** can be used to evaluate each mA station. A series of exposures is made at a particular kVp *using the same mAs value at each mA station,* with exposure time adjusted to maintain a constant mAs. The resultant step-wedge images should be identical. Performance of this test on properly calibrated equipment is a good illustration of the reciprocity law. ***Linearity*** of mA is frequently evaluated using a digital dosimeter (ionization chamber). Exposures are made at a particular mAs with various combinations of mA and time; x-ray output is measured in mR/mAs, and should be accurate to within 10%.

C. *Timer*

Timer accuracy is related to patient dose and the production of expected radiographic densities. ***Spinning-top tests,*** for determination of timer accuracy, have been described in an earlier chapter. The use of the digital dosimeter, however, is favored by many as a more simple and accurate measure of timer accuracy. The selected exposure time should be within 5% of the actual exposure time. Similar tests are used to evaluate the accuracy of automatic exposure devices (AECs).

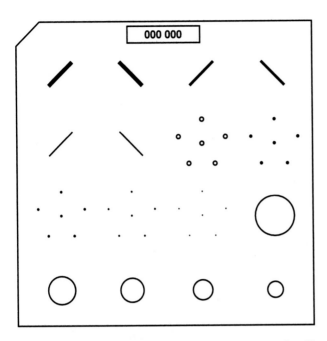

Figure 16–1. A mammographic phantom contains mylar fibers, simulated masses, and specks of simulated calcifications. ACR accreditation criteria states that a minimum of 10 objects (4 fibers, 3 specks, 3 masses) must be visualized on test films. (Courtesy of Gamex/RMI.)

D. REPRODUCIBILITY

This test evaluates consistency of tube output. A particular group of technical factors is selected and a series of consecutive exposures (at least five) are made. The factors are changed between exposures and then changed back to the original technique. The digital radiation meter should register radiation output that does not vary more than 5%. If a radiographer notices an exposure fluctuation while using a particular group of technical factors, the **reproducibility** test is performed using those factors, but alternately changing to other technical factors between exposures.

E. HALF-VALUE LAYER (HVL)

HVL testing provides beam quality information that is different from that obtained from kVp testing. HVL is defined as the thickness of any absorber that will reduce x-ray beam intensity to one-half its original value. HVL is determined by measuring the beam intensity without an absorber, then recording the intensity as successive millimeters of aluminum are added to the radiation field. HVL is influenced by the type of rectification, total filtration, and kVp. An x-ray tube HVL should remain almost constant. If HVL decreases, it is an indication of a decrease in the actual kVp. If the HVL increases, it indicates the deposition of vaporized tungsten deposits on the inner surface of the glass envelope (as a result of tube aging) or an increase in the actual kVp.

F. FOCAL SPOT SIZE

Focal spot size accuracy is related to the degree of geometric blur, ie, edge gradient or penumbra. Manufacturer tolerance for new focal spots is a surprisingly large 50%, ie, a 0.3 mm focal spot may actually be 0.45 mm (that can significantly impact magnification radiography). Additionally, the focal spot can increase in size as the x-ray tube ages; hence the importance of testing newly arrived focal spots and periodic testing to monitor focal spot changes.

▶ Focal spot size can be measured with a ***pinhole camera*** or
▶ ***star pattern*** type *resolution device*. The pinhole camera is rather difficult to use accurately and requires the use of excessive tube (heat) loading. The star pattern, or similar resolution device, can measure focal spot size as a function of geometric blur and is readily adaptable in a QC program to monitor focal spot changes over a period of time. It is recommended that focal spot size be checked on installation of a new x-ray tube and annually thereafter.

II. RADIOGRAPHIC AND FLUOROSCOPIC ACCESSORIES

A. CASSETTES

The exterior of all cassettes should be checked periodically for damage and signs of wear. Loose latches or hinges, damaged frames, or deteriorated felt or sponge should be repaired or replaced.

B. INTENSIFYING SCREENS

Intensifying screens should first be visually inspected for abrasions, stains, and other signs of wear. Screens need regular periodic cleaning according to the manufacturer recommendations. In general, a nonabrasive, lint-free cloth is used with a special antistatic screen cleaner. Care must be taken not to use excessive solution and to allow the screens to dry thoroughly before use.

Adequate screen care includes periodic screen and film contact tests using the special wire-mesh test device. The cassette to be tested is placed on the x-ray table, the wire-mesh device on top of the cassette, and an exposure made of about 5 mAs and 40 kVp. The processed film should be viewed at a distance of at least 6 feet. Any blurry areas are indicative of poor screen to film contact and representative of diminished image detail. Cassettes having areas of poor screen and film contact must be repaired or replaced, as poor contact will seriously impair recorded detail.

Grid cassettes should be evaluated periodically to identify any damage to the fragile lead strips within. The film-loaded grid cassette is slightly exposed, just enough to make the lead strips visible. The processed radiograph is examined for any areas of uneven density or evidence of damaged, misaligned lead strips.

C. ILLUMINATION

One of the most frequently overlooked components of an adequate QC program is radiographic illumination. Radiographic density and contrast can be significantly misrepresented on illuminators providing different degrees of brightness. A radiographic image viewed by the QC technologist in the processor room can look very different on the radiologist's illuminator. A simple light meter, held the same distance from each illuminator (about 3 feet), will reveal any differences in illumination.

Illuminator surfaces need to be cleaned periodically to remove build-up of dust and grime. When one bulb in a bank of illuminators requires changing, all the bulbs should be changed to guarantee uniform brightness.

D. LEAD APRONS AND GLOVES

Personal fluoroscopic shielding apparel such as lead aprons, gloves, and thyroid shields should be fluoroscoped annually to detect any cracks that may have developed in the leaded vinyl.

Proper care is required to help prolong the useful life of lead apparel. If soiled, it can be cleaned with a damp cloth. Lead aprons should not be folded or carelessly dropped to the floor, for that facilitates the development of cracks in the leaded vinyl. Lead aprons and gloves should be hung on appropriate racks when not in use.

Summary

- The function of QC is to provide consistent high quality radiographs, thus reducing patient dose and increasing cost effectiveness.
- QC programs involve evaluation and documentation of all imaging components from the x-ray tube to automatic processor.
- Kilovoltage accuracy can be determined using a Wisconsin test cassette or digital meter, and must be accurate to within 5 kVp (plus or minus 10%).
- Milliamperage accuracy is determined using an aluminum step wedge or digital dosimeter, and must be accurate to within 10%.
- Timer accuracy is evaluated using a manual spinning top (for Sϕ) or synchronous spinning top (for 3ϕ), and must be accurate to within 5%.
- Reproducibility refers to tube output consistency, and must not vary more than 5%.
- HVL is tested periodically to evaluate x-ray beam quality; HVL should remain almost constant.
- Focal spot size is tested, using a pinhole camera or star test pattern, on installation and every year thereafter.
- Cassette exteriors and interiors should be inspected periodically.
- Intensifying screens must be cleaned regularly and screen and film contact tests performed periodically.
- Grid cassettes should be tested for damaged lead strips.
- Illuminators must be cleaned and checked for uniformity.
- Lead gloves and aprons must be fluoroscoped annually to detect any cracks; they should be properly hung when not in use.

Chapter Exercises

 Congratulations! *You have completed your review of the entire chapter. If you are able to answer the following group of very comprehensive questions, you should feel confident that you have really mastered this section. You are then ready to go on to "Registry-type" questions that follow. For greatest success, do not go to these multiple choice questions without first completing the short answer questions below.*

1. Describe the value of a QC program *(pp. 457–458)*.

2. Identify the method used for kV calibration and the required degree of accuracy *(p. 458)*.

3. Describe the method of evaluating mA calibration using an aluminum-step wedge *(p. 458)*.

4. Describe how mA linearity is usually evaluated and identify the required degree of accuracy *(p. 458)*.

5. Describe how Sφ and 3φ timer accuracy is evaluated, identify the appropriate tool for each, give examples of acceptable results, and identify the degree of accuracy required *(p. 458)*.

6. Explain what is meant by reproducibility and identify the degree of accuracy required *(p. 459)*.

7. Define HVL and list the three factors that influence it *(p. 459)*.

8. Explain how tube aging can result in increased HVL *(p. 459)*.

9. Identify when the focal-spot size should be checked and the two devices that can be used *(p. 460)*.

10. Describe the kinds of things cassettes and intensifying screens should be visually checked for *(p. 460)*.

11. Explain the need for, and proper method of, periodic screen cleaning *(p. 460)*.

12. Describe the purpose and method of a screen and film contact test *(p. 460)*.

13. Explain how to check the condition of a grid *(p. 460)*.

14. Explain the necessity of QC checks on illumination *(p. 460)*.

15. Describe the proper care, storage, and checking of lead apparel *(p. 461)*.

A&U Chapter Review Questions

1. Proper care of leaded apparel includes:
    1. periodic check for cracks
    2. careful folding following each use
    3. routine laundering with soap and water
   (A) 1 only
   (B) 1 and 2 only
   (C) 1 and 3 only
   (D) 1, 2, and 3

2. Which of the following contribute(s) to inherent filtration?
    1. x-ray tube glass envelope
    2. x-ray tube port window
    3. aluminum between tube housing and collimator
   (A) 1 only
   (B) 1 and 2 only
   (C) 1 and 3 only
   (D) 1, 2, and 3

3. The spinning top test can be used to evaluate:
    1. timer accuracy
    2. rectifier failure
    3. effect of kVp on contrast
   (A) 1 only
   (B) 2 only
   (C) 1 and 2 only
   (D) 1, 2, and 3

4. Poor screen to film contact can be caused by which of the following:
    1. damaged cassette frame
    2. foreign body in cassette
    3. warped cassette front
   (A) 1 only
   (B) 2 only
   (C) 1 and 3 only
   (D) 1, 2, and 3

5. A quality control program includes checks on which of the following radiographic equipment conditions?
    1. reproducibility
    2. linearity
    3. positive beam limitation
   (A) 1 only
   (B) 1 and 2 only
   (C) 1 and 3 only
   (D) 1, 2, and 3

6. Periodic equipment calibration includes testing of the:
    1. focal spot
    2. mA
    3. kVp
   (A) 1 only
   (B) 1 and 3 only
   (C) 2 and 3 only
   (D) 1, 2, and 3

7. Which of the following tests is performed to evaluate screen contact?
   (A) spinning top test
   (B) wire mesh test
   (C) penetrometer test
   (D) star pattern test

8. Which of the following refers to a regular program of evaluation that ensures proper functioning of x-ray equipment, thereby protecting both patients and radiation workers?
   (A) sensitometry
   (B) densitometry
   (C) quality assurance
   (D) modulation transfer function

9. Excessive anode heating can cause vaporized tungsten to be deposited on the port window. This can result in:
    1. decreased tube output
    2. tube failure
    3. electrical sparking
   (A) 1 only
   (B) 2 only
   (C) 1 and 2 only
   (D) 1, 2, and 3

10. Radiographs from a particular three-phase, full-wave rectified x-ray unit were underexposed, using known correct exposures. A synchronous spinning top test was performed using 100 mA, 1/20 sec, and 70 kVp, and a 12° arc is observed on the test film. Which of the following is MOST likely the problem?
    (A) the 1/20 sec time station is inaccurate
    (B) the 100 mA station is inaccurate
    (C) a rectifier is not functioning
    (D) the processor needs servicing

Answers And Explanations

1. (A) Protective lead aprons and gloves are made of lead-impregnated vinyl or leather. They should be checked for cracks radiographically from time to time. Otherwise, minimal care is required. Lead aprons and gloves should always be hung on appropriate hangers. Glove supports permit air to circulate within the glove. Apron hangers provide convenient storage without folding. If lead aprons are folded (or just left in a heap!)

cracks are more likely to form. If lead aprons or gloves become soiled, cleaning with a damp cloth and appropriate solution is all that is required. Excessive moisture should be avoided.

2. (B) Inherent filtration is that which is "built into" the construction of the x-ray tube. Before exiting the x-ray tube, x-ray photons must pass through the tube's glass envelope and port window; the photons are filtered somewhat as they do so. This inherent filtration is usually the equivalent of 0.5 mm Al. Aluminum filtration *placed* between the x-ray tube housing and collimator is added in order to contribute to the total necessary requirement of 2.5 mm Al equivalent. The collimator itself is considered part of the added filtration (1.0 mm Al equiv) because of the silver surface of the mirror within. It is important to remember that as aluminum filtration is added to the x-ray tube, the half-value layer (HVL) increases.

3. (C) The spinning top test is used to evaluate *timer accuracy* or *rectifier failure.* With single-phase, full-wave rectified equipment (120 pulses per sec) for example, 12 dots should be visualized when using the 1/10 sec station. A few more or less indicates timer inaccuracy. If the test demonstrated five dots, one might suspect rectifier failure. With three-phase equipment a special synchronous spinning top (or oscilloscope) is used and a solid black arc is obtained rather than dots. The length of this arc is measured and compared with the known correct arc.

4. (D) Perfect contact between the intensifying screens and film is essential in order to maintain image sharpness. Any separation between them allows diffusion of fluorescent light and subsequent blurriness and loss of detail. Screen and film contact can be diminished if the cassette frame is damaged and misshapen, if the front is warped, or if there is a foreign body between the screens elevating them.

5. (D) The accuracy of all three are important to ensure adequate patient protection. *Reproducibility* means that repeated exposures at a given technique must provide consistent intensity. *Linearity* means that a given mAs, using different mA stations with appropriate exposure time adjustments, will provide consistent intensity. *Positive beam limitation (PBL)* is automatic collimation and must be accurate to 2% of the SID. Light-localized collimators must be available and must be accurate to within 2%.

6. (D) Radiographic results should be consistent and predictable not only in positioning accuracy but with respect to exposure factors and image sharpness as well. X-ray equipment should be calibrated periodically as part of an ongoing QA program. The quantity (mAs) and quality (kVp) of the primary beam have a big impact on the quality of the finished radiograph. The focal spot should be tested periodically to evaluate its impact on image sharpness.

7. (B) Perfect film and screen contact is essential to sharply recorded detail. Screen contact can be evaluated with a wire-mesh test. A spinning top test is used to evaluate timer accuracy and rectifier operation. A penetrometer (aluminum step wedge) is used to illustrate the effect of kVp on contrast. A star pattern is used to measure resolving power of the imaging system.

8. (C) Sensitometry and densitometry are used in evaluation of the film processor, just one part of a complete quality assurance (QA) program. Modulation transfer function (MTF) is used to express spatial resolution, another component of the QA program. A complete QA program includes testing of all components of the imaging system: processors, focal spot, x-ray timers, filters, intensifying screens, beam alignment, and so on.

9. (D) Vaporized tungsten may be deposited on the inner surface of the glass envelope at the tube (port) window. It acts as an *additional filter,* thereby *reducing tube output.* The tungsten deposit may also attract electrons from the filament, *creating sparking* and *causing puncture* of the glass envelope and subsequent tube failure.

10. (A) A synchronous spinning top test is used to test timer accuracy or rectifier function in three-phase equipment. Since three-phase, full-wave rectified current would expose a 360° arc per second, a 1/20 second exposure should expose an 18° arc. Anything more or less indicates timer inaccuracy. If exactly one half the expected arc appears, one should suspect rectifier failure.

BIBLIOGRAPHY

Adler A, Carlton R. *Introduction to Radiography and Patient Care* (2nd ed). Philadelphia: WB Sanders Co. 1999.

Ballinger PW. *Merrill's Atlas of Radiographic Positions and Radiologic Procedures* (8th ed). St. Louis: CV Mosby, 1995.

Bontrager KL, Anthony T. *Textbook of Radiographic Positioning and Related Anatomy* (4th ed) St. Louis: CV Mosby, 1997.

Burns, EF. *Radiographic Imaging: A Guide for Producing Quality Radiographs* (1st ed). Philadelphia: WB Saunders Co, 1993.

Bushong SC. *Radiologic Science for Technologists* (5th ed). St. Louis: CV Mosby, 1993.

Carlton RR, Adler AM. *Principles of Radiographic Imaging: An Art and a Science* (2nd ed), Delmar, 1996.

Chusid JG. *Correlative Neuroanatomy & Functional Neurology* (19th ed). East Norwalk, CT: Appleton & Lange, 1985.

Cornuelle et al. *Radiographic Anatomy and Positioning.* Stamford, CT; Appleton & Lange, 1998.

Cullinan AM. *Optimizing Radiographic Positioning* (1st ed). Philadelphia: JB Lippincott, 1992.

Cullinan AM. Cullinan JE. *Producing Quality Radiographs* (2nd ed). Philadelphia: JB Lippincott, 1994.

Curry, Dowdey, Murry. *Christensen's Introduction to the Physics of Radiology* (4th ed). Philadelphia: Lea and Febiger, 1990.

Ehrlich RA, McCloskey ED. *Patient Care in Radiography* (5th ed). St. Louis: CV Mosby, 1999.

Eisenberg RL, Dennis CA. Comprehensive Radiographic Pathology (1st ed). St. Louis: CV Mosby, 1990.

Gurley LT, Callaway WJ. *Introduction to Radiologic Technology* (4th ed). St. Louis: CV Mosby, 1996.

Hames CC, Joseph DH. *Basic Concepts of Helping* (2nd ed). East Norwalk, CT: Appleton-Century-Crofts, 1986.

Haus, Arthur G and Jaskulski SM. *Film Processing in Medical Imaging* (1st ed). Madison, WI: Medical Physics Publishing, 1997.

Hopp JW, Rogers EA. *AIDS and the Allied Health Professions* (1st ed). FA Davis, 1989.

Kent TH, Hart MN. *Introduction to Human Disease* (2nd ed). East Norwalk, CT: Appleton-Century-Crofts, 1987.

Laudicina P. *Applied Pathology for Radiographers* (1st ed). Philadelphia: WB Saunders, 1989.

Linder HH. *Clinical Anatomy* (1st ed). East Norwalk, CT: Appleton & Lange, 1989.

Mace JD, Kowalczyk N. *Radiographic Pathology for Technologists* (3rd ed). St. Louis: CV Mosby, 1998.

Martini FH. *Fundamentals of Anatomy & Physiology* (3rd ed). Englewood Cliffs, NJ: Prentice Hall, 1995.

McKinney WEJ. *Radiographic Processing and Quality Control* (1st ed). Philadelphia: JB Lippincott, 1988.

Miller RD. *Problems in Hospital Law* (5th ed). Aspen Publishers, 1986.

Mill WR. The relation of bodily habitus to visceral form, tonus, and motility. *Am J. Roentgengr* 1917;4:155–169.

Muma RD, Lyons BA, Borucki MJ et al. *HIV Manual for Health Care Professionals.* East Norwalk, CT: Appleton & Lange, 1994.

NCRP Report no. 102: *Medical X-ray, Electron Beam and Gamma Ray Protection for Energies up to MeV (Equipment Design, Performance and Use).* NCRP, 1989.

NCRP Report no. 105: *Radiation Protection for Medical and Allied Health Personnel.* NCRP. 1989.

NCRP Report no 116: *Recommendations on Limits for Exposure to Ionizing Radiation.* NCRP, 1987.

Purtilo R. *Health Professional and Patient Education* (4th ed). Philadelphia: WNB Saunders Co, 1990.

Rice J. *Medical Terminology with Human Anatomy* (4th ed). East Norwalk, CT: Appleton & Lange, 1999.

Saia DA. *Appleton & Lange's Review for the Radiography Examination* (3rd ed). East Norwalk, CT: Appleton & Lange, 1997.

Selman J. *The Fundamentals of X-ray and Radium Physics* (8th ed). Springfield, IL: Charles C. Thomas Publisher, 1994.

Sherer, Visconti, Ritenour. *Radiation Protection in Medical Radiography* (3rd ed). St. Louis: CV Mosby, 1993.

Simon RR, Koenigsknecht SJ. *Emergency Orthopedics—The Extremities* (3rd ed). East Norwalk, CT: Appleton & Lange, 1995.

Sprawls P. *Principles of Radiograhy for Technologists* (1st ed). Aspen, 1990.

Taber's Cyclopedic Medical Dictionary (18th ed), FA Davis, 1997.

Thompson, Hattaway, Hall, et al. *Principles of Imaging Science and Protection* (1st ed). Philadelphia: WB Saunders Co, 1994.

Torres, LS. *Basic Medical Techniques and Patient Care for Radiologic Technologists* (5th ed). Philadelphia: JB Lippincott, 1997.

Tortora GJ, Grabowski SR. Principles of Anatomy and Physiology (8th ed). New York: Harper Collins, 1996.

Wallace, Jerry Ellen. *Radiographic Exposure: Principles & Practice* (1st ed). Philadelphia, PA: FA Davis, 1995.

Way LW. ed *Current Surgical Diagnosis & Treatment* (10th ed). East Norwalk, CT: Appleton & Lange, 1994.

Wolbarst, AB. *Physics of Radiology* (1st ed). East Norwalk, CT; Appleton & Lange, 1993.

Index

Page numbers followed by an *f* indicate a Figure. Page numbers followed by a *t* indicated a Table.

Directions for Installing MICROSTUDY®

MICROSTUDY® V3.2 FOR WINDOWS® FEATURES

1. Quizzes consisting of chapter questions may be taken in the authors' original order or in a randomly scrambled order.
2. Follow-up tests are composed of missed-questions.
3. Electronic notebook enables students' comments to be entered and saved while studying, then recalled later for review, modifying or printing.
4. Customized comprehensive exams may be automatically built. These exams may be presented under NAPLEX simulation or in the standard MICRO-STUDY simulated exam format.
5. Performance is monitored and a report card is assembled after each work session. Comprehensive exam statistics are tabulated and displayed for exam performance comparisons.
6. Digital timer shows elapsed study time.
7. Audio feedback that signals responses may be used.
8. A four-function memory calculator is available while studying.

MICROSTUDY® V3.2 FOR WINDOWS® INSTALLATION AND STARTUP

1. Hard Disk Installation from Run in Windows® 3.1 or 3.11
   a. Once the computer is started, insert the MICRO-STUDY disk marked INSTALL into the appropriate floppy drive.
   b. Select Run from under the File Menu. Type **A:\INSTALL** or **B:\INSTALL** in the Command Line of Run, then press OK.
   c. INSTALL copies all required files from the designated floppy drive to the designated hard drive and its subdirectories, then creates a MICRO-STUDY icon within a MICROSTUDY program group.
   d. Start MICROSTUDY by double clicking with a mouse on the MICROSTUDY program icon in the MICROSTUDY group.

2. Hard Disk Installation from File Manager in Windows® 3.1 or 3.11
   a. Once the computer is started, insert the MICRO-STUDY disk marked INSTALL into the appropriate floppy drive.
   b. From File Manager, click on the floppy drive symbol where the MICROSTUDY INSTALL disk was inserted. Find the program file INSTALL.EXE and double click on it to start the installation.
   c. INSTALL copies all required files from the designated floppy drive to the designated hard drive and its subdirectories, then creates a MICRO-STUDY icon within a MICROSTUDY program group.
   d. Start MICROSTUDY by double clicking with a mouse on the MICROSTUDY program icon in the MICROSTUDY group.

3. Hard Disk Installation from Start in Windows® 95
   a. Once the computer is started, insert the MICRO-STUDY disk marked INSTALL into the appropriate floppy drive.
   b. Select Run from the Start Menu. Type **A:\INSTALL** or **B:\INSTALL** in the Command Line of Run, then press OK.
   c. INSTALL copies all required files from the designated floppy drive to the designated hard drive and its subdirectories, then creates a MICRO-STUDY icon within a MICROSTUDY program group.
   d. Start MICROSTUDY by double clicking with a mouse on the MICROSTUDY program icon in the MICROSTUDY group.

4. Hard Disk Installation from Explorer in Windows® 95
   a. Once the computer is started, insert the MICRO-STUDY disk marked INSTALL into the appropriate floppy drive.
   b. From Explorer, click on the floppy drive symbol in which the MICROSTUDY INSTALL disk was inserted. Find the program file INSTALL.EXE and double click on it to start installation.
   c. INSTALL copies all required files from the designated floppy drive to the designated hard drive and its subdirectories, then creates a MICRO-STUDY icon within a MICROSTUDY group.
   d. Start MICROSTUDY by double clicking with a mouse on the MICROSTUDY program icon in the MICROSTUDY group.